Revealing Nursing Expertise Through Practitioner Inquiry

Edited by

Sally Hardy
Angie Titchen
Brendan McCormack
Kim Manley

Foreword by Patricia Benner

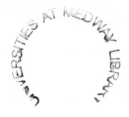
ⓌWILEY-BLACKWELL

A John Wiley & Sons, Ltd., Publication

This edition first published 2009
© 2009 Blackwell Publishing Ltd

Blackwell Publishing was acquired by John Wiley & Sons in February 2007. Blackwell's publishing programme has been merged with Wiley's global Scientific, Technical, and Medical business to form Wiley-Blackwell.

Registered office
John Wiley & Sons Ltd, The Atrium, Southern Gate, Chichester, West Sussex, PO19 8SQ, United Kingdom

Editorial offices
9600 Garsington Road, Oxford, OX4 2DQ, United Kingdom
2121 State Avenue, Ames, Iowa 50014-8300, USA

For details of our global editorial offices, for customer services and for information about how to apply for permission to reuse the copyright material in this book please see our website at www.wiley.com/wiley-blackwell.

The right of the author to be identified as the author of this work has been asserted in accordance with the Copyright, Designs and Patents Act 1988.

Wiley also publishes its books in a variety of electronic formats. Some content that appears in print may not be available in electronic books.

Designations used by companies to distinguish their products are often claimed as trademarks. All brand names and product names used in this book are trade names, service marks, trademarks or registered trademarks of their respective owners. The publisher is not associated with any product or vendor mentioned in this book. This publication is designed to provide accurate and authoritative information in regard to the subject matter covered. It is sold on the understanding that the publisher is not engaged in rendering professional services. If professional advice or other expert assistance is required, the services of a competent professional should be sought.

Library of Congress Cataloging-in-Publication Data
    Revealing nursing expertise through practitioner inquiry / edited by
Sally Hardy ... [et al.].
        p. ; cm.
    Includes bibliographical references and index.
    ISBN 978-1-4051-5178-8 (pbk. : alk. paper)   1. Nursing.   2. Nursing—Research.
I. Hardy, Sally, RGN.
    [DNLM: 1. Nursing Care—methods.   2. Professional Competence.
3. Nursing Research. WY 16 R449 2009]
    RT42.R45 2009
    610.73072—dc22

                                                                    2009006626

A catalogue record for this book is available from the British Library.

Set in 9.5/11.5 pt Palatino by Aptara® Inc., New Delhi, India
Printed and bound in Malaysia by KHL Printing Co Sdn Bhd

1   2009

Revealing Nursing Expertise Through Practitioner Inquiry

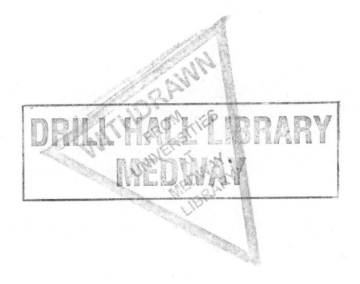

Contents

Contents

Contents

Section Three: Methods and Resources for Revealing Practice Expertise

Contents

Contributors

Angela Brown, Associate Head, University of Wollongong, Wollongong, Australia

Margaret Conlon, Lecturer in Mental Health, Napier University, Edinburgh, UK

Dr Cheryl Crocker, Consultant Nurse, Nottingham University Hospital, Nottingham, UK

Alison Greggans, Student of Conservation and Countryside Management. Formerly Nurse Lecturer, Queen Margaret University, Edinburgh, UK

Dr Sally Hardy, Professor of Mental Health Nursing, Head of Mental Health & Learning Disabilities, City University London, UK; Honorary Associate Professor, Monash University, Melbourne, Australia

Karen Harrison, Consultant Admiral Nurse, Barnet, Enfield and Haringey Mental Health NHS Trust and The National Council for Palliative Care, UK

Liz Henderson, Lead Cancer Nurse, Northern Ireland Cancer Network, UK

Dr Nancy Jane Lee, Associate Head of School (Research), University of Salford, Salford, UK

Dr Kim Manley, Manager Resources for Learning and Improving/Lead for Quality and Standards, Royal College of Nursing, London, UK; Visiting Professor, Bournemouth University, Bournemouth, UK

Professor Brendan McCormack, Professor of Nursing Research, University of Ulster, Northern Ireland, UK; Adjunct Professor of Nursing, Monash University, Melbourne, Australia; Visiting Professor, University of Northumbria, Newcastle, UK

Maeve McGinley, Clinical Nurse Specialist in Bladder and Bowel Dysfunction, Foyle Health & SS Trust, Northern Ireland, UK

Sarah Ryan, Nurse Consultant in Rheumatology, Haywood Hospital, Staffordshire, UK; Honorary Senior Clinical Lecturer, Keele University, Staffordshire, UK

Contributors

Professor Angie Titchen, Clinical Chair, Fontys University of Applied Sciences, Eindhoven, The Netherlands; Visiting Professor, University of Ulster, UK; Adjunct Professor, Charles Sturt University, Sydney, Australia, Associate Fellow, University of Warwick, UK; Independent Practice Development & Research Consultant.

Dr Jonathan Webster, Consultant Nurse for Older People, University College London Hospitals NHS Foundation Trust, London, UK; Associate Fellow, Gerontological Nursing, Royal College of Nursing, London, UK; Faculty Fellow, University of Brighton & Honorary Visiting Fellow, City University London, UK.

Foreword

This book is the culmination of many years of research and development of action-oriented research on practice development. It is the necessary companion and often marginalised major means required to achieve the person-centred outcomes in today's extremely rationalised 'bottom line health care'. These authors have taught practitioners how to uncover their own best practice, and to critically examine areas of their practice where they do not live up to their own views of best practice and literally engage in self and practice transformation.

Today's measurement-oriented work cultures insist on evaluation primarily based upon outcomes. An outcomes-oriented approach is designed based upon a narrow rationality that separates *means* and *ends*. This process of separation unwittingly devalues and fragments the means. I am thinking of nurses' work as the means for achieving improved safety and quality outcomes in Health Care Systems. But in many areas of health care, means and ends are inextricably bound together, for example, in the attentiveness and care required to achieve worthy person-centred outcomes in birthing, rescuing and helping patients recover and helping people to die with dignity.

I consider the work of Hardy, Titchen, McCormack and Manley groundbreaking work in practice, practice-based learning, research and organisational development. These researchers recognise that emancipatory inquiry as well as appreciative inquiry that captures existing expertise and artistry are both essential for practice and organisational development. Emancipatory inquiry is required to identify, critique and change oppressive personal and organisational impediments to good practice. This is an essential freedom from organisational and personal strictures, impediments and oppressive behaviours, processes and structures. But their project requires 'freedom' to engage in artistry and creative practice bringing new possibilities into the practice and organisational communities, articulating them, making them public, accessible and more researchable.

This work is also groundbreaking in articulating the different levels and possibilities of practice-based learning and research. This work focuses on:

- facilitating learning and a work-based learning culture;
- facilitating inquiry, evaluation and evidence use in practice;
- facilitating a culture of effectiveness through leadership;
- using consultancy approaches that foster self-sufficiency in problem-solving across teams and organisations (refer to chapter 1).

All of these practice-based forms of inquiry and development are essential to re-form and form self-improving practices of nursing. Nursing as a practice cannot thrive nor survive in institutions that are literally not fit for good practice. It is tempting for organisational leaders to overlook and devalue the organisational policies, structures and rules necessary for enhancing a self-improving and learning organisation that not only meets outcome measures of effectiveness but also makes them happen and then continually improve upon them.

This work is innovative and groundbreaking in developing action-oriented and reflexive pedagogies that foster personal and organisational development. Their development of the consummate coach as a *critical companion* is central to the methodology of this work. The critical companion offers situated teaching and coaching that also helps the practitioner actively develop their own community of learning through seeking counsel from other team members and stakeholders. These authors recognise that both learning and knowledge work are social, public and community based. A companion is defined as 'a partner on a journey of dis-covery, someone who is reliable, an advocate, supporter who has genuine interest in development and growth' (Royal College of Nursing, 2000, *Expertise in Practice Project Glossary*, RCN, London, p. 1). The creative and critical companion has the following guiding aims:

1. to endorse and evidence patient-centred practices;
2. to enable a shared vision of practice between facilitator and practitioner;
3. to challenge how power can be used in positive and enabling ways;
4. to advocate the *insider* and *outsider* perspective;
5. to encourage deep learning which is significant for the individual and the or-ganisation in which they work (refer to chapter 6).

We all need such critical companion coaches to help develop best practices of nurs-ing care. To become organisations of learning, growth and ongoing improvement, one cannot get past either the individual practitioner, the community of practi-tioners and finally the organisational culture, vision and structures and process. These authors recognise this and have taken up the labour-intensive work of prac-tice development in all the relevant spheres including knowledge development of nurses as knowledge workers in their context. Current health care contexts with-out intervention can be almost void of positive, reflective evaluation, critique and continuous improvement. This book gives us ways out of this entropy and blind-ness.

Patricia Benner, PhD, FAAN, FRC, Hon.

Introduction

Preparation for this book could be marked as commencing back in the 1990s, when Kim Manley and Brendan McCormack developed a master's module on practice expertise at the Royal College of Nursing (RCN), London (Manley & McCormack, 1997). They had come to work together from different paths, Kim having worked at the Chelsea & Westminster in London, and Brendan at Oxfordshire Community Health Trust/National Institute for Nursing, where Angie Titchen was also working (with Sue Pembrey, Alison Binnie and others) on a new understanding of clinical practice development.

I [Sally Hardy] came to meet my fellow book editors whilst employed as a research associate, at the RCN in 2001, for an innovative, complex and ambitious research project exploring nursing practice expertise. The RCN's Expertise in Practice project (Manley *et al.*, 2005) was how we met the various contributors in this book. Friendships were formed, as project participants met together with colleagues, academics and researchers to discuss, debate, critique and unravel the complexity that is health care practice expertise. Undertaking the process enabled people to share intimate details of their values, beliefs and consequent behaviours. Yet it went further than that. People were engaging in a process of human flourishing. Within relationships of openness, honesty and exploration, trust was created that overturned conventional working and research relationships. Meeting regularly across England, Scotland, Northern Ireland and Wales, we began to look forward to the 'luxury' of our action learning meetings, or the regular critical companionship conversations, where anything and everything became of interest; as excitement for practice was renewed, new levels of interest and understanding gained, forward thinking and plans for the future could all be brought to the table without fear of retribution, judgement or blame.

Long after the project came to an end, and participants had completed their portfolios of evidence, the relationships continued. We met at conferences, work events and at each other's houses to continue the discussions, as the impact of the project continued to reveal itself. Two people left the health system altogether, realising their ambitions laid elsewhere, as their personhood came into stark contrast to the imposition of prominent values they experienced in health care culture.

Within this book, you will read about nursing practice expertise, from why and what practice expertise is, to the where and how expertise takes place, but, most importantly, the impact of working from a value system of person-centeredness. Section One offers the context within which nursing practice expertise is being refined and honed, and processes to continue to refine our understanding. Section Two acts as a core section for the book, providing valuable insight into the reality nurses experience when striving to achieve excellence in health care practice. The final section offers additional resources for further revealing, articulating and expanding understanding of expertise and its development, in addition to offering principles for nurturing professional artistry, human flourishing and person-centred practices.

Collectively, this book provides a contemporary insight into practice at the summits of health care. It has taken many years to get there, but each time others wish to follow the trail, it will become a more well-trodden path.

Sally Hardy
Angie Titchen
Brendan McCormack
Kim Manley
March 2009

Abbreviations

AGREE	Appraisal of Guidelines for Research and Evaluation
ALS	Action learning sets
BPH	Benign prostatic hyperplasia
CINAHL	Cumulative Index for Nursing and Allied Health Literature
CNS	Clinical nurse specialist
EAR	Emancipatory action research
ePD	Emancipatory practice development
EPP	Expertise in Practice Project
IPL	Interprofessional learning
NP	Nurse practitioner
PCR	Practitioner-centred research
PNF	Professional Nursing Forum
RA	Rheumatoid arthritis
RCN	Royal College of Nursing
WBL	Work-based learning

Section One

The Context

1. From Artistry in Practice to Expertise in Developing Person-Centred Systems: A Clinical Career Framework

Kim Manley, Angie Titchen and Sally Hardy

Introduction

Throughout this book, we aim to provide a broad, interwoven vision of what is possible in nursing practice. This introductory chapter places nursing practice expertise within a clinical career framework that encompasses five interdependent domains. The first domain is about achieving professional expertise and artistry in the nurse–patient relationship. The other four domains are about developing expertise in implementing and sustaining person-centred systems. The development of person-centred systems requires expertise that includes the facilitation of individuals, teams, systems, learning, research, inquiry, evaluation and change in practice, so as to enable a culture of effectiveness to develop in the workplace. Other chapters of this book provide more detailed examples that illustrate expertise across some or all of the domains outlined in this chapter.

This chapter will focus on the following:

1. The domain of nursing practice expertise within the nurse–patient relationship.
2. The four domains associated with developing person-centred systems, namely,
    (i) facilitating practice change and a culture of effectiveness in the workplace through leadership;
    (ii) facilitating inquiry, evaluation and evidence use in practice;
    (iii) facilitating learning and a work-based learning culture, where learning in and from practice is the norm and all learning feeds into practice transformation;
    (iv) using consultancy approaches that foster self-sufficiency in problem-solving across teams and organisations.

3. Identifying the relationships between various roles that encompass expertise in nursing practice and person-centred systems. For example advanced, specialist and consultant nurse practice and other clinically related career opportunities beyond the consultant nurse role.

The context of nursing practice expertise

Inherent in all nursing practice career frameworks is a spectrum of expertise that spans the range of domains above. This spectrum is necessary for practice teams and cultures to be experienced as person centred and evidence based. The establishment of person-centred systems enables patients and users to receive person-centred and evidence-based care, regardless of whether the most immediate provider of care has expertise or not. The reason for this is that such systems create cultures that enable a consistently high quality of nursing to be experienced by patients and users from the whole team. In other words, this spectrum or span of expertise is underpinned by an assumption that nursing is about both the relationship with the person who has health or illness needs, and also, the context in which nursing takes place (Manley, 2000) (Box 1.1).

The context for nursing practice therefore extends from that most immediate to the nurse–patient relationship, through to the health care team and onto the patient's journey, which may cross a number of interfaces. It is at these interfaces that nursing practice expertise has most potential for developing person-centred systems (McCormack *et al.*, 2008a, 2008b). This is not to deny that nursing does and should not have influence at other levels, such as the organisational level – it does (Aiken *et al.*, 2002; McCormack *et al.*, 2008b), or that other levels of organisation aren't important – they are (McCormack *et al.*, 1999) but the predominant focus here is on the workplace rather than the organisation.

Expertise: a lifetime's journey

Although there is an interdependence in the development of expertise across the five domains, it is recognised that individuals follow different career trajectories

---

Box 1.1   Context for nursing practice (*Source*: This box was published in *Surgical Nursing: Advancing Practice*, K. Manley & L. Bellman, p. 4. Copyright Elsevier, 2000.)

Nursing is about
- caring values;
- focusing on relationships with individuals, groups and populations;
- managing/facilitating the context of care;
- enabling coordination and continuity of care;
- using knowledge of patients as people with concepts and implications of health and illness to inform assessment, interventions, evaluation, patient education and health promotion.

(Manley, 2000)

and that these are not necessarily linear. By focusing on the different domains that constitute the spectrum of nursing expertise from that located within the in-dividual nurse–patient relationship through to that related to implementing and sustaining person-centred systems, it is hoped that different starting points and professional experiences are recognised and greater fluidity in career progression is valued. Expertise doesn't develop overnight. It happens through using work-place experiences as the main resource for learning and inquiry. These experiences are combined with an impetus and desire for refining everyday practice, through structured and supported reflection that has potential to transform practice, the individual and the team, within an everyday culture that supports this transfor-mation (Manley, 2004). This is a lifetime's journey within the context of lifelong learning, one that requires us working with others and exposing our practice to critique. Working with and exposure to critique were characteristics of the Royal College of Nursing's (RCN's) Expertise In Practice Project (EPP; Manley & Gar-bett, 2000; Hardy *et al.*, 2002; Manley *et al.*, 2005; Hardy *et al.*, 2006, 2007) in which participants, who were recognised by their colleagues as having expertise, were involved in trying to understand and articulate their nursing expertise and its outcomes. Through the process of portfolio development and with the help of a critical companion (Titchen, 2004), participants, by the end of the research, could explain not only why they had expertise, but also what the outcome of this exper-tise was on patients, colleagues and the service. This study led to the recognition that even experts needed help with unpicking and articulating their expertise, as well as the processes for developing it further in themselves and others. A set of standards emerged that would assist others in their development of not just clinical expertise but also person-centred systems (RCN, 2004a, 2004b). The four domains associated with developing these systems will be described later once the domain of person-centred expertise has been considered in more depth.

Nursing practice: person-centred expertise

Expertise in person-centred practice

The contemporary understanding of nursing expertise presented here (Box 1.2; Figure 1.1) is based on the findings of the RCN's EPP (Manley & Garbett, 2000; Hardy *et al.*, 2002; Manley *et al.*, 2005; Hardy *et al.*, 2006, 2007) and can be clearly traced to the original research of Benner (1984), Benner and Wrubel (1989) and Benner *et al.* (1996). Chapter 3 discusses these and other early works and sets out the literature landscape concerned with expertise in nursing and its development. This chapter focuses on the EPP which spanned a period from May 1998 and continued through to 2004. It included six cohorts of practising nurses working in four countries of England, Wales, Scotland and Northern Ireland. The project aimed to develop a deep and rich understanding of nursing practice expertise across diverse clinical specialities, through the identification and verification of its attributes and enabling factors. Derived from insights and augmented by a comprehensive analysis of the literature, these attributes and enabling factors formed the conceptual framework for the project (Manley & McCormack, 1997).

Box 1.2 'The attributes of expertise'

Holistic practice knowledge is concerned with:
- using all forms of knowledge in practice;
- ongoing learning and evaluation from new situations;
- drawing from the range of knowledge bases (alongside experiential learning to assess situations and inform appropriate action with consideration of consequences);
- embedding new knowledge and accessing this in similar situations as they occur.

Saliency related to:
- picking up cues (that can be missed or dismissed by others) to inform the situation;
- observation of non-verbal cues to understand the person's individual situation;
- listening and responding to verbal cues;
- regarding the patient as a whole (i.e. recognising their uniqueness) to inform treatment process;
- ability to recognise the needs of the patient colleagues and others in the actions taken.

Knowing the patient is about:
- respect for people and their own view of the world (ontology);
- respecting patients unique perspective on their illness/situation;
- willingness to promote and maintain a persons' dignity at all times;
- conscious use of self to promote a helping relationship;
- promoting the patients own decision-making;
- willingness to relinquish 'control' to the patient;
- recognising the patient's/other's expertise.

Moral agency is concerned with:
- providing information that will enhance people's ability to problem solve and make decisions for themselves;
- working at a level of consciousness that promotes another person's dignity, respect and individuality;
- a conscientious awareness in one's work of integrity and behaving impeccably;
- working and living one's values and beliefs, whilst not enforcing them on others.

Skilled know-how refers to:
- enabling others through a willingness to share knowledge and skills;
- adapting and responding with consideration to each individual situation;
- mobilising and using all available resources;
- envisioning a path through a problem/situation and inviting others on that journey.

Benner and her colleagues used phenomenology to interpret and illustrate nursing expertise through a number of paradigm cases and exemplars that showed overarching and specific aspects of expertise, respectively. In contrast, the EPP drew on emancipatory action research (Grundy, 1982) and fourth generation evaluation (Guba & Lincoln, 1989). The latter is an approach to social research that integrates action in the workplace with the concerns, claims and issues of

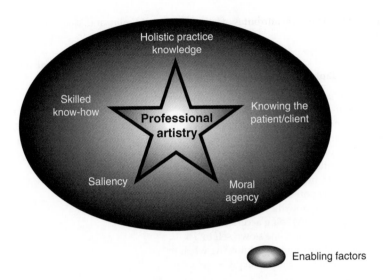

Enabling factors

Figure 1.1 A conceptual framework for nursing expertise in the UK. (*Source*: Reproduced with kind permission of the Royal College of Nursing from *Changing Patient's Worlds through Nursing Practice Experience* (Manley *et al.*, 2005).)

stakeholders. Schratz and Walker (1995) suggest that social research is about enabling practitioners to become more critical about their practice through identifying and evaluating their actions and decisions. Whilst supporting this notion, the EPP went way beyond it by inviting practitioners to become practitioner researchers who, simultaneously, investigated and developed their own expertise. To help participants to develop the necessary skill sets for practitioner research, participants and their critical companions were invited to join monthly action learning sets facilitated by two members of the research team. Participants also met regularly with their chosen critical companion (Titchen, 2001) in the workplace, in addition to collaboratively gathering evidence of and about the nurse participants' practice. The methodology of this study is further described in Chapter 3.

The outcomes of this project included a framework of expertise that offers a language for nurses to articulate and share with others what constitutes their practice expertise, thus providing a greater level of insight and articulation of what occurs between the expert practitioner and the people they care for. Table 1.1 sets out refinements and additions to the attributes identified in the original concept analysis conducted by Manley and McCormack (1997). Refinements and additions were established through an overall analysis of the nurse participants' portfolios of evidence and review of literature since 1997.

Analysis of the portfolios in the EPP also supported the three enabling factors of expertise identified in the original concept analysis, that is, reflective ability (reflexivity), organisation of practice (capacity to critically control all of their interactions to impact on the organisation through being able to see the bigger picture)

Table 1.1 Support for the attributes of expertise since Manley and McCormack's (1997) concept analysis

Attributes (Adapted from Manley *et al.*, 2005)	Examples of empirical support in the literature since 1997
1. *Knowing the patient/client/colleague/organisation* Seeing patients as people who are unique, recognising and respecting their view of their illness or situation; getting to know the patient as person in the context of their own life to enable unique interventions and care that meet the needs of patients and their carers as they see them; recognising patients' patterns of behaviour and understanding how they are likely to react; forming rapport easily, being accessible on a personal level and using one's own self to promote helping relationships; knowing when to relinquish control to patients/clients	Binnie and Titchen, 1999; Titchen, 2001; Titchen and McGinley, 2003; Bonner and Greenwood, 2006; McCormack and McCance, 2006
2. *Holistic practice knowledge* Integrating and using all kinds of knowledge in practice (e.g. theory, research, practical know-how, praxis, experiential, intuitive, aesthetic, personal); ongoing evaluation of, and learning from, new situations and embedding this knowledge for future use; using generic knowledge appropriately to individuals, groups, organisations or circumstances	Titchen, 2000; Titchen and McGinley, 2003; Donnelly, 2003; Judd, 2005; Kennedy, 2004; McCormack and McCance, 2006
3. *Saliency: knowing what matters and acting on it* Recognising intuitively and rationally what matters quickly and responding with immediate, seamless action; using skills appropriately and at the right time; listening and picking up verbal and non-verbal cues that can be missed by others; recognising patients', colleagues' and others' needs and reflecting these in action taken	Binnie and Titchen, 1999; Titchen, 2001 (skilled companionship); Taylor, 2002; Foley *et al.*, 2002
4. *Moral integrity* Consciously promoting others' dignity and individuality and respecting their values and actions without passing judgement; working and living one's values and beliefs without pushing them on others; providing information which enhances people's ability to solve problems and make decisions; being aware of one's own integrity and of setting the highest standards; aspiring to promote human flourishing for all involved in the clinical encounter through one's actions	Ersser, 1997; Binnie and Titchen, 1999; Titchen, 2000; Judd, 2005; Johnston and Smith, 2006; McCormack and McCance, 2006; McCormack and Titchen, 2006

Table 1.1 *(Continued)*

Attributes (Adapted from Manley *et al.*, 2005)	Examples of empirical support in the literature since 1997
5. *Skilled know-how* Adapting and responding skilfully and with consideration to each situation; enabling others through a willingness to share knowledge and skills; mobilising and using all available resources; seeing a path through a problem and inviting others on that journey	Binnie and Titchen, 1999; Titchen, 2001; Titchen and McGinley, 2003; Judd, 2005; Bonner and Greenwood, 2006
6. *Acting as a catalyst* Creating harmony and understanding, enabling new ways of working, and influencing colleagues' practice for better patient care, through education and role modelling 'Being a catalyst' describes the activities undertaken and considered necessary to keep the momentum of development continuing as well as the personal communication with individuals that enabled inclusivity	Binnie and Titchen, 1999; Titchen, 2001; Manley, 2001; Titchen and McGinley, 2003; Manley *et al.*, 2005
7. *Creative, innovative and challenging behaviour* Pursuing person-centred improvement relentlessly; being willing to take informed risks, that is, working ethically in a non-standard way, to achieve the best outcome for patients/clients; challenging practices and organisations to improve practices; encouraging others to develop a shared vision	Binnie and Titchen, 1999; Manley *et al.*, 2005; Bonner and Greenwood, 2006
8. *Self-awareness* Exploring and recognising one's own strengths and weaknesses; recognising one's scope of influence and impact; seeking self-improvement; articulating one's expertise and passion for nursing Being self-aware and attuned to others	Manley, 2001; Manley *et al.*, 2005; McCormack and McCance, 2006

and autonomy and authority (capacity for making decisions, taking responsibility for any arising consequences and willingness to challenge whole teams and senior colleagues if patient care was compromised). In addition, the EPP demonstrated that nurses with expertise effect change and facilitate both performance and organisational development.

Apart from Titchen's (2000, 2001) study, the processes of encouraging and supporting practitioners to deconstruct and then reconstruct their practice have not occurred before in an investigation of practice expertise. Indeed, the conclusion of other research undertaken to date (e.g. from our search of the literature related to practice expertise between 1996 and 2008) is that supporting nurses with expertise as practitioner researchers is puzzling and problematic. This study, therefore, makes another contribution in relation to setting out the practical know-how of enabling practitioner research. Thereby, it offers a unique framework for helping practitioners to inquire, critique and, perhaps most importantly, continue to learn from the process of investigating their practice, ongoing development and the articulation of their practice expertise as illustrated by participants in the EPP (e.g. Richmond, 2003; Titchen & McGinley, 2003; Brown & Scott, 2004; McCormack & Henderson, 2007).

Originally presented as a typology (as in Table 1.1), we concluded that the dynamic relationships between the attributes were not articulated and how nurses use them in a holistic way within their practice were not shown. So building on Titchen's (2001) and Titchen and McGinley's (2003) findings, we re-presented the typology as shown in Figure 1.1 and introduced professional artistry as the overarching enabling factor into our framework. Professional artistry enables the blending and melding of the attributes into unique configurations for each unique patient and context. The dimensions of professional artistry include, for example, different kinds of knowledge, ways of knowing, multiple intelligences, creative imagination and therapeutic use of self. These dimensions and the processes of professional artistry are described in Chapters 3 and 12. Whilst further research is required, we propose that professional artistry includes the reflexive and metacognitive processes that underlie the three enabling factors above.

Although the EPP primarily focused on what happened within the nurse–patient relationship, it was also evident that expert nurses impacted on their colleagues and the organisations in which they were located. This illustrates how expertise in nursing spans and is interdependent with expertise in the other domains necessary for developing person-centred systems. As nurses progress through the clinical career ladder, they develop expertise that extends beyond the world of the nurse–patient relationship to the immediate systems in which care provision is located.

Expertise in developing person-centred systems

Kitwood defines person-centredness as

> a standing or status that is bestowed upon one human being, by others, in the context of relationship and social being. It implies recognition, respect and trust.
>
> *Kitwood, 1997, p. 8*

Person-centred systems are characterised in the workplace, regardless of setting, by the presence of structures, processes and patterns of behaviour that are embedded in the principles of person-centred care and are manifested in a culture that is person-centred (McCormack *et al.*, 2008b). These principles include maximising opportunities for enabling continuity and integration of services by keeping the person at the centre of decision-making, minimising discontinuity through systems re-design, helping individuals and teams to work effectively, and the building of social capital (McCormack *et al.*, 2008b).

Social capital refers to the connections between individuals and is located in the relationships and social networks identified by the norms of reciprocity and trustworthiness that arise from these connections (Putnam, 1993; Adler & Kwon, 2002). Just like economic capital, social capital can be accumulated for distribution among society based on the idea that the more connected a citizen is to his or her social networks, the more social capital or resource that is available for citizens to draw upon in order to improve their lives. The extent to which social capital exists in a given context critically influences the success of collective and collaborative work (Putnam, 1993). Social capital leads to greater potential for networking and commitment to cooperative action (Cohen & Prusak, 2001) and therefore contributes to creating workplace cultures where people flourish through trust, shared values, mutual understanding and respect. Manley (2000, 2004) and Manley *et al.* (2007) describe the culture arising from such principles as an *effective workplace culture*, one that is associated with specific attributes that include the values, patterns of behaviours, structures and processes necessary for achieving social capital, person-centredness, evidence-based care, and individual and team effectiveness.

Person-centred systems through their structures and processes therefore actively support practitioners and practice teams to deliver on key values. This characteristic is demonstrated well by the Magnet Hospital Programme and the outcomes it achieves (Aiken *et al.*, 2002). In Magnet Hospitals, nursing is highly valued and supported and this is reflected in the quality of care experienced by patients. Enabling person-centred systems to develop in practice requires a specific skill set that builds on nursing practice expertise located in the nurse–patient relationship. This skill set is outlined in Box 1.3, but for greatest effect, needs to be located as near to the interface of care between health care providers and recipients as possible (Manley & Webster, 2006).

These skills were derived from a set of methods, for example, agreeing ethical processes, analysing stakeholder roles and ways of engaging stakeholders, being person centred, clarifying the development focus, collaborative working relationship, continuous reflective learning, and developing a shared vision, among others known to be influential in developing practice (McCormack *et al.*, 2006). This

Box 1.3   The skill set required for developing person-centred systems (*Source*: From Manley and Webster (2006).)

- Working collectively with users and others, and representing different stakeholder groups.
- Developing an effective culture, including transformational leadership.
- Work-based learning encompassing approaches that include reflective practice.
- Using and developing knowledge and policy.
- Evaluating practice at individual and team levels.
- Helping individuals and teams achieve the above skill set.

skill set underpins the following four domains necessary for developing person-centred systems:

- facilitating learning and a work-based learning culture;
- facilitating inquiry, evaluation and evidence use in practice;
- facilitating a culture of effectiveness through leadership;
- using consultancy approaches that foster self-sufficiency in problem-solving across teams and organisations.

The four domains build on the first – nursing practice expertise in the nurse–patient relationship – that captures the scope of the clinical career framework in nursing. Developing expertise in the four domains is now considered from the perspectives and the frameworks that currently exist to describe them.

Four domains of person-centred expertise

Facilitating learning and a work-based learning culture

Fundamental to the EPP and the development and articulation of nursing practice expertise was the creation of a learning culture that helped participants to learn from and in their practice, and in parallel for some, to re-create such a culture in their own workplace. This was achieved in two ways: first, through the nurse with expertise and their critical companion, and second, through action learning sets (McGill & Beaty, 2001) involving both nurse with expertise and critical companions so as to facilitate group learning about work and critical companionship (Titchen, 2004) that could be mirrored in the workplace. Both sets of learning processes were designed to help each participant to become more effective in their own work as well as develop the facilitation skills needed to help others with their learning and development in the workplace (Dewar & Walker, 1999; Ogrinc *et al.*, 2004).

Central to this approach is the concept of work-based learning with its potential to transform health care services so as to improve patients' and users' experiences, provide value for money, improve productivity and achieve continued modernisation (Manley *et al.*, 2009). Developing expertise in the facilitation of learning in and from practice, therefore, meets the needs of not only the learner but also the organisation (Flanagan *et al.*, 2000; Gallagher & Holland, 2004). Using experiential learning in health care organisations requires educators and managers to be aware of the need for skilled facilitation, and for that facilitation to be provided by practitioners who are prepared for their role (Green & Holloway, 1997; Walker & Dewar, 2000; Manley *et al.*, 2009) as an internal facilitator of it (e.g. Manley, 1997, 2001, 2002).

Work-based learning requires active learners who are motivated and have potential for learning and development. However, active learners span a continuum, and this continuum provides insights into practitioners' ability to learn themselves, as well as facilitate learning in others. Whilst it is possible to use active learning processes in practice to promote learning and a learning culture (Dewing,

12

2008), developing expertise in the facilitation of others' learning and an ability to process learning, in terms of what is happening in the learning process, cognitively and metacognitively, is an additional asset. Manley *et al.* (2009), in an analysis and synthesis of the literature, develop a contemporary framework for work-based learning and identify a continuum that describes the journey of the active learner. At one end of the continuum, active learners may be recognised as listening and learning from others, taking the initiative in identifying self-deficits, setting their own learning objectives and goals, and learning from their own work experience. The development of professional artistry marks the other end of the continuum, one that characterises the pinnacle of professional practice, one that integrates and appreciates learning with inquiry and encompasses a number of characteristics described in more detail in Chapter 12.

Hence, within the domain of *facilitating learning in and from practice*, artistry in the practice of nursing provides the building block for developing expertise in the enablement of others' learning in the workplace. This expertise includes the ability to: recognise where individuals are on a continuum of active learner characteristics; deconstruct and reconstruct what is learnt in a meaningful way at several levels that integrate inquiry; and, simultaneously, develop a genuine learning culture in the workplace, one where work-based learning is valued and acted upon. Developing a learning culture requires that the characteristics of active learning and the skills to develop these be nurtured in and used by others, with regard to not only individual learning, but also group- and team-based learning (Manley *et al.*, 2009). A learning culture would therefore be recognised when the everyday work of health care, whatever a person's position, forms the basis for learning and inquiry in the workplace, and varied learning and development activities involving others are evident (see Chapter 12).

A set of evidence-based standards informed by frameworks, such as critical companionship (Titchen, 2004), have been developed to help practitioners to show their readiness for career progression with regard to facilitating others in their learning in and from practice both formally and informally, individually and in groups (RCN, 2004b). These standards are underpinned by a range of processes that would constitute the everyday repertoire of practitioners with expertise in facilitating, not only learning and development, but also person-centred systems (see Box 12.2). This range is important because these processes integrate and underpin all four of the domains identified for developing person-centred systems integral to nursing's career framework.

The domain of *facilitating learning and a work-based learning culture* is interdependent with *facilitating inquiry, evaluation and evidence use* – the next domain. This is because both domains require expertise in the same processes of facilitation.

Facilitating inquiry, evaluation and evidence use

Facilitating the integration of learning with inquiry, as argued above, is a characteristic that would be expected of those at the pinnacle of their career framework in practice. Some practitioners develop this expertise as a result of being exposed to the type of culture and processes described above; others come to this understanding from a different pathway that may have started with more traditional approaches to research. Practitioners at the pinnacle of their career framework, however, in addition to facilitation expertise, need expertise and an understanding in research approaches that cross different paradigms and inform different purposes. These purposes range from informing technical interventions through to developing practical understanding of patients' and users' experiences, as well as action-based participatory approaches in the workplace relevant to the context (Manley & McCormack, 2003). In addition, there are varying perspectives that extend from the use of evidence in practice, the development of evidence from practice and theorising from practice (Bucknall *et al.*, 2008) through to enabling others to contribute to the knowledge base through original practice-based research using a range of different research approaches.

Using the facilitation skills and processes referred to above (Manley *et al.*, 2009), and expanded in Chapter 12 (see Box 12.2), combined with an understanding of different research approaches as part of an action research study operationalising the consultant nurse role, Manley (2001) was able to make research real through using it in practice, facilitating research critique and application and helping practitioners undertake research and evaluation in their everyday work. The way the consultant nurse worked with and facilitated practitioners (as co-researchers) in developing research expertise resulted in not only a positive valuing of research by all, but also enabled care to be up to date, for example, through nearly all nursing interventions being informed by evidence-based standards. In turn, these results enabled the development of a strong research culture.

The practitioners, as co-researchers in the work, were able to contribute to a programme of research in the workplace (Manley, 1994; Manley *et al.*, 1996, 1997), informed further by masters and undergraduate theses. This research increased the staff's understanding of practice and the needs of patients and families within the workplace and helped them to use a range of different research approaches that led to benefits for patients, relatives and staff (Mills, 1993, 1997; Welch, 1993; Creasey, 1996; Cruse, 1996; Pinnock, 1998).

In another action research study (Down, 2004), the full range of research approaches, combined with facilitation expertise and work-based learning, were used to implement person-centred systems by developing, implementing and evaluating an organisation-wide practice development strategy. The skills involved in facilitating the implementation of person-centred systems drew extensively from those identified in the consultant nurse action research study but extended them to the organisational level. In the organisational study, practitioners were enabled to use work-based learning approaches, become practitioner researchers and develop research skills that augmented and strengthened their everyday practice. This resulted in research products, namely, research protocols developed by practitioners for patient stories, staff stories, observation of practice, qualitative 360-degree feedback, using the RiCH tool as a research culture benchmarking tool (Fox & Feasey, 2001) and the Appraisal of Guidelines for Research and Evaluation (AGREE) instrument (AGREE Collaboration, 2001) to enable the use of evidence from practice (RCN, 2007), thus improving practice through a climate of inquiry.

The facilitation of transformational research that involves shared action drawing on critical and phenomenological approaches is a feature of research in the workplace that includes genuine involvement of stakeholders in the research process (Titchen & Manley, 2007). Facilitators of transformational research, that is, research that transforms individuals, teams and organisations through the process of the research, will need to develop expertise in a number of strategies, specifically:

- creating a transformational research culture;
- holistic facilitation that enables stakeholders to develop research skills and to sustain these (Binnie & Titchen, 1999; Manley, 2001);
- promoting authentic collaboration;
- overcoming the obstacles to genuine collaboration in the workplace so that decision-making is democratic and stakeholders are not marginalised.

Titchen and Manley (2006) identify a range of principles necessary to guide the achievement of authentic collaboration and also tools that can be used to enable it, such as, values clarification, claims, concerns and issues, thematic analysis and interpretation, and collaborative theory generation (Titchen & Manley, 2007); these are expanded further in Chapter 13.

The practitioner at the pinnacle of the clinical career framework would therefore be expected to develop expertise in using these tools in a range of different settings; different kinds of knowledge, using different methodological assumptions within action research for different purposes; and 'critical, creative communities that are mindful of the practicalities of being rigorous with audit trails, the critiquing of claims and findings, making explicit the many complex spirals of related activity that take place, as well as more consciously and collectively surfacing the barriers to action and promoting human flourishing' (Titchen & Manley, 2006, p. 345).

One repeated theme throughout this chapter is that of integration – and how the development of practice expertise is integrated with developing expertise in the other domains. Facilitation too has been an integrating theme with facilitation pivotal in the EPP (Manley *et al.*, 2005), and work-based learning (Manley *et al.*, 2009), helping others to both become inquirers of their own practice, as well as a prerequisite to achieving evidence-based practice (Rycroft-Malone, 2004). Three factors enable research to be implemented in practice: the quality of the evidence, the need for skilled facilitation and a context that includes a conducive culture, leadership and evaluation (Rycroft-Malone, 2004) highlighting again how the domains of practice expertise are integrated.

Facilitating a culture of effectiveness through leadership

Earlier, a culture of effectiveness was stated as the purpose of person-centred systems. A culture of effectiveness is recognised by five attributes (Box 1.4).

Whilst both organisational and individual enabling factors have been identified as influential in developing such a culture (Manley *et al.*, 2007), this chapter in

Box 1.4 Five attributes of an effective workplace culture (*Source*: Adapted from Manley *et al.* (2007).)

1. Specific values promoted in the workplace, namely:
   - person-centredness
   - lifelong learning
   - support and challenge
   - leadership development
   - involvement and participation by stakeholders (including service users)
   - evidence use and development
   - positive attitude to change
   - open communication
   - teamwork
   - safety (holistic).
2. All the above values are realised in practice; there is a shared vision and mission and individual and collective responsibility.
3. Adaptability, innovation and creativity maintain workplace effectiveness.
4. Appropriate change is driven by the needs of patients/users/communities.
5. Formal systems and skilled facilitation exist to continuously enable and evaluate learning, performance and shared governance.

the context of the clinical career framework will focus on individual enabling factors as these are most relevant for developing expertise in facilitating an effective workplace culture. The individual enablers include transformational leadership, skilled facilitation and role clarification (Manley *et al.*, 2007). Skilled facilitation has already been identified as an important skill set for developing expertise in practice, learning in and from practice, as well as for promoting a culture of inquiry that is evidence based.

Role clarity with clear expectations and responsibilities is recognised as a prerequisite for enabling evidence-based practice and critical thinking (Davies *et al.*, 2000, Newman *et al.*, 2000), the implementation of Total Quality Management (Huq and Martin, 2000) and also an effective culture (Jones & Redman, 2000; Bevington *et al.*, 2004). Role clarity is something that can be achieved through using tools such as qualitative 360-degree feedback (see Chapter 13) and so the focus here will be primarily on leadership.

Leadership and practice expertise

Leadership has long been identified as the key to culture change (Bate, 1994; Brown, 1998) and the main approach to developing a culture of effectiveness in the workplace (Kouzes & Posner, 1987; Manley, 1997). Transformational leadership is a clear and well-researched concept that encompasses paying attention to culture (Jones & Redman, 2000; Manojlovich & Ketefian, 2002), role-modelling shared values (Haworth, 2000; Bevington *et al.*, 2004) and achieving a common vision through engaging hearts and minds (Davies *et al.*, 2000).

Leadership and management are different activities that are related (Marquis & Huston, 1996), but it is leadership expertise that is essential for cultural change. Kotter (1990) identifies the specific mechanisms through which leaders achieve action:

- creating a perceived need to change;
- clarifying the vision of what change was needed;
- challenging the status quo but marshalling a lot of evidence to support this;
- communicating a new vision in words and deeds;
- motivating many others to provide the leadership to implement the vision.

As this chapter focuses on the clinical career framework, it is pertinent to consider both the advantages and disadvantages of including an operational management component to senior clinical posts (Manley, 1993). Whilst benefits include having legitimate power and influence to change practice through authority from position power (Handy, 1993), the disadvantages relate to the time and energy consumed in administration and operational management, reducing dramatically the time available for developing practice (Lathlean, 1995; Fulbrook, 1998). Past arguments are that without the position power of an operational management role, it may be more difficult to influence and change practice (Manley, 1997), although this is unproblematic if values and beliefs are shared (Manley, 1993; Fulbrook, 1998) and everyone takes responsibility for making values live. Within a culture that is collaborative, therapeutic and participative, sources of power are devolved. Credibility is from expertise, power of argument and critique, power to enable others, and shared values and beliefs.

Whilst it may be argued that formal management is not a core component of advanced practice (Fulbrook, 1998), there is an argument for emphasising the strategic aspects of management and management skills, rather than the operational aspects (Goodman, 1998). The need for strategic vision, having a good sense of direction and 'seeing the possibilities' (Manley, 2001) is integral to leadership expertise, with the ability to work within strategic frames of reference a necessity for developing practice (McCormack *et al.*, 1999).

Being a political leader is one of the five dimensions of cultural leadership (Bate, 1994) (Box 1.4). Bate argues that political leaders focus on interaction and assign meaning by putting ideas into words and giving ownership of the idea to the organisation or community; they bring about cultural change through changing people's frames of reference (see Box 1.4). For example, translating the concerns of practitioners who provide care at the interface with users to those responsible for executive decisions is a highly developed skill recognised in successful executive nurses who are described as translators and interpreters (Antrobus, 1999). At a micro-politics level, Ward *et al.* (1998) identify the importance of addressing stakeholders' concerns before undertaking practice development activity, identifying the need to consider the impact that activities will have on one's own work practices, as well as relationships with significant others. In addition, he identifies the need for strategies to deal with possible negative organisational attributes because lack of ownership of practice initiatives by all stakeholders negatively influences project outcomes. Political leadership aims to influence policy through positioning key ideas, getting stakeholders on board and developing and using influencing strategies that will have an impact on the development and uptake of local as well as national policy (Antrobus, 2003).

Effective cultures are characterised by being strategically appropriate and adaptable and involve leadership that mediates between a changing context and the providers of the service, constantly drawing this changing context to the notice of practitioners so that they can respond. An example of this is seen in advanced practitioner roles where nursing expertise is augmented by a specific set of competencies to enable changing health care needs to be met.

Bate (1994) comprehensively identifies the five dimensions necessary for cultural leadership, but considers not all would be present in any one person arguing, the need for balance between them at different times (Box 1.4). Expertise in this domain would include developing expertise in some areas whilst recognising how the expertise of others can complement the full range of leadership dimensions required.

Transformational leadership is emphasised in enabling a culture of effectiveness to develop (Manley, 2004), but leadership expertise at the pinnacle of the nursing career framework needs to integrate clinical and strategic leadership with transformational and political approaches (Manley, 1997, 2002; Redfern, 2003; Hayes, 2003).

In helping consultant nurses in older peoples nursing to explicate their clinical leadership role, through a cooperative inquiry, the need to appreciate leadership as influencing others was a focus. As practising nursing expertly may not positively influence others if there is no one to experience and observe nursing expertise other than the patient (Manley *et al.*, 2008). This inquiry set out to identify that which was taken for granted in the consultant nurses' everyday leadership practice. A complex picture emerged that was multifaceted and multidimensional, one that involved working across levels, seeing connections between teams, interacting policy strategy decisions with an impact on clinical decisions. Clinical leadership strategies at three levels of influence resulted and these were directed at the:

- *immediate care of the patient*, for example an active judgement was made to lead patient care because of the complexity of the patient, or, working across boundaries to benefit the patient;
- *team*, for example by being opportunistic and intentional in using any situation that emerged to work with staff to develop their practice, planting seeds, facilitating participation of stakeholders in developing a common vision;
- *organisation*, for example building relationships at a strategic level, developing networks for engaging in and building on at a later date, using governance frameworks to influence practice.

In this fourth domain, *facilitating a culture of effectiveness*, facilitation expertise, role clarity and a number of leadership dimensions have been identified that are essential requirements for nurses at the pinnacle of their career framework if both a culture of effectiveness is to be achieved in practice and nursing is to influence the broader health care agenda. The final domain focuses on consultancy approaches in clinical practice.

Consultancy approaches to foster self-sufficiency in problem-solving

The provision of specialised help reflects consultancy practice in its commonest form, that of, providing expertise and advice to a consultee. Growth in consultancy has arisen across society from increasing demand for social and technical knowledge and skills (Gallessich, 1982) also reflected in increasing specialism within nursing (ICN, 1999). Gallessich (1982) differentiates the role of consultancy from other roles considering it an emerging professional in its own right. She argues that innovative consultancy practice crosses traditional professional boundaries and spans three developmental levels, suggesting that the knowledge base informing consultancy practice is broader than the original focus of a discipline and extends to drawing extensively on knowledge from other fields such as organisational change, development and learning.

Caplan's (1970) consultancy model is health specific, was developed in mental health, and is driven by the assumption that consultancy is about disseminating as much expertise as possible to the widest number of people requiring access to it. Caplan's model includes both direct and indirect consultancy focused at either the individual patient or health care provider through to the system, programme or organisational level (Table 1.2). This model therefore provides a framework for understanding and developing consultancy practice and expertise across the career framework for nursing (Manley, 1996, 1997):

> Expertise in nursing consultancy would include the ability to operate within all four types, so that, the potential of nursing practice expertise can be realised at strategic levels as well as clinical levels.
>
> *Manley, 1996, 1997*

Consultancy is not about developing dependence on the consultant. Although, in the past, expert specialist nurses acting in a consultancy function may have unwittingly caused dependency. For example, in being asked to provide help and advice (client-centred consultancy) about a patient's leaking stoma bag, the specialist nurse would have attended to the challenge, drawing on years of experience to provide a completely leak-proof bag to the satisfaction of the patient, with the consequence that other practitioners became deskilled and dependent on the expert. In Caplan's model, the focus of the consultant is on enabling such expertise to develop in others. Helping others to become self-sufficient in their own decision-making and problem-solving, and continuing to be self-critical is essential to achieving a sustainable culture of effectiveness across any service. This approach to consultancy is termed process consultancy.

Schein (1988) differentiates *process consultancy* from other approaches to consultancy, namely, the *purchase of expertise model* and the *doctor–patient model*, where consultancy tends to be underpinned by the premise that the expert knows best and that others will accept their advice without question. Whilst there will be

Table 1.2 Examples of consultancy activity using Caplan's (1970) consultancy model

Type of consultancy	Direct/indirect	Focus of consultancy	Examples
Client-centred consultancy	Direct to the patient/client/user and sometimes the care provider	Focus is on the client (i.e. the patient/user) and their health and illness issues. Although the request may come from a consultee (the care provider)	Specific patient-centred issues, for example assessment, diagnosis, intervention, evaluation and review
Consultee-centred consultancy	Indirectly focused on patients/clients	The consultee (health provider – individual /team) is the main focus of attention and is helped with their own activity, knowledge and learning	Improving knowledge and skills of health care providers as individual practitioners and teams
Program-centred administrative consultancy	Direct focus on a programme of activity	The focus is on developing, implementing and evaluating a programme/system of activity across an organisation	Implementing and evaluating, for example, critical care outreach or infection surveillance systems across directorates or organisations
			Implementing directorate-wide and organisation-wide programmes of, for example, practice development, systems for monitoring and maintaining patient safety, clinical governance, clinical effectiveness
Consultee-centred administrative consultancy	Indirect	Focus is on supporting the consultee who is implementing a programme of activity	Helping individuals (consultees) to implement and evaluate programmes/systems across directorates and organisations through, for example, mentoring, coaching and supervision

times when experts' advice and guidance are required, the importance of working predominantly within a process consultancy model is important. This is because it fosters individuals and teams to develop their own skills in problem-solving activities so that they become self-sustaining. Process consultancy is also consistent with the facilitation approaches previous described and would be necessary for both developing and sustaining person-centred systems. Process consultancy is underpinned by values about collaboration and how others develop. Successful use of process consultancy and also Caplan's model involves:

- being able to work in a truly collaborative way with others;
- helping others to become self-sufficient in their thinking, learning and development processes by using approaches that enable ongoing reflection and critique;
- drawing on a number of tools which facilitate the development of a common vision and the giving and receiving of feedback.

> The consultant is often viewed by the consultee as an expert. He or she may be expected to pass along relevant information and knowledge to the person of lesser expertise. While such a perception may benefit the consultant by increasing the likelihood that he or she will be listened to, it also negates the strength of the consultee and ignores the need of the consultee for assistance in the diagnostic process. To achieve the best resolution to the consultee's problem the consultant must work in collaboration with the consultee.
>
> *Hansen et al., 1991, p. 31*

Developing expertise in a consultancy approach that enables self-sufficiency in ongoing problem-solving marks the final domain linked to the clinical career framework. At the beginning of the chapter, it was stated that nurses will be on different journeys in their development across the domains of the clinical career framework and will have different starting points. Whilst this is the case, for those at the pinnacle of their clinical career pathway, expertise in nursing practice and expertise in the other four domains necessary for developing person-centred systems would be a necessary requirement.

The clinical career framework

Differing emphasis of expertise

The clinical career picture in nursing has undergone a period of change internationally (Schober & Affara, 2006). Nursing practice has moved from one that has been uncoordinated, underdeveloped, undersupported, with little options for the practitioner beyond the clinical manager role, to a position where it is now possible to progress coherently within a practice-based framework that enables the expertise of practitioners to remain in practice but still grow and develop the scope of their expertise (Rolfe & Fulbrook, 1998; Manley, 2001). There is now a much clearer vision for practitioners in their clinical career pathways; where they can go, as well as how to get there.

During recent years, there has been an emergence of different roles linked to advancing the practice of nursing and health care in response to changing health care needs and demand, for example nurse practitioners, clinical nurse specialists, generalist health care practitioners, lecturer practitioners and practice development facilitators as well as consultant nurses – within an international dimension, these roles all have subtlety different meanings. The challenge now is how these roles can be linked and integrated more clearly to the concepts of nursing expertise across the career framework in a coherent way that enables clear public accountability as well as transparent career progression, and an explicit contribution to a modern and effective health care service.

Currently, there are tensions between a focus on developing generalists and specialists. Increasing specialism is a movement pervading all activities within a growing technological society, one where there is a knowledge explosion with new knowledge, technological advances, and increasing public needs and demands (International Council of Nurses, 1999). On the other hand, there is political interest in having a more generic worker with flexible skills to work within any health care setting; however, there lies the dilemma if one is seldom practising the skills one has learnt, then competency becomes questionable (Eraut, 1994). Within nursing, it is possible to have both expertise in terms of a specific client group such as the older person with mental health needs, and also generalist expertise in leadership, facilitation of cultural change and the development of a learning and research culture. Therefore, the career framework needs to reflect these two parameters:

- *A growing expertise and specialism with a specific client group,* for example as seen in nurse practitioners who work in general medical practices, or emergency nurse practitioners working within a minor injuries unit, or clinical nurse specialist working with patients with acute or chronic pain. Such practitioners are associated with predominantly client-centred care in the majority of their professional role.
- *A growing expertise in the domains necessary to develop person-centred systems* where patients and users experience care that is both person centred and evidence based; for example team or clinical leaders and managers who develop their managerial and leadership expertise in addition to their practice expertise; practice developers who develop their skills in enabling service teams to provide person-centred and evidence-based care and may be working either across organisations or within particular clinical directorates; lecturer practitioners and clinical facilitators who work with specific client groups but are developing their roles as facilitators, educators and enablers; and some clinical nurse specialists who are developing teams and services across whole organisations and sectors. This parameter is associated with a split in the time spent directly and indirectly with actual practice, although all activities are practice focused and interdependent.

These two parameters may have a different emphasis within any one job role, but one could argue that expertise in the primary role of practising one's discipline is an essential prerequisite to progressing through a clinical career ladder in nursing, although the achievement of expertise in practice of caring for one's client group may not be a prerequisite to progressing along other career pathways such as health care management, higher education and traditional research pathways. The focus of the clinical career pathway is the integration of the clinical aspects of these functions within practice and for some the first and second parameters run sequentially and for others they develop in parallel. Within the UK, the consultant nurse is the pinnacle of the clinical career ladder in nursing and requires the achievement of expertise in all the domains necessary to develop person-centred systems. The consultancy function of the consultant nurse role integrates consultancy on nursing practice and practice development with consultancy on research and education in practice settings as well as consultancy on consultancy itself (Manley, 1996).

Consultant nurses use their expertise in nursing practice combined with expertise in the other domains to develop a workplace culture dedicated to providing quality care across the patients' journey, regardless of who provides care (Manley, 2001; Manley & Dewing, 2002). Clinical nurse specialists, like consultant nurses, are also usually expert nurses for a specific client group; however, they may be on their own journey of developing expertise in the other domains expected of the consultant nurse. Advanced practitioner roles are growing in number, whether they are generic or specialist; these too have nursing expertise at their core. However, advanced practitioner roles are associated with a specific set of competencies that will enable health care services to 'mind the gap' in the patients journey. Such competencies are informed by the technical interventions previously associated with different disciplines and in the future will also be integral to other roles in the nursing career framework. However, there is a perceptual difference between demonstrating such competencies at a level that is safe and confident and integrating them into a pattern of behaviour that can be described as expertise. Through explicating frameworks, standards and skills across the five domains, it is hoped that there is greater clarity about how to both achieve and recognise nursing practice expertise with regard to both the nurse–patient relationship and the development of person-centred systems.

Pathways beyond the consultant nurse role: where next?

Once the pinnacle of the clinical career pathway has been reached, it is important to reflect on the opportunities that may be available that places nursing practice expertise at their centre. Can nursing practice still be a part of one's role beyond a consultant nurse post? To answer this question, those posts that would build on the clinical achievements of the consultant nurse rather than posts that take practitioners away from the world of practice and the provision of direct services to patients and users are highlighted. Such posts fall into three areas; all are currently immature but have the potential for further development and would appear to be a natural progression for those who have developed their expertise across all the key domains of the consultant nurse but wish to influence health care practice and services more broadly:

1. *Clinical chairs*. These are posts that bridge health care organisations and universities with most of the post's emphasis being based in the health care organisation rather than the university. Clinical chairs would be leading an organisation-wide strategic programme of practice-related research and practice development where they would be supporting consultant nurses, senior practice developers and practitioner researchers in a corporate way contributing to the goals of the health care organisation. Clinical chairs are likely in the future to be the main supporters, coaches and mentors of consultant nurses across the organisation and would be a resource to the university in ensuring that Higher Education Institutions provide programmes relevant to the world of practice. The clinical chair would continue to practise nursing with possibly a small caseload within a specific area but predominantly their generic expertise would be used to support organisation-wide activity and would be strategically focused.

2. *Executive clinical leads/directors*. These are posts that in the future would be occupied by people who have progressed through the clinical career ladder and who have considerable experience as consultant nurses or practice developers rather than through the general management route. Their role would encompass providing expertise in nursing and service development as a member of the organisation's executive team in addition to leadership. They provide a strategic executive opportunity similar to executive medical directors and would still continue with a small caseload, thus keeping them in touch with the realities of practice and service delivery at the patient interface.

3. *Clinical deans*. These posts again bridge the health care organisation and the university similarly to the clinical chairs, although the time in the university would be much higher in proportion than with their clinical chair counterparts. These posts would mediate between the Workforce Confederations, health care providers, strategic health authorities and the universities providing clinical educational leadership with a focus on clinical education.

Summary

This chapter has set out to help readers to develop a broad vision for a clinical career pathway that is focused on nursing practice expertise. It has provided a vision for a clinical career pathway that focuses on two parameters: the development of expertise in the practice of nursing for a specific client group through the nurse–patient relationship, as well as, developing expertise in all the other areas necessary for providing quality services to patients – the four domains required to develop person-centred systems, regardless of national context.

Through considering the frameworks presented, readers are encouraged to assess themselves and their readiness to proceed through a clinical career framework, to decide where they are, where they want to be and to have some understanding about what they need to do to move in the direction of their vision. Many of the contributors to this book have been on this journey and are shining lights for what nursing expertise can offer – they are living models for the impact nursing expertise can have on contemporary health care.

References

Adler, P. & Kwon, S. (2002) Social capital: arospects for a new concept. *Academy of Management Review* **27**(1), 17–40.

AGREE Collaboration (2001) *Appraisal of Guidelines for Research and Evaluation (AGREE) Instrument*. Available from www.agreecollaboration.org.

Aiken, L.H., Clarke, S.P. & Sloane, D.M. (2002) Hospital, staffing, organization and quality of care: cross-national findings. *Nursing Outlook* **50**(5), 187–194. (Reprinted from *International Journal for Quality in Health Care*, 2002, Volume 14.)

Antrobus, S. (1999) *Reconstructing Nursing Management*. MPhil Critical Management. Management School, Lancaster University.

Antrobus, S. (2003) What is political leadership? *Nursing Standard* **17**(43), 40–44.

Bate, P. (1994) *Strategies for Cultural Change*. Butterworth Heinemann, Oxford.

Benner, P. (1984) *From Novice to Expert: Excellence and Power in Clinical Nursing Practice*. Addison-Wesley, Menlo Park, CA.

Benner, P., Tanner, C.A., Chesla, C.A., Dreyfus, H.L., Dreyfus, S.E. & Rubin, J. (1996) *Expertise in Nursing Practice: Caring, Clinical Judgement, and Ethics*. Springer, New York.

Benner, P. & Wrubel, J. (1989) *The Primacy of Caring: Stress and Coping in Health and Illness*. Addison-Wesley, Menlo Park, CA.

Bevington, J., Halligan, A. & Cullen, R. (2004) Culture vultures. *Health Service Journal* **114**, 30–31.

Binnie, A. & Titchen, A. (1999) *Freedom to Practice*. Butterworth Heinemann, Oxford.

Bonner, A. & Greenwood, J. (2006) The acquisition of nephrology nursing expertise: a grounded theory study. *Journal of Clinical Nursing* **15**(4), 480–489.

Brown, A. (1998) *Organisational Culture*, 2nd edn. Financial Times Pitman Publishing, London.

Brown, A. & Scott, G. (2004) Art & artistry in practice: a reflective account. In: *Delivering Cancer & Palliative Care Education* (eds L. Foyle & J. Hostad), Chapter 8. Radcliffe, Oxon.

Bucknall, T., Kent, B. & Manley, K. (2008) Evidence use and evidence generation in practice development. In: *International Practice Development in Health Care* (eds K. Manley, B. McCormack & V. Wilson), pp. 84–104. Blackwell, Oxford.

Caplan, G. (1970) *The Theory and Practice of Mental Health Consultation*. Tavistock, London.

Cohen, D. & Prusak, L. (2001) *In Good Company. How Social Capital Makes Organizations Work*. Harvard Business School Press, Boston, MA.

Creasey, J. (1996) A phenomenological study of the lived experience of family members, of patients who are nursed in a general intensive care unit. Unpublished MSc Thesis. North-East Surrey College of Technology, Ewell.

Davies, H., Nutley, S.M. & Mannion, R. (2000) Organisational culture and quality of health care. *Quality in Health Care* **9**, 111–119.

Dewar, B.J. & Walker, E. (1999) Experiential learning: issues for supervision. *Journal of Advanced Nursing* **30**, 1459–1567.

Dewing, J. (2008) Becoming and being active learners and creating active learning workplaces: the value of active learning in practice development. In: *International Practice Development in Health Care* (eds K. Manley, B. McCormack & V. Wilson), pp. 273–294. Blackwell, Oxford.

Donnelly, G. (2003) Clinical expertise in advanced practice expertise: a Canadian perspective. *Nurse Education Today* **233**, 168–173.

Down, J. (2004) 'From Conception to Delivery' A journey towards a trust-wide strategy to develop a culture of patient-centredness. In: *Practice Development in Nursing* (eds B. McCormack, K. Manley & R. Garbett), pp. 267–287. Blackwell, Oxford.

Eraut, M. (1994) *Developing Professional Knowledge and Competence*. Falmer Books, London.

Ersser, S.J. (1997) *Nursing as a Therapeutic Activity: An Ethnography*. Avebury, Aldershot.

Flanagan, J., Baldwin, S. & Clarke, D. (2000) Work based learning; as a means of developing and assessing nursing competence. *Journal of Clinical Nursing* **9**, 360–368.

Foley, B.J., Kee, C.C., Minick, P., Harvey, S. & Jennings, B. (2002) Characteristics of nurses and hospital work environments that foster satisfaction and clinical expertise. *Journal of Nursing Administration* **32**(5), 273–282.

Fox, C. & Feasey, S. (2001) *Evidence-Based Care Benchmark Research in Child Health (RiCH) Network*. Royal College of Nursing, London.

Fulbrook, P. (1998) Advancing practice: the advanced practitioner perspective. In: *Advancing Nursing Practice* (eds G. Rolfe & P. Fulbrook), Butterworth Heinemann, Oxford.

Gallagher, A. & Holland, L. (2004) Work based learning: challenges and opportunities. *Nursing Standard* **4**(19), 39–42.

Gallessich, J. (1982) *The Profession & Practice of Consultation*. Jossey-Bass, San Francisco.

Goodman, I. (1998) Developing advanced practice. In: *Advancing Nursing Practice* (eds G. Rolfe & P. Fulbrook), Butterworth Heineman, Oxford.

Green, A.J. & Holloway, D.G. (1997) Using a phenomenological research technique to examine student nurses' understandings of experiential teaching and learning a critical review of methodological issues. *Journal of Advanced Nursing* **26**, 1013–1019.

Grundy, S. (1982) Three modes of action research. *Curriculum Perspectives* **2**(3), 23–34.

Guba, E.G. & Lincoln, Y.S. (1989) *Fourth Generation Evaluation*. Sage, Newbury Park, CA.

Handy, C. (1993) *Understanding organisations*, 4th edn. Penguin, Harmondsworth.

Hansen, J.C., Himes, B.S. & Meier, S. (1991) *Consultation: Concepts and Practices*. Prentice-Hall, Englewood Cliffs, NJ.

Hardy, S., Garbett, R., Titchen, A. & Manley, K. (2002) Exploring nursing expertise: nurses talk nursing. *Nursing Inquiry* **9**(3), 196–202.

Hardy, S., Titchen, A. & Manley, K. (2007) Patient narratives in the investigation and development of nursing practice expertise: a potential for transformation *Nursing Inquiry* **14**(1), 80–88.

Hardy, S., Titchen, A., Manley, K. & McCormack, B. (2006) Re-defining nursing expertise in the United Kingdom. *Nursing Science Quarterly* **19**(3), 260–264.

Haworth, S. (2000) New management culture in the NHS. *Nursing Management* **7**(3), 16–17.

Hayes, N. (2003) Consultancy – the future for nursing roles? In: *Nursing Practice and Health Care* (eds S. Hinchliff, S. Norman, & J. Schober), 4th edn, pp. 443. Hodder Arnold, London .

Huq, Z. & Martin, T.N. (2000) Workforce cultural factors in TQM/CQI. Implementation in hospitals. *Health Care Management Review* **25**(3), 80–93.

International Council of nurses (1999) Guidelines on specialisation. ICN.

Johnston, B. & Smith, L. (2006) Nurses' and patients' perceptions of expert palliative nursing care. *Journal of Advanced Nursing* **6**, 700–709.

Jones, K. & Redman, R. (2000) Organizational culture and work design: experiences in three organizations. *Journal of Nursing Administration* **30**(12), 604–610.

Judd, J. (2005) Strategies used by nurses for decision-making in the paediatric orthopaedic setting. *Journal of Orthopaedic Nursing* **9**(3), 166–171.

Kennedy, C.M. (2004) A typology of knowledge for district nursing assessment practice. *Journal of Advanced Nursing* **45**(4), 401–409.

Kitwood, T. (1997) On being a person. In: *Dementia Reconsidered: The Person Comes First* (ed. T. Kitwood), pp. 7–19. Open University Press, Milton Keynes.

Kotter, J.P. (1990) *A Force for Change: How Leadership Differs from Management*. Free Press, New York.

Kouzes, J.M. & Posner, B.Z. (1987) *The Leadership Challenge*. Jossey-Bass, San Francisco.

Lathlean, J. (1995) *The Implementation and Development of Lecturer Practitioner Roles in Nursing* [Thesis]. University of Oxford, Oxford.

Manley, K. (1993) The clinical nurse specialist. *Surgical Nurse* **6**(3), 21–25.

Manley, K. (1994) Primary nursing in critical care. In: *Critical Care Nursing: Care of the Critically Ill* (eds B. Miller & P. Burnard). Balliere Tindall, London.

Manley, K. (1996) *Consultancy*. MSc Nursing. Distance Learning Module. RCN Institute, London.

Manley, K. (1997) A conceptual framework for advanced practice: an action research project operationalising: an advanced practitioner/consultant nurse role. *Journal of Clinical Nursing* **6**, 179–190.

Manley, K. (2000) The role of the surgical nurse and knowledge for practice. In: *Surgical Nursing; Advancing Practice* (eds K. Manley & L. Bellman). Churchill Livingstone, Edinburgh.

Manley, K. (2001) *Consultant Nurse: Concept, Processes, Outcomes*. Unpublished PhD Thesis. University of Manchester/RCN Institute, London.

Manley, K. (2002) Commentary on critique of consultant nurse framework. *Nursing in Critical Care* **7**(2), 84–87.

Manley, K. (2004) Transformational culture: a culture of effectiveness In: *Practice Development in Nursing* (eds B. McCormack, K. Manley & R. Garbett), pp. 51–82. Blackwell, Oxford.

Manley, K., Cruse, S. & Keogh, S. (1996) Job satisfaction of intensive care nurses practising primary nursing and a comparison with those practising total patient care. *Nursing in Critical Care* **1**(1), 31–41.

Manley, K. & Dewing, J. (2002) The consultant nurse role NHS. *Journal of Healthcare Professionals*. May 8–9.

Manley, K. & Garbett, R. (2000) Paying Peter and Paul: reconciling concepts of expertise with competency for a clinical career structure. *Journal of Clinical Nursing* **9**, 360–368.

Manley, K., Hamill, J.M. & Hanlon, M. (1997) Nursing staff's perceptions and experiences of primary nursing practice in intensive care 4 years on. *Journal of Clinical Nursing* 6(4), 277–287.

Manley, K., Hardy, S., Titchen, A., Garbett, R. & McCormack, B. (2005) Changing patients' worlds through nursing practice expertise. Exploring nursing practice expertise through emancipatory action research and fourth generation evaluation. *A Royal College of Nursing Research Report 1998–2004*, RCN Institute, London.

Manley, K. & McCormack, B. (1997) *Exploring Expert Practice*. MSc Nursing Distance Learning Module, RCN Institute, London.

Manley, K. & McCormack, B. (2003) Practice development: purpose, methodology, facilitation and evaluation. *Nursing in Critical Care* 8(1), 22–29.

Manley, K., Sanders, K., Cardiff, S., Davren, M. & Garbarino, L. (2007) Effective workplace culture: a concept analysis. In: *RCN Workplace Resources for Practice Development*. RCN Institute, London, p. 6–10.

Manley, K., Titchen, A. & Hardy, S. (2009) Work based learning in the context of contemporary UK healthcare education and practice: a concept analysis, *Practice Development in Health Care*, in press.

Manley, K. & Webster, J. (2006) Can we keep quality alive? *Nursing Standard* 21(3), 12–15.

Manley, K., Webster, J., Hale, N., Hayes, N. & Minardi, H. (2008) Leadership role of consultant nurses working with older people: a co-operative inquiry. *Journal of Nursing Management* 16, 147–158.

Manojlovich, M. & Ketefian, S. (2002) The effects of organisational culture on nursing professionalism: implications for health resource planning. *Canadian Journal of Nursing Research* 33(4), 15–34.

Marquis, B. & Huston, C. (1996) *Leadership Roles and Management Functions in Nursing: Theory and Application*, 2nd edn. Lippincott, Philadelphia.

McCormack, B., Dewar, B., Wright, J., Garbett, R., Harvey, G. & Ballantine, K. (2006) *A Realist Synthesis of Evidence Relating to Practice Development: Executive Summary*. NHS Quality Improvement. Scotland. Available from www.nes.scot.nhs.uk/.

McCormack, B. & Henderson, E. (2007) Critical reflection and clinical supervision: facilitating transformation. In: *Clinical Supervision in Practice: Some Questions, Answers and Guidelines for Professionals in Health and Social Care* (ed. V. Bishop). Palgrave, Basingstoke.

McCormack, B., Manley, K., Kitson, A., Titchen, A. & Harvey, G. (1999) Towards practice development – a vision in reality or a reality without vision? *Journal of Nursing Management* 7, 255–264.

McCormack, B., Manley, K. & Walsh, K. (2008) Person-centred systems and processes. In: *International Practice Development in Health Care* (eds K. Manley, B. McCormack & V. Wilson), pp. 17–41. Blackwell, Oxford.

McCormack, B. & McCance, T. (2006) Development of a framework for person-centred nursing. *Journal of Advanced Nursing* 56(5), 1–8.

McCormack, B., McCance, T., Slater, P., McCormick, J., McArdle, C. & Dewing, J. (2008) Person-centred outcomes and cultural change. In: *International Practice Development in Health Care* (eds K. Manley, B. McCormack & V. Wilson), pp. 189–214. Blackwell, Oxford.

McCormack, B. & Titchen, A. (2006) Critical creativity: melding, exploding, blending. *Educational Action Research: An International Journal* **14**(2), 239–266. Available from http://www.tandf.co.uk/journals.

McGill, I. & Beaty, L. (2001) *Action Learning: A Guide for Professional Management and Educational Development*, 2nd edn. Kogan Page Ltd, London.

Mills, C. (1993) The lived experience of families whose family member is transferred from an intensive care unit practising primary nursing to a ward that is not. Unpublished BSc Dissertation. Institute of Advanced Nursing, Royal College of Nursing (Manchester University), London.

Mills, C. (1997) Presence in critical care nurses: an action research study. Unpublished MSc Thesis. RCN Institute (Manchester University), London.

Newman, M., Papadopoulos, I. & Melifonu, R. (2000) Developing organisational systems and culture to support evidence-based practice: the experience of the Evidence-Based Ward Project. *Evidence-Based Nursing* **3**, 103–105.

Ogrinc, G., Headrick, L., Morrison, L.J. & Foster, T. (2004) Teaching and assessing resident competence in practice based learning and improvement. *Journal of General Internal Medicine* **19**, 496–500.

Pinnock, D. (1998) The skills of critical care nurses can use to appropriately include significant others in the care of patients. An action research study. Unpublished MSc Dissertation. RCN Institute (Manchester University), London.

Putnam, R.D. (1993) *Making Democracy Work. Civic Traditions in Modern Italy*. Princeton University Press, Princeton, NJ.

RCN (2004a) Expertise in practice standards. RCN Accreditation Unit, RCN Institute, London.

RCN (2004b) Standards for becoming a RCN Accredited Facilitator. RCN Accreditation Unit, RCN Institute, London.

RCN (2007) Workplace resources for practice development. RCN Institute, London.

Redfern, L. (2003) Clinical pinnacle. *Nursing Standard* **22**(17), 96.

Richmond, J. (2003) *Maximising Nursing Expertise within Oncology (Perspective)*. Cancer Nursing Practice. Available from http://www.highbeam.com/Cancer+Nursing+Practice/publications.aspx?date=200304.

Rolfe & Fulbrook (1998) *Advancing Nursing Practice*. Butterworth Heinemann, Oxford.

Rycroft-Malone, J. (2004) Research implementation: evidence, context and facilitation – the PARIHS framework. In: *Practice Development in Nursing* (eds B. McCormack, K. Manley & R. Garbett), pp. 118–147. Blackwell, Oxford.

Schein, E.H. (1988) *Process Consultation (Volume I): Its Role in Organizational Development*, 2nd edn. Addison-Wesley, Reading, MA.

Schratz, M. & Walker, R. (1995) *Research as Social Change. New Opportunities for Qualitative Research*. Routledge, London.

Taylor, C. (2002) Assessing patients needs: does the same information guide expert and novice nurses? *International Nursing Review* **49**(1), 11–19.

Titchen, A. (2000) *Professional Craft Knowledge in Patient-Centred Nursing and the Facilitation of Its Development*. D.Phil., Linacre College, University of Oxford. Ashdale Press, Oxfordshire.

Titchen, A. (2001) Critical companionship: a conceptual framework for developing expertise. In: *Practice Knowledge and Expertise in Health Professions* (eds J. Higgs & A. Titchen). Butterworth Heinemann, Oxford.

Titchen, A. (2004) Helping relationships for practice development: critical companionship. In: *Practice Development in Nursing* (eds. B. McCormack, K. Manley & R. Garbett), pp. 148–174. Blackwell, Oxford.

Titchen, A. & Manley, K. (2006) Spiralling towards transformational action research: philosophical and practical journeys. *Educational Action Research* **14**(3), 333–356.

Titchen, A. & Manley, K. (2007) Facilitating research as shared action and transformation. In: *Being Critical and Creative in Qualitative Research* (eds J. Higgs, A. Titchen, H. Byrne Armstrong & D. Horsfall). Hampden, Sydney.

Titchen, A. & McGinley, M. (2003) Facilitating practitioner-research through critical companionship. *NT Research* **8**(2), 115–131.

Walker, E. & Dewar, B.J. (2000) Moving on from interpretivism: an argument for constructivist evaluation. *Journal of Advanced Nursing* **32**(3), 713–720.

Ward, M., Titchen, A., Morrell, C., McCormack, B. & Kitson, A. (1998) Using a supervisory framework to support and evaluate a multiproject practice development program. *Journal of Clinical Nursing* **7**(1), 29–36.

Welch, J. (1993) Nurse's perceptions of alarm sounds. Unpublished BSc Dissertation. Birkbeck College University of London.

2. Practitioner Research

Brendan McCormack

Introduction

Contemporary practice emphasises the importance of practitioners reflecting on practice, developing practice and engaging in systematic inquiry about practice in order to ensure effective, efficient and safe care. In order for expertise to be revealed, explored, analysed, developed and maximised in practice, there is a need for processes that support and enable systematic inquiry into practice. However, the need for systematic inquiry into practice extends beyond utilitarian needs plus there is a need for methodological developments that enable the artistry of practice to be revealed. In this chapter, the concept of practitioner research will be explored as one such development that has much to offer the advancement of expertise in nursing, as revealed in the other chapters of this book. In this chapter, the relationship between systematic inquiry through practitioner research and the development of expertise will be articulated through an exploration of methodologies and methods for practitioner inquiry.

Practitioner research – the context

The dominant position of nursing as a practice-based profession means that the challenge to nursing research is to find ways of generating, disseminating and using knowledge that inform and are informed by practice itself. Plato makes a distinction between 'those who know and do not act and those who act and do not know'. What Plato is suggesting here is that there are those who strive to know but do not engage in acting on the basis of that knowing and those who act but do not always have the knowledge to underpin their reasoning for acting in a particular way. This argument could be seen to underpin the traditional divide that exists between researchers (those who strive to 'know') and practitioners (those who 'act'). Further, the reasons why practitioners view researchers as being in their 'ivory tower' become clear as there is a perceived hierarchy between the bearers of the knowledge and those who need the knowledge to support their practice. The hierarchical relationship that exists between the knowledge bearers and the knowledge users is one that has greatly influenced the development of knowledge in nursing and indeed has been an inherent barrier to the way that research is perceived among clinical nurses.

Many studies have been published concerning ways of creating a 'research culture' in health and social care organisations (e.g. Parahoo, 1999, 2000; Perälä, 2000; Rodgers, 2000; Thomas, 2000; McCormack, 2003; Meyer *et al.*, 2003; Gerrish & Clayton, 2004). Many of these studies have moved away from a more traditional view of research culture in terms of it being synonymous with 'research awareness' and have instead identified creative means of engaging clinicians in 'critical inquiry'. More recently, McCormack and Crisp (2008) have proposed that inquiry among nurses can happen at three levels:

- Inquiry that involves critical engagement with everyday practice, through formal and informal models of reflection and action.
- Inquiry that involves collaborative and ongoing evaluation of local nursing practices through audit.
- Inquiry that involves the advancement of nursing's knowledge base through research.

These levels are not mutually exclusive and indeed each overlaps with and informs the other. The potential to harness a disparate collection of approaches to 'local' inquiry, development and research into one strategy that generates substantial knowledge for and about practice can be realised through an integrated approach to practice inquiry. This can have the added benefit of 'demystifying research'. McNiff (1998) asserts, '[W]e have grown so accustomed to the idea of the solitary and wilful creator that we find it difficult to see the deeper ecology of creation.' McNiff argues that we need to look at how things are created and not rely solely on externally derived knowledge and forces to shape our experiences. In order to see what is around us, we need to be able to find systematic and rigorous ways of exploring and making sense of such experiences. One way of doing this is to adopt principles of 'practitioner research' in health care research strategies. The focus of inquiry and the research processes adopted in a practitioner research agenda are those of everyday experiences of practitioners integrated with more formalised research processes, with seen as neither more systematic nor rigorous than the other. Therefore, research processes can be seen by practitioners to be useful and a part of everyday practice.

Practitioner research – what is it?

It is widely contended in the literature that the term 'practitioner research' is problematic (cf. Bartlett & Burton, 2006). Whilst the term is often used by researchers to mean research that is focused on the work of practitioners, in reality, it is associated with multiple meanings, world views and methods of inquiry. The diversity of opinion about what counts as practitioner research has resulted in it being used as a 'catch-all' phrase to be used by researchers as a means of suggesting a direct connection between their research and its relevance to practice, when at best such connection is often tenuous. Rolfe (1998), in drawing on the work of Laurence Stenhouse (cf. Rolfe, 1998, pp. 66–68), argues that research has imposed its own agenda on practice in terms of what counts as valid knowledge in and for practice. Rolfe argues that judgements of quality in research have overridden judgements of quality in practice and as a result knowledge is used in practice based on the quality of the methodology of the research rather than on the credibility of the findings for practice. Rolfe asserts, '[I]f there are no flaws in the design and conduct of the study, then we are compelled to accept the findings as applicable to practice' (p. 66). Whilst it is largely indisputable that there is a direct link between methodological rigour and quality of research findings, Rolfe does make an important point about the decontextualised acceptance of research findings without due consideration for the socio-cultural implications of their implementation and the behavioural and cultural barriers to their acceptance. Rolfe argues for a need to shift criteria for accepting research findings for practice away from a critique of the methodology to a critique of the findings themselves.

Practice is contextually located and embedded in multiple cultures that are created and re-created by the 'actors' in that context. Individuals can influence the context of practice but this influence can only be translated into sustainable change when the culture is receptive to it (Argyris, 1999). Cultural change happens from 'within' and Manley (2000) refers to this as 'workplace culture', that is, the multiple cultures that make up the setting of practice (i.e. the workplace or context). Accessing these cultures enables the release of the practice knowledge that is embedded in experience, contextually bound and rarely reproduced in propositional form (Titchen & Higgs, 2001). This approach values knowledge that is both inductively and deductively derived (Kitson *et al.*, 1996). So bearing in mind that if knowledge is to be embedded in practice culture, there is a need for new paradigmatic perspectives that take us away from either/or positions – for example either technical or emancipatory, either quantitative or qualitative. In reality, practitioner research needs to transcend such arguments and focus on utilising approaches that enable the achievement of its primary purpose – the systematic critique of practice and self as practitioner, in order to generate new understandings about practice and its social, cultural, discursive and relational dimensions that enable or hinder clinical effectiveness. Thus, the definition of practitioner research adopted in this chapter is:

> [P]ractitioner research is a formal and systematic attempt made by practitioners either alone, or in collaboration with others, to understand their work, with the intended purpose of making public new knowledge about the transformation of self, colleagues and work contexts.
>
> *Adapted from McCormack, 2003*

This definition is deliberately inclusive in terms of paradigm, methodology and method, that is, it does not attempt to dictate acceptable forms of knowledge, methodological approaches or data collection methods. Within this definition, various interpretations of what constitutes 'research' are possible. However, it emphasises the building on knowledge generated through the systematic inquiry into practice experiences and research into *self* as practitioner. 'Experience' is the foundation stone for the development of new knowledge (Higgs & Titchen, 2007). Recognising and learning from the development of nurses' experience in a particular practice context is an essential route towards the development of 'expertise' in practice (Hardy *et al.*, 2006). The definition also makes reference to the type of role as researcher that the practitioner might adopt. For example, the practitioner may be conducting research alone and focusing on their own practice; the practitioner's work may be the focus of research that is coordinated by others; or the practitioner's work may be the focus for research conducted in some form of collaborative arrangement between the practitioner and others. In all cases, the practitioner is somebody engaged in the planning, management or delivery of health and social care. However, despite these differences, some common principles do exist. Practitioner research:

- utilises research processes that are negotiated and that are an integral component of practice development;
- adopts processes that are based in practice and supported by a variety of potential supervisory frameworks (e.g. academic supervision, clinical supervision, mentorship, external facilitation, appraisal and action learning);
- focuses on personal and professional effectiveness;
- enables the systematic development of practice and an integrated approach to the evaluation of the effectiveness of structures, processes and outcomes;
- considers knowledge to be contextually bound and therefore new knowledge is derived from an engagement with the context of practice.

Rolfe (1998, p. 75) asserts that for practitioner research to be embraced, we need to be explicit that we are meaning 'practitioner-*centred* research':

It is practitioner-centred rather than practitioner-based because it is research undertaken by the practitioner into herself and her own practice; and it is research rather than inquiry to emphasise the point that it should be seen as a serious alternative to the traditional scientific research paradigm.

Whilst Rolfe's perspective is useful in ensuring that the distinguishing feature of practitioner research (i.e. research conducted with and by practitioners into one's own practice) are overtly maintained, there is the danger of polarising research paradigms. Practitioner research is not an 'alternative' to other research paradigms but is instead a paradigm with a specific purpose, focus and thence methodologies that enable it to be realised in practice. Further, whilst practitioner research is *centred* on the practitioner, it should not be seen as a 'naval-gazing' self-indulgent introspective activity. Rather, the focus on the practitioner emphasises and makes explicit the interconnected and synergistic relationship between the practice (of practitioners), care outcomes for patients and development outcomes for teams and workplaces. The danger lies in practitioner research being seen as a solitary and individualistic activity and as such has the potential to separate (rather than integrate) practitioner research from other forms of knowledge

Box 2.1   Example 1: Level 1, practitioner-led research

A group of nurses want to set up a clinical supervision group in their ward. A facilitator is appointed to work with the group. The group do not have any specific development agenda but agree that they are interested in exploring and developing their working relationships, their team functioning and increasing their effectiveness in practice. A research practitioner works with the group and the facilitator (who could be the research practitioner) to establish the supervision contract, agreement for the supervision data to be used as 'process data' for informing an overall clinical supervision strategy evaluation and for understanding how the practitioners make sense of evidence in practice. The participants are aware of and agree to the data being used as part of a practitioner research collaborative. This is formally agreed through a contract including ethical issues and concerns. Over a period of 6 months, the supervision sessions are recorded. The practitioners and the research practitioner work together to collect and analyse the data and identify outcomes for themselves (own growth in expertise), the team(s) with whom they work (the development of team expertise), service users (outcomes arising from growth in expertise) and their organisation (translation of knowledge into organisational targets and strategy). Individual nurses may choose to use questions and issues arising from the practitioner research to formulate proposals for further research that may lead to academic award.

generation. To prevent such an occurrence, it can be proposed that practitioner research operates at three modes of *practitioner engagement:*

Mode 1: Practitioner led (Box 2.1). In this model, the practitioner is actively engaged in research and development work, including the planning of the work, data collection, analysis and publication. The focus of the research is the practitioner's own work. The practitioner manages changes arising from the work set within a framework of organisational support and informed by health and social care strategy. The role of a 'research practitioner'[1] in this approach is to provide the support infrastructure for the practitioner to engage in the work, including research resources, critical companionship (Titchen, 2001), supervision and a culture of challenge and support. The work undertaken can be supported by a range of academic work-based accreditation processes at a variety of academic levels.

Mode 2: Practitioner collaborative (Box 2.2). In this model, the practitioner is actively engaged in research and development work, but not leading the whole work from planning through to publication. The focus of the work is the

---

[1] The term 'research practitioner' is being used in this chapter to represent the various roles that exist in organisations to support research in practice. Across the world, there exist a variety of models of joint academic-practice appointments, clinical academic positions, lecturer practitioner, research practitioner and senior nursing positions that have research as a role function. All these roles exist to support research in practice and generate new knowledge in and from practice.

Box 2.2 Example 2: Level 2, practitioner collaborative research

Nurses across a number of wards and departments in a hospital identify the meeting of patients oral hygiene needs as being a significant problem across the organisation. Practice is inconsistent, relatives often complain about the 'state of their relative's mouth' when they visit and it is generally a neglected area of practice. Pharmacy departments have identified that anti-fungal agents are used inappropriately, and that if oral hygiene was given greater priority, these agents would not be needed. The group agree to undertake a development project in each ward and department addressing this issue by working together over a 4-month period to develop a formal research and development proposal. The group formally contract with a nurse researcher from the local University who facilitates the development of the research and development proposal set within an action research methodology and utilising realistic evaluation (Pawson & Tilley, 1998). Different group members take on responsibility for the development of different parts of the proposal, including the review of the available evidence, the formalisation of the research questions, developing the ethical approval process, establishing the research protocol and access issues. The group collectively agree the methodology and data collection methods, and a 1-year project is established. An explicit part of the methodology will be the collection of data concerning mechanisms for bringing about changes in practice (M), the contextual issues needed for getting the evidence into practice (C) and the resulting outcomes (O) (after Pawson & Tilley, 1998). All the data is 'pooled' and analysed to explore the relationship between M, C and O. On the basis of this work, three sets of data are developed. Firstly, data to inform the need for practice developments at an individual ward and department level. Secondly, data concerning the contextual changes needed to support this practice, team developments needed, professional development issues and the effectiveness of the processes used to bring about this change, and thirdly, information about the success (or not) of developing a consistent approach to one area of practice.

practitioner's own work, the work of colleagues or own work in an organisational context. The practitioner may be working as a part of a community of researchers who are focusing on a particular part of work or on creating a culture that sustains particular practice developments. The practitioner may have a formal collaborative and/or supervisory relationship with a research practitioner or a researcher from a higher education institution who may have a more active role in leading the research project, managing the collaborative inquiry and creating a support infrastructure. Part of this infrastructure may include action-learning sets, group and individual supervision, literature searching and analysis, computer support, publication support and enabling the accreditation of the learning achieved through a variety of work-based learning pathways.

Mode 3: Practitioner focused (Box 2.3). In this model, the practitioner is not actively engaged in the research and development work, but is the focus of the work. In this model, a research practitioner or a researcher from a higher education institution leads the research and development and the degree of engagement by the practitioner is negotiated as a part of the overall research

Box 2.3   Example 3: Level 3, practitioner-focused research

A university-based professor of Nursing Research with a particular interest in exploring the way in which expert nurses use their expertise to develop practice at micro (team) and macro (organisation) levels brings together senior nurses from six health care facilitates to discuss the topic. Twelve nurses (nurse consultants, nurse specialists, advanced practice nurses and nurse practitioners) come together, each of whom has been engaging in practitioner-centred research into aspects of their own practice. They agree to work with the Professor of Nursing Research as participants who will be the 'focus' of her research. As a part of the agreed methodology, process data through supervision notes, reflective diaries, action-learning notes, peer-review (for example) are maintained by the individual nurses. This data is 'pooled', and as a result, a large data set is generated that allows for the detailed analysis of nursing expertise, the contextual factors that enable expertise to flourish and the impact of expertise on patient outcome. In addition, secondary data analysis is performed to explore process and organisational issues to do with practitioner effectiveness in undertaking research.

design. The level of engagement can range from participation in shaping the research design, agreeing data collection methods through to participation in elements of data collection, analysis, publication and dissemination.

It is anticipated that in any organisation, the three levels of practitioner engagement would be in operation simultaneously. However, it can also be suggested that in order for the full potential of practitioner research activities to be realised, an organisational framework for the coordination of practitioner research needs to exist in health care organisations. Figure 2.1 proposes one such framework. It highlights how the different modes of engagement in a model of practitioner research could all be located within a coherent strategic framework for the organisation, management and funding of the research activity. The framework places reflective inquiry as the central focus of research question generation that proceed through a systematic approach to the translation of questions into research activity. The coordination of the practitioner research activity would ensure that an organisation can draw on a 'data pool' to demonstrate outcomes for patients and teams that can be linked to key performance indicators. Figure 2.1 further illustrates how each element of the framework informs the other and thus no part exists in isolation of the other.

The transformative potential of practitioner research

As suggested earlier, practitioner research seeks to understand and generate knowledge about practice in context and the resulting outcomes. However, critics suggest that many accounts of practitioner research are little more than stories and recollections that have important meanings to the author but whose meanings are

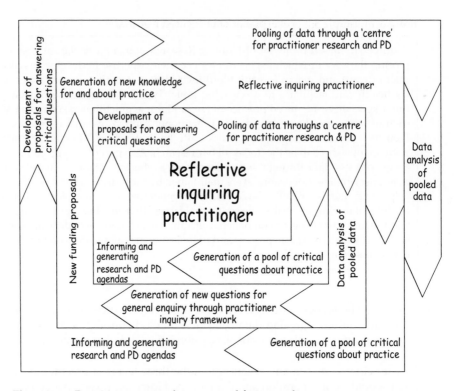

Figure 2.1   Practitioner research conceptual framework.

lost to the reader as they fail to connect to the subtle meanings inherent in the story (Brooker & Macpherson, 1999) or as Fine (1994) suggests when the research accounts are innocent moments of experience that have a romantic, uncritical and an uneven handling of the multiple voices inherent in the story. If practitioner research is to be more than the telling of 'romantic uncritical recollections and stories', then it needs to adopt a 'critical' perspective. A perspective that understands that:

> changing practices is not just a matter of changing ideas of individual practitioners alone, but also discovering, analysing and transforming the social, cultural, discursive and material conditions under which their practice occurs.
>
> *Kemmis, 2006, p. 474*

McCormack and Titchen (2006) have argued that for transformation to occur, there is a need for clarity of understanding. They referred to this systematic inquiry into understanding as 'hermeneutic praxis'. It emerges from the philosophical tradition of hermeneutics and the transformation of understanding can lead to the transformation of self, teams, organisations and communities. Locating practitioner research in a critical framework provides a vehicle for understanding the social, cultural, discursive and material conditions of practice and the potential for transformation. Thus, practitioner research can be located within an interpretive paradigm but with an intent of transformation through the taking of action from clarity of understanding. Research methodologies that have a focus on 'taking action' (e.g. action research, emancipatory practice development and transformational practice development) are typically located within the critical paradigm. Traditionally, many approaches to bringing about changes to practice have relied on pedagogical methods (knowledge inputs to increase understanding of the need for change and/or knowledge about the new change to be implemented) and/or interpretive methods (knowledge derived from interpretations of practice and its effectiveness through the use of social science methods). The idea being that once practitioners have acquired this knowledge, then their practice will change. Action-orientated methodologies of research and development, including emancipatory action research, emancipatory practice development and transformational practice development reject pedagogical and interpretive methods (as stand-alone methods) because of the naïve assumption that having an understanding of a situation leads to action. Habermas (1972) calls this knowledge that is focused on 'practical interest', that is, knowledge that is concerned with understanding and clarifying how others see their worlds. For example, Brown and McCormack (2006) demonstrated that although nurses in a surgical setting had an in-depth understanding of the need for systematic assessment of pain among older people having abdominal surgery and indeed were aware of the evidence-based protocols in existence to guide their practice; little of this knowledge was used in practice. Even though Brown undertook a systematic and rigorous ethnography of the existing practices and discussed these in detail with the ward staff, practice did not change, that is, having a greater understanding of patients' and users' experiences may have been achieved, but this did not result in a change in the way nurses practice.

It is the action component that is addressed by critical social science, that is, emancipatory interest. Critical social science argues that achieving understanding is necessary in order to identify possibilities for action, but it is only through the processes of taking action (acting on shared interpretations) and the learning that results that true emancipation (i.e. freedom from previous forces of domination that hinder effective action) can be achieved.

Critical social science is derived from critical theory. Critical theory may be distinguished from other forms of theory in its explicit intent towards emancipation. With its roots in a Western European Marxist tradition, the aim of emancipation is 'to liberate human beings from the circumstances that enslave them' (Horkheimer, 1982, p. 244). Thus, critical theory goes beyond interpretation and understanding, in the sense that it does not just set out to explain and understand social contexts but instead aims to free people from social and contextual circumstances that may limit effectiveness. Emancipation arises from critique undertaken by individuals or groups concerned with exposing contradictions in the rationality or justice of social actions. Critical social science is concerned with the kind of action that arises from raised awareness or increased understanding that leads to a desire by individuals or groups to redress contradictions, oppressions or domination, rather than action resulting from power or coercion. 'Action' is concerned with changing practice (Carr & Kemmis, 1986). Practitioner research from a critical social science perspective, therefore, is concerned with challenging and reframing established practices, opening up and showing tensions in language use and generating new knowledge about the processes and outcomes arising from the inquiry processes used. These processes encourage productive dialogue with the intention of encouraging new ways of thinking and acting (emancipation).

Fay (1987) developed a comprehensive framework of critical theory. Fay suggested that a comprehensive critical social scientific theory is necessarily comprised of a complex of 8 theories and 20 sub-theories (Table 2.1).

Fay argues for the centrality of reflection in emancipatory processes. He suggests that reflection is important not as a means of learning *about* theory but as a means of learning about oneself *in terms* of the theory. Fay's theory of 'the body' is central to being reflective, that is, understanding how we inherit ways of being and the limits posed by these inherited dispositions on our freedom. To overcome many of these limitations of critical social science, Fay argues that all eight theories (Table 2.1) need to be kept in balance in order to achieve emancipation because 'our world is marked by continual tension in human life between illumination and activity on the one hand, and concealment and dependency on the other' (p. 215). He suggests that it is a mistake to focus on one side of the tension at the exclusion of the other and that by integrating the eight theories into the critical social science project, a balance can be achieved:

> A proper critical social theory is one which possesses a stereoscopic vision which recognizes every situation as one of both gain and loss, of change and stasis, of possibility and limit. The amended scheme [eight theories] is meant to incorporate this dual vision.
>
> *Fay, 1987, p. 215*

A number of methodologies exist that operationalise critical theory and in this chapter three of these will be explored – emancipatory action research, emancipatory practice development and transformational practice development.

Emancipatory action research

The purposes of emancipatory action research are threefold:

- Develop practice, introduce a change, respond to a need or problem (Elliott, 1991; Binnie & Titchen, 1999).
- Enable practitioners/participants to learn/develop/become empowered (Grundy, 1982; Kemmis & McTaggart, 1988; Titchen & Binnie, 1993a).
- Contribute to or refine theory (Lewin, 1947; Elliott, 1991; McNiff, 1988; Whyte, 1991; Titchen & Binnie, 1993b, 1994; Greenwood, 1994).

These purposes integrate the development of practice and practitioners with contributing to a public knowledge base. Emancipatory action research has

Table 2.1 The theories and sub-theories of critical social science

Theory	Sub-theory
1. *False consciousness*	1. Demonstrates the ways in which the self-understandings of a group of people are false or incoherent or both
	2. Explains how the members of this group came to have these self-misunderstandings and how they are maintained
	3. Contrasts them with an alternative self-understanding; showing how this understanding is superior
2. *Crisis*	4. Spells out what a 'crisis' is
	5. Indicates why the particular crisis exists
	6. Provides a historical account of the development of this crisis in terms of structures and processes
3. *Education*	7. Offers an account of the conditions necessary and sufficient for enlightenment to happen
	8. Shows how these conditions are satisfied in a given context
4. *Transformative action*	9. Isolates those aspects of a society that must be altered if the dissatisfaction of a group's members is to be lessened
	10. Details a plan of action indicating how people who are to carry out social transformation are to carry this out
5. *The body*	11. Develops an explicit account of the nature and role of inherited dispositions and the ways in which knowledge is embodied
	12. Points out how embodied knowledge is created without reaching consciousness
	13. Spells out the limits which inherited dispositions and embodied knowledge place on transformative action
6. *Tradition*	14. Identifies which parts of a particular tradition are, at any given time, changeable
	15. Identifies which parts of a particular tradition are, at any given time, not changeable or worthy of change
7. *Power*[a]	16. Develops an account of the conditions and use of power in a particular situation
	17. Explicitly recognises the limits and effectiveness of critical theory in certain situations of power
8. *Reflexivity*	18. Explains one's own historical tradition and makes explicit one's own biases and prejudices in particular contexts
	19. Does not pretend that any one change is able to capture the essence of emancipation
	20. Offers an account of the ways in which any change is contextual and incomplete

Source: From McCormack and Titchen (2006); adapted from Fay (1987).
[a] In Fay's (1987) original work, he used the word 'force' instead of power. For the purpose of this chapter and our understanding of critical social science in the context of the development of practice in healthy and social care contexts, we understand Fay to mean 'power' when he uses the word 'force'.

the development of self and others as a deliberate purpose, through enabling learning from critical reflection on experience (Binnie & Titchen, 1999; Manley, 2001; Titchen, 2001):

> The intention of action research is to give persons the power to act to bring about change (action) by generating knowledge through rational reflection on personal experience (research).
>
> *Grundy, 1982, p. 24*

As early as 1978, Susman and Evered articulated this purpose as developing the 'self-help competencies' of people facing problems. Carr and Kemmis (1986) propose that the focus of such development is on emancipation. For Fay (1987), practitioners pass along a continuum from enlightenment, through empowerment, to emancipation. Emancipation to Grundy (1982) is true praxis, an action freed from the dominating constraints of the environment. She argues it is the act itself, rather than the product of the act that is emancipatory. Like Fay, Grundy concludes that emancipation results from developing critical theorems and enlightenment. The development of such enlightenment is also present in Mezirow's (1981) concept of perspective transformation, specifically theoretical reflexivity which is achieved through structured reflection. Although sometimes a consequence of approaches underpinned by other world views, for critical theory, this purpose is a deliberate intention and unique to emancipatory action research.

The other two purposes of action research, those of developing practice and developing theory, have been shown to be shared by all world views in action research, although the nature of theory may differ.

Carr and Kemmis (1986) summarise the fundamental purposes of action research as 'to improve' and 'to involve' – thus providing a bridge to other characteristics of action research not evident in the three purposes above, by introducing some of the processes. First, they consider that action research improves practice through developing practitioners' understanding of both practice itself and the situation in which practice takes place; second, they emphasise involvement of practitioners in all phases. Action research is concerned with both the processes and outcomes. Outcomes are considered important but their exact nature may not be known in advance other than their general strategic direction or the presence of process outcomes such as enlightenment, empowerment and emancipation. The following processes are therefore the methods of emancipatory action research:

- development of critical intent of individuals and groups;
- working with values, beliefs and assumptions;
- developing moral intent;
- focusing on the impact of the context/system on practice as well as practice itself;
- using self-reflection and fostering reflection in others;
- fostering widening participation and collaboration by all involved.

Pivotal to an action research approach based on critical social science is the concept of 'practitioner researchers' – practitioners involving themselves in participatory research about their own practice, understandings and situations (Carr & Kemmis, 1986). Carr and Kemmis argue that if transformation of real practice situations is to occur, then the duality of research and practice roles need to be transcended.

Such an approach therefore involves the *participants themselves*, not 'critical investigators' as the source of programmes of education and action designed for enlightenment. Broadly, the source of such activity within emancipatory action research can be drawn from two interrelated areas of action/practice:

- One's own individual action and effectiveness as a practitioner, which may also include actions as a facilitator of group critical intent.
- Group actions (of which the facilitator is part) in achieving a deliberate and strategic purpose.

A consequence of action research involving groups will be that activities need to be facilitated, coordinated or assisted by an individual or a small group of researchers (Grundy, 1982; Stringer, 1996). Grundy considered that this role will require the facilitator to take greater responsibility for the practical organisation of the group's deliberative processes, such as preparing agendas and disseminating information. Stringer (1996) defines this role as 'research facilitator', providing leadership and direction to other participants and stakeholders in the research process. Caution would be required with the leadership approach selected in Grundy's (1982) emancipatory mode if manipulation and exploitation are to be avoided. Grundy recognises that if group critical intent exists then the facilitator who is likely to have a broader theoretical background would bring this to the group as a resource to draw on.

Stringer (1996) identifies a further issue when working with groups as an insider. He considers that the demands of professional or community life can actually prevent practitioners from taking on an active leadership role. Stringer therefore draws on outsiders such as consultants to provide facilitation and coordination functions. Drawing on the complementary strengths of insiders and outsiders, their relative and different disadvantages are minimised. In addition, Titchen and Binnie (1994) and Titchen and Binnie (1993b) found effective ways to overcome the inherent pitfalls and tensions of such insider–outsider relationships. Models of outsider-researcher and insider-practitioner have been successfully used in nursing to facilitate the development of patient-centred care through an action research study where the outsider acted as a critical companion (Titchen, 2001). Critical companionship is similar to Carr and Kemmis's (1986) 'critical friend' but is augmented by Campbell's (1984) notion of 'skilled companionship' which accentuates the helping relationship within which critical companionship occurs. This framework can also be used where the critical companion is an insider (Titchen, 2001).

However, the action researcher as an insider, researching and evaluating his or her own role and practice as an individual and member of a group, poses particular issues for traditional science and its understandings of truth and reality. Susman and Evered (1978) indirectly challenge the notion of an 'independent reality' considering it incompatible with action research, highlighting again the roles of values and moral consequences in guiding means and ends. In addition, the processes used by the action researcher are suggested:

> The positivist assumption of a detached, neutral, independent, objective researcher is incompatible with the requirements of action research. Once one accepts organisations as artefacts, created by humans for the purpose of serving human needs, then one cannot escape the realization that actions in an organization have moral consequences that must be faced. The success of action research hinges on understanding the values of the relevant actors since such values guide the selection of means and ends for solving problems and develop the commitment of the actors to a particular solution. Empathy, taking the role of the other, participant observation, etc. may be the most effective means for making the theoretical or practical knowledge the researcher possesses really useful and accepted by clients.
>
> *Susman and Evered, 1978, pp. 598–599*

The notion that action research belongs to practitioners does not mean that methods can be ignored because in learning significantly from experiences, practitioners use skills that can be improved and methods that can be described (Winter, 1989). The action research process provides a schema for guiding the collection and analysis of data in relation to both fact finding and evaluation, which in turn influences action and provides the means of establishing if action has led to an improvement (Hart & Bond, 1995). It is argued that action researchers are more inclined to use more qualitative data such as that arising from participant observation and unstructured interviews. However, the use of both quantitative and qualitative data as a strategy for achieving methodological triangulation is now commonplace.

Approaches to analysis must be faithful to and not distort the views and opinions of co-researchers. Analysis in action research is more likely to run concurrently with data collection than following it. Preliminary analysis is shared with participants and the traditional boundaries between the roles of researcher and researched are muddied. In emancipatory action research, all stakeholders should be engaged in the processes of investigation: collecting data, theorising, acting and evaluating (Grundy, 1982).

To summarise, emancipatory action research enables the processes involved in developing practice to be explored for the purposes of continually improving the quality of care to patients and developing theory about such processes. It is collaborative and participative, supporting a research *with* rather than research *on* philosophy. This is congruent with the values underpinning practitioner research. It is also an approach enabling maximum stakeholder involvement, has the potential through emancipatory approaches to develop practice, enable participants to become empowered to research and transform their own practices, and develop theory about practice.

Emancipatory practice development

In previous work, Manley and McCormack (2003, 2004) have outlined the purpose, aims and methodology of emancipatory practice development (ePD). PD is defined as a continuous process of improvement towards increased effectiveness in patient-centred care. This is brought about by helping health care teams to develop their knowledge and skills and to transform the culture and context of care. It is enabled and supported by facilitators committed to systematic rigorous continuous processes of emancipatory change that reflect the perspectives of service users and service providers' (Garbett & McCormack, 2002). This definition makes explicit the purpose of ePD as being that of 'increased effectiveness in patient-centred care', and the means to achieving this is through:

- developing knowledge and skills;
- enabling nurses/health care teams to transform the culture and context of care;
- skilled facilitation;
- systematic, rigorous and continuous process of emancipatory change.

PD activities are directly targeted at practice and impact on how practitioners work with patients, discriminating it from professional development which may or may not indirectly impact on practice. PD includes using evidence in practice as well also generating evidence from practice. The knowledge base that results from and informs decision-making in PD is eclectic, comprising policy, traditional propositional theory in addition to local theory, concerning the specific context, personal theory encompassing professional craft knowledge, and also patients' personal knowing including their preferences. McCormack *et al.* (1999) added that there is a need for matched activity at the organisational and strategic interfaces to optimise PD activity at the client/patient interface.

The *raison d'etre* of PD is to improve some aspect of patient care or service directly. Improvement is a key reason for justifying the establishment of PD roles in organisations (Garbett & McCormack, 2001; McCormack *et al.*, 2006), with an explicit desire to enable practitioners to change practice, rather than just their knowledge base, which is a more indirect focus. In ePD, the development and empowerment of staff is a deliberate purpose interrelated with creating a specific type of culture – termed a *transformational* culture (Manley, 2001) – one where quality becomes everyone's business, positive change becomes a way of life, everyone's leadership potential is developed, and where there is a shared vision, investment in and valuing of staff (Manley, 2000). Therefore, ePD is concerned with enabling practitioners to become empowered to develop their individual and collective service and fostering the development of an integrative and transformational culture (Manley, 2001).

ePD relies on skilled holistic facilitation   (Harvey *et al.*, 2002; Manley & McCormack, 2003, 2004; Shaw *et al.*, 2008). Facilitators aim to help participants become aware of and freed from taken-for-granted aspects of their practice and the organisational systems constraining them. Facilitators foster a climate of critical intent through reflective discussion involving various 'ideas' of group members and assist the groups' enlightenment through nurturing a culture which enables individuals and groups to act. Responsibility for action rests with the practitioners/group (Grundy, 1982). This approach is consistent with emancipatory action research (EAR). Through pursuing an interest in the external climate and broader social system in which care is provided, collective insight, understanding and ownership develops through practitioners' own actions, rather than the actions of others, thus enabling the first steps towards action through developing enlightenment. The facilitator is responsible for enabling a culture to develop where such enlightenment is possible – a culture of critique – and in addition its administrative organisation (Grundy, 1982). Also, the facilitator does have technical expertise to share but his or her contribution is of no greater or lesser importance than that of other group members.

Evaluation of the outcomes of ePD would be concerned then with specific technical interventions and with demonstrating the impact of such interventions on the service or client care showing that they made a difference. Additionally, however, evaluation would focus on personal/collective enlightenment, empowerment and emancipation, and evaluation of the culture in relation to the attributes of a transformational culture (Manley, 2001), one where change had become a way of life with a proactive stance to meeting changing health care needs, and one where all key stakeholders have been involved in developing criteria by which evaluation was undertaken. Evaluation processes would be transparent and underpinned by explicit values and beliefs in recognition that different types of knowledge are interwoven with the human interests they serve. Habermas proposes a much more open focus on values, not as goals to be judged in terms of absolute truth but for enabling the examination of the process of negotiation (Wuthnow *et al.*, 1984, p. 183). Such processes constitute the main work of practice developers using critical social science approaches.

ePD is concerned with the medium of power, so, when selecting evaluation approaches, it is important to select those underpinned by similar premises and aims. Evaluation in ePD serves two purposes – determining the success of the PD in bringing about a change in practice culture and contributing to theory. Two particular approaches to evaluation are compatible with ePD – EAR (Grundy, 1982) and Fourth Generation Evaluation (Guba & Lincoln, 1989).

Theory in ePD is concerned with personal theory arising from action – praxis – the knowledge that informs action, and reflexivity – a theorising spiral in practice, with personal theories evolving constantly from critiquing action, and where action further informs personal theories. So, ePD results in both personal theory, as well as contributing to the public knowledge base with regard to the phenomenon being addressed. This may be local theory, concerned with the local context, although there will be aspects of this, which can be transferred to other contexts and therefore *generalisable* in the sense that the same theory arises from different contexts. In this sense, good PD contributes to theory and its refinement through the evaluation approaches it uses.

In summary, ePD has as its explicit intent the development of cultures that can sustain continuous processes of practice improvement and innovation with a focus on the development of person-centred cultures. The explicit intention of ePD is the empowerment of all practitioners to take responsibility for the quality of their practice, develop practice, learn about the processes involved, and (as a practitioner researcher) inform theory development. The latter is not a primary purpose of ePD in the way that it is in EAR.

Transformational practice development[2]

McCormack and Titchen (2006), whilst acknowledging how critical theory informed their research and development practice, identified gaps within Fay's (1987) eight critical theories for practice and ways in which these gaps hindered the full potential of critical social science to achieve transformation in the way it is espoused. Through critical exploration, they began to address these gaps, by combining the assumptions of the critical world view with their experiences of using creative imagination and expression in their ePD work. Then through a critical review of their work, they created a new synthesis for transformational development and research to add to the critical world view called *critical creativity*.

In their first paper articulating their reflexive journey towards developing critical creativity, McCormack and Titchen (2006) critiqued assumptions underpinning the critical world view and articulated the unique philosophical, theoretical and methodological assumptions of critical creativity. As a result, they proposed a substantial elaboration of Fay's sub-theory 10 (a sub-theory of his theory 4 – *transformative action*) (see Table 2.1). They called this elaboration of sub-theory 10, *creativity* (see McCormack & Titchen, 2006). The critical approach, as elaborated by Fay, does not sufficiently explain or direct attention to the issue of how a critical theory can be turned into actual practice. McCormack and Titchen (2006) identified that even within *transformative action* (theory 4), sub-theory 10 of Fay's model (a plan of action that indicates how people are to carry out a social transformation) leaves the impression that the movement from the level of abstract theory to the level of practice is nothing more than application. But this is misguided; practical activity involves skills, sensitivities and capacities that require an artistry that involves far more than knowing the contents of a theory. This is why they elaborated sub-theory 10 and named it *creativity*.

Practical activity involves praxis through which practitioners learn how to pick out significant features of their environment, develop insightful responses to these features, and adjust and adapt themselves to the particularities of a given situation. Of course, praxis can be informed by theory, but genuine praxis requires that practitioners go far beyond learning this theory in order to be effective practitioners, that is, we need to place ourselves in the context of theory by how we live, feel and know the environment/landscape of practice. In particular, in trying to implement a critical theory, practitioners need to employ a kind of creative activity whereby they enable themselves to perform in particular situations. Practising

---

[2] This section on 'transformation practice development' is a synthesis of the original paper by McCormack and Titchen (2006).

this creative activity and developing practical knowing will enable practitioners to develop a professional artistry without which their interventions or transformative actions in the practical world would be clumsy, routine or unresponsive. McCormack and Titchen (2006) identified that what was needed to augment Fay's critical model, then, was a *praxis spiral* that focuses attention on the important creative work in which practitioners must engage if they are to be effective in taking or facilitating transformative action. Recently, Titchen and McCormack (2008) demonstrated how the methodology of critical creativity operationalised this praxis spiral through the use of creative methods grounded in nature. Titchen and McCormack (2008) suggest therefore that creativity enables holistic engagement of mind, heart, body and spirit at the heart of critical social science which has, traditionally, centred on using the mind for critiquing historical, social, political and cultural contexts of practice. Thus the sub-theory of *creativity* blends and melds all the other sub-theories as set out by Fay. Without such creativity, the knowing that is at the heart of transformative action cannot be fully realised through the professional artistry of practice. We set out the sub-theory of *creativity* as:

> the blending and weaving of art forms and reflexivity (critical consciousness) located in the critical [worldview]. Blending and weaving occur through professional artistry in order to achieve the ultimate outcome of human flourishing. Thus this theory has critical, moral and sacred dimensions.
>
> *McCormack and Titchen, 2006, p. 259*

This sub-theory has a critical dimension because it builds on critical theory, a moral dimension because it encompasses praxis and a spiritual dimension because we use our spiritual intelligence to make meaning, uplift ourselves and to take or facilitate transformative action. Figure 2.2 presents the theoretical framework for transformational PD within a critical creativity world view.

The praxis spiral is the central spiral of the framework. It represents the journey from wherever we are now towards human flourishing as the ends and means of transformational development and action research. The journey is facilitated through the processes of blending, connecting, energising, reflecting, practising, learning and becoming. Praxis has been placed centrally because it is through this spiral that we tap our paradigmatic foundation, that is, critical creativity, shown in Figure 2.2 as dynamic energy or 'Catherine Wheel'. This spiral then connects with the theory spirals at the centre of the figure when we engage in praxis. Thus, critical creativity flows throughout the framework. Through a blend of cognitive and artistic critique, transformational development workers and researchers are able to turn the nine critical practice theory spirals into informed, transformed and transforming action with the moral intent of social justice, equity and human flourishing for all stakeholders. Professional artistry enables the continual reconstruction of theory in and on practice.

Little work has been undertaken to develop theoretical frameworks that integrate creative expression with systematic approaches to research and development in order to achieve transformation. The use of critical creativity as philosophical, theoretical and methodological bases for practitioner research enables

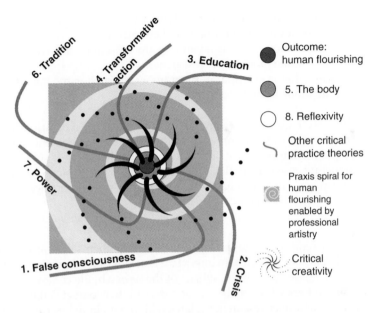

Figure 2.2 A theoretical framework for human flourishing located in the critical creativity world view. (*Source*: From Titchen and McCormack (2008).)

the integration of traditional paradigms with different methods of practitioner research in order for the taken-for-granted assumptions to be challenged and transformed. The new theoretical framework of critical creativity underpins transformational PD and action-orientated research and offers direction for practitioner researchers interested in working with a creative methodology through the integration of cognitive and artistic methods.

Operationalising methods of practitioner research through reflexivity

The methods of practitioner research are multifaceted and numerous. Practitioner research, like all research, needs to adopt a systematic and rigorous process of inquiry that clearly demonstrates a direct linkage between the methodological approach used to frame the question(s) being asked, the methods used to operationalise the methodology, answer the research question(s) and the data analysis processes. However, given the position adopted in this chapter, that practitioner research is usually located within a critical paradigm, then the methods used are focused on achieving transformation of self (as practitioner) and practice (processes and people) through engagement in action-oriented methodologies. Thus, the purpose of research undertaken by practitioner researchers is to achieve transformation. The methods of research need to reflect this purpose, and thus it is not the methods themselves that will differ from other research purposes but the way in which they are operationalised. Unstructured interviews, reflective diaries, practice observation, individual and group reflection, and creative engagement are all 'tools' of the practitioner researcher.

However, what is essential in practitioner research is the operationalisation of research methods through reflexivity:

> Reflexivity requires an awareness of the researcher's contribution to the construction of meanings throughout the research process, and an acknowledgment of the impossibility of remaining 'outside of' one's subject matter while conducting research. Reflexivity then, urges us to explore the ways in which a researcher's involvement with a particular study influences, acts upon and informs such research.
>
> *Nightingale and Cromby, 1999, p. 228*

Reflexivity requires the researcher to be aware of themselves as the instrument of research. This is a particularly important issue for practitioner researchers who are intimately involved with the subject of the research, the context in which it takes place and others who may be stakeholders in that context. Taking account of the way the practitioner researcher relates with others in the research context is thus critical to a rigorous and ethically sound research endeavour. Thus, how one considers issues associated with (say) interviewing staff, receiving feedback on performance and observations of practice is different for the practitioner researcher than the external (disengaged) researcher. Nightingale and Cromby (1999) suggest that the researcher needs to be reflexive from two perspectives – personal reflexivity and epistemological reflexivity.

Personal reflexivity involves the researcher reflecting upon how their beliefs, values, experiences, interests, beliefs, political commitments, wider aims in life and social identities have shaped the research. As well as that, they suggest that a reflexive researcher will also reflect on ways in which the research itself may have changed us as a researcher and as a person. Titchen *et al.* (2007) suggest that this is like a dance whereby each research experience is a unique personal journey that is concerned with action, liberation, illumination, transformation and ultimately human flourishing.

Epistemological reflexivity requires the researcher to consider decisions about the research question(s), the chosen methodology, the data collection and analysis methods, and ways in which these create 'boundaries' in the research. Reflecting on the way the question has shaped the study, how the data collection methods were operationalised and how theory was generated makes explicit the assumptions made by the researcher about knowledge and the place of knowledge in the specific research context and the implications of these assumptions for the research findings and the communication of these findings to others. As Titchen *et al.* (2007, p. 285) suggest, '[C]ritical-creative researchers are watchful for flaws, tangles and holes in the emerging tapestry of the knowledges and practices they are co-creating.' So, in essence, an eclectic approach needs to be applied to decision-making about what data collection methods to use. The important issues are, firstly, ensuring that the methods answer the questions asked and serve to illuminate the transformational processes and outcomes of the research itself, and secondly, applying both person and epistemological reflexivity to the operationalisation of the methods in order to ensure rigour.

Conclusions

In this chapter, the principles, processes and methodologies of practitioner research have been articulated. Practitioner research is at the heart of a systematic approach to articulating the expertise embedded in nursing. Rich descriptions of expertise and 'outcomes' from practice expertise through stories have much to offer the study of nursing practice. However, we need to be cautious about the presentation of uncritical self-reported stories of expertise that are uncorroborated. A systematic approach to practitioner research enables the avoidance of this pitfall. Further, it demonstrates the potential for transformation in collaborative, participatory and inclusive action and contributes to theory development – theory about nursing practice and its effectiveness, theory about the context of practice and theory about methodologies for effective practitioner inquiry. Developing critically creative methodologies that integrate established philosophical, theoretical and methodological perspectives is crucial to the engagement of practitioners in research in a health care arena that is increasingly pressurised, economically driven and professionally challenging. As further chapters in this book will illustrate, drawing on practitioner research methodologies enables 'critical spaces' to be created within which windows of opportunity can be opened for the growth of human potential.

References

Argyris, A. (1999) *On Organizational Learning*, 2nd edn. Blackwell, Oxford.

Bartlett, S. & Burton, D. (2006) Practitioner research or descriptions of classroom practice? A discussion of teachers investigating their classrooms. *Educational Action Research – An International Journal* **14**(3), 395–405.

Binnie, A. & Titchen, A. (1999) *Freedom to Practice: The Development of Patient Centred Nursing*. Butterworth Heinemann, Oxford.

Brooker, R. & Macpherson, I. (1999) Communication – the processes and outcomes of practitioners research: an opportunity for self-indulgence or a serious professional responsibility? *Educational Action Research* **7**(2), 207–220.

Brown, D. & McCormack, B. (2006) Determining factors that have an impact upon effective evidence-based pain management with older people, following colorectal surgery: an ethnographic study. *Journal of Clinical Nursing* **15**(10), 1211–1351

Campbell, A.V. (1984) *Moderated Love: A Theology of Professional Care*. SPCK, London.

Carr, W. & Kemmis, S. (1986) *Becoming Critical: Education, Knowledge and Action Research*. Falmer Press, London.

Elliott, J. (1991) *Action Research for Educational Change*. Open University Press, Milton Keynes.

Fay, B. (1987) *Critical Social Science*. Polity Press, Cambridge.

Fine, M. (1994) Dis-stance and other stances: negotiations of power inside feminist research. In: *Power and Method: Political Activism and Educational Research* (ed. A. Gitlin). Routledge, London.

Garbett, R. & McCormack, B. (2001) The experience of practice development: an exploratory telephone interview study. *Journal of Clinical Nursing* **10**, 94–102.

Garbett, R. & McCormack, B. (2002) A concept analysis of practice development. *NT Research* **7**(2), 87–100.

Gerrish, K. & Clayton, J. (2004) Promoting evidence-based practice: an organisational approach. *Journal of Nursing Management* **12**, 114–123.

Greenwood, J. (1994) Action research: a few details, a caution and something new. *Journal of Advanced Nursing* **20**, 13–18.

Grundy, S. (1982) Three modes of action research. *Curriculum Perspectives* **2**(3), 23–34.

Guba, E.G. & Lincoln, Y.S. (1989) *Fourth Generation Evaluation*. Sage, Newbury Park, CA.

Habermas, J. (1972) *Knowledge and Human Interests* (Trans. J.J. Shapiro). Heinemann, London.

Hardy, S., Titchen, A., Manley, K. & McCormack, B. (2006) Re-defining nursing expertise in the United Kingdom. *Nursing Science Quarterly* **19**(3), 260–264.

Hart, E. & Bond, M. (1995) *Action Research for Health and Social Care: A Guide to Practice*. Open University Press, Buckingham.

Harvey, G., Loftus-Hills, A., Rycroft-Malone, J., Titchen, A., Kitson, A., McCormack, B. & Seers, K. (2002) Getting evidence into practice: the role and function of facilitation. *Journal of Advanced Nursing* **37**(6), 577–588.

Higgs, J. & Titchen, A. (2007) Becoming critical and creative in qualitative research. In: *Being Critical and Creative in Qualitative Research* (eds J. Higgs, A. Titchen, D. Horsfall & H. Armstrong), pp. 1–9. Hampden Press, Sydney.

Horkheimer, M. (1982) *Critical theory*. Seabury, New York.

Kemmis, M. (2006) Participatory action research and the public sphere. *Educational Action Research – An International Journal* **14**(4), 459–476.

Kemmis, S. & McTaggart, R. (1988) *The Action Research Planner*. Deakin University Press, Melbourne.

Kitson, A.L., Ahmed, L.D., Harvey, G., Seers, K. & Thompson, D.R. (1996) From research to practice; One organisational model for promoting research based practice. *Journal of Advanced Nursing* **23**, 430–440.

Lewin, K. (1947) Frontiers in group dynamics II: channels of group life; social planning and action. *Human Relations* **1**, 143–153.

Manley, K. (2000) Organisational culture and consultant nurse outcomes: Part 1, organisational culture. *Nursing Standard* **14**(36), 34–38.

Manley, K. (2001) Consultant nurse: concept, processes, outcome. Unpublished Doctoral Study, University of Manchester/RCN Institute, London.

Manley, K. & McCormack, B. (2003) Practice development: purpose, methodology, facilitation and evaluation. *Nursing in Critical Care* **8**, 22–29.

Manley, K. & McCormack, B. (2004) Practice development: purpose, methodology, facilitation and evaluation. In: *Practice Development in Nursing* (eds B. McCormack, K. Manley & R. Garbett). Blackwell, Oxford.

Meyer, J., Johnson, B., Bryar, R. & Procter, S. (2003) Practitioner research: exploring issues in relation to research-capacity building. *NT Research* **8**(6), 407–417.

Mezirow, J. (1981). A critical theory of adult learning and education. *Adult Education* **32**(1), 3–24.

McCormack, B. (2003) Knowing and acting: a strategic practitioner-focused approach to nursing research and practice development. *NT Research* **8**(3), 86–100.

McCormack, B. & Crisp, J. (2008) Engaging in critical inquiry and practice development. In: *Potter & Perry's Fundamentals of Nursing* (eds J. Crisp & C. Taylor), 3rd edn. Elsevier, Sydney.

McCormack, B., Dewar, B., Wright, J., Garbett, R., Harvey, G. & Ballantine, K. (2006) *A Realist Synthesis of Evidence Relating to Practice Development: Final Report To NHS Education for Scotland and NHS Quality Improvement Scotland*. Available from http://www.nhshealthquality.org/nhsqis/qis.

McCormack, B., Manley, K., Titchen, A., Kitson, A. & Harvey, G. (1999) Towards practice development: a vision in reality or a reality without vision. *Journal of Nursing Management* **7**, 255–264.

McCormack, B. & Titchen, A. (2006) Critical creativity: melding, exploding, blending. *Educational Action Research* **14**(2), 239–266.

McNiff, S. (1998) *Trust the Process: An Artist's Guide to Letting Go*. Shambhala Press, London.

McNiff, J (1988) *Action Research: Principles and Practice*. McMillan Education, Basingstoke.

Nightingale, D. & Cromby, J. (eds) (1999) *Social Constructionist Psychology*. Open University Press, Buckingham.

Parahoo, K. (1999) Research utilization and attitudes towards research among psychiatric nurses in Northern Ireland. *Journal of Psychiatric & Mental Health Nursing* **6**(2), 125–135.

Parahoo, K. (2000) Barriers to, and facilitators of, research utilization among nurses in Northern Ireland. *Journal of Advanced Nursing* **31**(1), 89–98.

Pawson, R. & Tilley, N. (1998) *Realistic Evaluation*. Sage, London.

Perälä, M. (2000) Recommendations for the integration of nursing research into practice. *International Journal of Nursing Practice* **6**(6), 354–355.

Rodgers, S.E. (2000) The extent of nursing research utilization in general medical and surgical wards. *Journal of Advanced Nursing* **32**(1), 182–193.

Rolfe, G. (1998) *Expanding Nursing Knowledge*. Butterworth Heinemann, Oxford.

Shaw, T., Dewing, J., Young, R., Devlin, M., Boomer, C. & Legius, M. (2008) Enabling practice development: delving into the concept of facilitation from a practitioner perspective. In: *Practice Development in Nursing: International Perspectives* (eds K. Manley, B. McCormack & V. Wilson). Blackwell, Oxford.

Stringer, E. (1996). *Action Research: A Handbook for Practitioners*. Sage, Thousand Oaks, CA.

Susman, G.I. & Evered, R.D. (1978) An assessment of the scientific merits of action research. *Administrative Science Quarterly* **23**, 582–603.

Thomas, K.K. (2000) Closing the gap between research and practice: strategies to enhance research utilization. *Research in Nursing & Health* **23**(2), 175.

Titchen, A. (2001). Critical companionship: a conceptual framework for developing expertise. In: *Practice Knowledge and Expertise in the Health Professions* (eds A. Higgs & A. Titchen). Butterworth Heinemann, Oxford.

Titchen, A. & Binnie, A. (1993a) A unified action research strategy in nursing. *Educational Action Research* **1**(1), 25–33.

Titchen, A. & Binnie, A. (1993b) Research partnerships: collaborative action research in nursing. *Journal of Advanced Nursing* **18**, 858–865.

Titchen, A. & Binnie, A. (1994) Action research. A strategy for theory generation and testing. *International Journal of Nursing Studies* **31**(1), 1–12.

Titchen, A. & Higgs, J. (2001) A dynamic framework for the enhancement of health professional practice in an uncertain world: the practice–knowledge interface. In: *Practice Knowledge and Expertise in the Health Professions* (eds J. Higgs & A. Titchen). Butterworth Heinemann, Oxford.

Titchen, A., Higgs, J. & Horsfall, D. (2007) Research artistry: dancing the praxis spiral in critical creative qualitative research. In: *Being Critical and Creative in Qualitative Research* (eds J. Higgs, A. Titchen, D. Horsfall & H. Armstrong), pp. 282–297. Hampden, Sydney.

Titchen, A. & McCormack, B. (2008) A methodological walk in the forest: critical creativity and human flourishing. In: *Practice Development in Nursing: International Perspectives* (eds K. Manley, B. McCormack & V. Wilson). Blackwell, Oxford.

Whyte, W.F. (ed.) (1991) *Participatory Action Research*. Sage, Newbury Park, CA.

Winter, R. (1989) *Learning from Experience: Principles and Practice in Action Research*. Falmer, Lewes.

Wuthnow, R., Davison Hunter, J., Bergesen, A. & Kurzweil, E. (1984) *Cultural Analysis*. Routledge, London.

3. A Kaleidoscope of Nursing Expertise: A Literature Review

Angie Titchen and Sally Hardy

Nursing practice expertise is like a spiralling kaleidoscope. With each turn, a nurse with expertise creates a unique moment; a creative response to, or intervention for, a patient, client or family that matches their needs, as they see them. As with the moving glass shards of a kaleidoscope, fundamental attributes of expertise make up new patterns for each distinctive moment. Turning the viewfinder of the kaleidoscope can also be likened to nurses with expertise engaging in inquiries of their own practice. Whilst the inquiry purpose might be to deepen understanding and enable articulation of their expertise to others, a remarkable thing occurs. Through the act of inquiry, expertise itself develops, deepening and widening. Thus, the imagery of a spiralling kaleidoscope can also be used to show the journey of becoming of a nurse with expertise.

This imagery emerged for us as research team members in the Royal College of Nursing (RCN) emancipatory action research study of nursing expertise in the UK, often referred to as the Expertise in Practice Project (EPP) (Manley *et al.*, 2005; Hardy *et al.*, 2006a). Together with the published literature presented in this chapter, the EPP showed why the understanding and articulation of expertise is central, not only to the giving and development of clinically effective, person-centred care, but also to the growth of expertise itself. Through the literature review, the attributes of expertise (shards of glass) are uncovered through research that has taken different approaches to the investigation of expertise. Some of these studies suggest that these attributes are brought together in moment-by-moment practices through professional artistry. Before examining these different approaches and building up an understanding of professional artistry in the literature, we point out overall patterns and colours in the literature kaleidoscope.

Patterns and colours

The nursing expertise literature

A search for professional, published literature on expertise and its elements yields a vast literature (see Table 3.1). Critical reviews of some of this literature are published elsewhere (e.g. Manley & McCormack, 1997; Titchen, 2000). Here, we make

Table 3.1 CINAHL search 23.4.07

Search history	Results (numbers of papers)
Patient education	32 846
Caring	14 956
Competency	4103
Comfort	4022
Patient participation	1988
Empathy	1711
Intuition	646
Clinical leadership	481
Nurse patient relationship	380
Nursing expertise	137
Higher level practice	38
Nursing attributes	2
Practitioner inquiry	0
Investigating nursing practice	0
Total	61 310

overall sense of the literature and give examples of studies that have been seminal to the contemporary understanding of nursing expertise.

The professional published literature from 1996 to 2006 was searched using the term EXPERT-NURSES, with all topic subheadings (as the synonymous thesaurus term for clinical expertise) in the Cumulative Index for Nursing and Allied Health Literature (CINAHL). Elements of expertise were also searched in CINAHL using the following terms: NURSE–PATIENT RELATIONSHIP, INTUITION, CARING, EMPATHY, COMFORT, PATIENT PARTICIPATION and PATIENT EDUCATION. In addition, MEDLINE, PSYCHLIT and PUBMED were searched for CARING. Research papers with rigorous methodologies were selected for review. Rigorous studies of expertise reported in books or doctoral theses were also included.

This literature search was extended for this chapter by undertaking another CINAHL search moving beyond our previous restriction to research papers. This time, we were looking for keywords in the title, keywords or texts of all published papers from 1982 to April 2007. From the 61 310 papers identified, interesting patterns and intensity of colour in the 'glass shards' are shown in Table 3.1. It is interesting that only 137 references relating to nursing expertise were identified, in comparison, for example, to 32 846 references relating to patient education.

Looking a little more closely, a large proportion of material relating specifically to expertise was published from late 1980 to late 1990. According to Adams *et al.* (1997), it was Patricia Benner's (1984) earliest work, exploring the nature of nursing practice expertise that had influenced and contributed to a steady increase in the number of publications about practice expertise. However, later publications tended to look at separate elements of expertise, using Benner's domains as benchmarks. Interest in publications about nursing expertise became paler towards the end of the 1990s, as colour intensified in the examination of higher levels of practice, advanced practice or extended and then expanded roles of the nurse. This change of palette seemed to be a response to nurses beginning to undertake technical tasks, previously the province of junior doctors. We see this literature as more concerned with singling out the technical skills of practice expertise and in contrast to a view of expertise as a dynamic of different elements. Today, there is still very little written about the nature of practice expertise. Rather, the intensity of colour is focused on competency-based approaches to skills development. As such approaches tend to compartmentalise expertise, the danger remains that expertise is not considered as a complex, dynamic whole.

Peering down the kaleidoscope to view only the research literature, this pattern is repeated. There are still more publications that look at the individual elements of expertise, for example studies of the decision-making or supportive role of expert nurses (for instance, Orme & Maggs, 1993; Radwin, 1995), than there are investigations that examine expertise as an entity in itself. Whilst investigations of individual elements increase our understanding and intensify the colour of the glass shards or attributes, such studies get at neither the essence nor the complexity of expertise in nursing practice. Whilst there has been a revived interest recently in studies of expertise, these studies have focused on specific roles or areas of nursing practice (see, for example Donnelly, 2003; Bonner & Greenwood, 2006). Such studies tend to strengthen the generic findings of earlier studies whilst offering new, more specific insights.

We focus, therefore, in our short review of the literature, on critiquing a few studies in-depth, primarily conducted in the eighties and nineties, plus our own research in the new millennium which looks at the nature of expertise as a dynamic whole. Examples of nursing research from 1997 to 2006 investigating the parts of nursing expertise have been presented in Chapter 1 (Table 1.1).

The works reviewed were inductive in nature; they did not impose a theoretical framework on the study, which means that the findings were not shaped by predetermined theoretical views of what nursing is. Studies with a priori theoretical frameworks tend to conceptualise expertise in different ways, for example the nurse as: user and tester of theory through nursing interventions; decision-maker/problem-solver; reflective practitioner (Titchen, 2000), evidence-based practitioner or intuitive worker (cf. Purkis & Bjornsdottir, 2006). By setting boundaries, such studies fail to address the complexity and comprehensiveness of nursing expertise and the ambiguities that come into play.

The studies reviewed here fall into three main patterns formed by the methodological approaches they used:

1. hermeneutic phenomenological studies of *expertise and its acquisition*,
2. *the lived experience of nursing* using ethnographic, phenomenological and critical science approaches and
3. *practitioner-inquiry* studies.

Expertise and its acquisition

Coming in closer now, we turn the kaleidoscope to examine investigations of expertise undertaken by Benner (1984), Benner and Tanner (1987), Benner and

Wrubel (1989), MacLeod (1990), Tanner *et al.* (1993) and Titchen (2001). These studies are primarily based on notions of what is good in practice and on the knowledge embedded in the expert practice of nursing. Predominantly, they compare nurses with different levels of proficiency, operating at different levels, to identify the characteristics of expertise and how it develops.

In her study of hospital nurses, Benner (1984) revealed six areas of an expert's practical knowledge: (1) graded qualitative distinctions, (2) common meanings, (3) assumptions, expectations and sets, (4) paradigm cases, (5) maxims and (6) unplanned practices. Thirty-one competencies located in seven domains of nursing practice were also uncovered: (1) the helping role, (2) the teaching–coaching function, (3) the diagnostic and patient-monitoring function, (4) effective management of rapidly changing situations, (5) administering and monitoring therapeutic interventions and regimens, (6) monitoring and ensuring the quality of health care practices and (7) organisational and work-role competencies. Benner stresses that these competencies are by no means comprehensive and further studies support this conclusion (cf. Steele & Fenton, 1988). We note that it is these competencies that other researchers and practitioners tend to refer to in their work, rather than the more abstract areas of practical knowledge.

Benner also identified the differences between the situation appraisal and clinical performance of novice and expert nurses. She found that the nurse develops expertise by passing through the five levels of proficiency identified in the Dreyfus model of skill acquisition (Dreyfus & Dreyfus, 1985). As the nurse progresses through the levels, there is broad movement from a reliance on abstract principles to the use of a large repertoire of past, concrete experiences, a passage from a detached to an involved stance, from a reliance on theoretical knowledge to practical knowledge and on rational action to intuitive judgement and a developing sense of saliency (knowing what matters and acting on it). For Benner and Tanner (1987), intuitive judgement is the hallmark of expertise, but when nurses with expertise meet situations in which they have no previous experience or when they incorrectly grasp the situation and expected behaviours and events do not occur, they use highly skilled analytical thinking. Benner asserts that 'expertise develops when the clinician tests and refines propositions, hypotheses, and principle-based expectations in actual practice situations' (Benner, 1984, p. 3).

There are several methodological and theoretical limitations in Benner's early study. The methodological limitations include the tendency in the data towards crisis situations, the dramatic and poignant at the expense of the mundane. This predominance is a considerable problem in a study of nurses' transparent coping in the ordinary, everyday world (a problem that Benner recognised and dealt with in later work). Other limitations are that the potential of participant observation for studying nurses' ways of being (rather than doing) does not appear to have been maximised and that only the nurses' perspective of the patient's experience is examined. The theoretical limitations are that evidence for the different levels in the model, apart from the fifth, expert level, is rather thin and Benner's development of a taxonomy of domains and competencies does not show the relationships between the different domains and competencies within them. For example, several competencies from different domains might be displayed in the same nursing action, but the form of the taxonomy makes that difficult to see. Her narratives are much more effective in showing such relationships.

Building on this work to address the care of specific groups of patients, Benner and Wrubel (1989, p. 7) developed 'an interpretive theory of nursing practice as it is concerned with helping people cope with the stress of illness'. They examine the relationships between caring, coping, stress and health, claiming that caring is a primary requirement for 'expert human practice'. Nurses attend to patients' stories of their illnesses and lives and to their interpretations of their symptoms. They seek to understand the meaning of the illness for the patient and for that patient's life, believing that such understanding can be used to facilitate healing. Nurses engage with their patients – they feel connected to them. They have a care and concern for them; their patients matter to them. They seek to establish a relationship based on respect and equality and to be with their patients in a way that acknowledges their shared humanity. Attention to the patient's personhood is total. Nurses help patients to gain a sense of control and active participation in their recovery. The attributes of the nurse are imaginative identification with the other person, creativity and therapeutic use of self. In further work, Benner and Tanner (1987) and Benner *et al.* (1996) proposed descriptors of expertise as shown in Box 3.1.

A number of studies have revealed a practical discourse of *knowing the patient* which nurses use to describe their patients' demeanour, self-presentation, everyday habits, practices and preferences (e.g. Jenny & Logan, 1992; Radwin, 1995). Tanner *et al.* (1993, p. 275) found that *knowing the patient* requires 'an immediate grasp, an involved, rather than detached understanding of the patient's situation and the patient's responses, an understanding that is directly apprehended, and

Box 3.1 Characteristics of expertise according to Benner and colleagues

---

- Expert practice is characterised by increased intuitive links between seeing the salient issues in the situation and ways of responding to them.
- Intuitive judgement is seen as the hallmark of expertise.
- The links between patient condition and action are sufficiently strong that the focus shifts to actions taken rather than the problems recognised.
- Practice is characterised through engaging practical reasoning, which relies on mature and practised understanding and perceptual grasp of distinctions and commonalities in particular situations.
- Expert practitioners are open to whatever the situation presents.
- Actions reflect attunement to the situation in that they are shaped by patients' responses and do not rely on conscious deliberation.
- Performance is fluent and seamless.
- Emotional involvement is matured to the extent that it varies according to the needs and openness of patients and their families.
- Moral agency, a concern for responding to patients as people, respecting their dignity, protecting their personhood in times of vulnerability, helping them feel safe, providing comfort and maintaining integrity in the relationship.

(Benner & Tanner, 1987; Benner *et al.*, 1996)

---

that may remain largely ineffable'. *Knowing the patient* is situated knowledge, specific to what can be known from the nurse/patient/family interaction and the clinical context. The researchers argue that knowing the patient is central to skilled clinical judgement and is part of clinical learning.

A methodological criticism of Tanner *et al.'s* study (and of those other existential phenomenological inquiries undertaken by Benner and her colleagues above) is that the researchers do not articulate their own contributions to the making of the data[1] in the form of their own conceptual leanings and interpretive backgrounds. Moreover, accounts of expert consensual validation to guard against the importation of meanings into the interpretation that are not supported by the text suggests that they saw the validator researchers as objective participants in the research process, rather than as involved, connected participants who were likely to have their own interpretations. Ignoring the impact of the researcher, particularly when using hermeneutic phenomenology, is flawed, as interpretation in this tradition is achieved through the researcher undertaking a process of critique and synthesis within the hermeneutic circle.

In the first British study in this set, MacLeod (1990) studied ten surgical ward sisters and set out specifically to explore the nature of everyday nursing practice in order to gain an understanding of how everyday experience contributes to the development of expertise. MacLeod placed far more emphasis on participant observation than the earlier existential phenomenological studies. In addition, the ward sisters were asked to describe their experiences with a focus on their moment-by-moment, taken-for-granted practices, rather than on situations that stood out for them, as Benner (1984) had done. MacLeod also discusses her application of the hermeneutic circle and contributes to making the data by including herself in the report.

MacLeod was able to discern Benner's (1984) seven domains of practice in the ward sisters' practices, but claims that by analysing and presenting her data in relation to the ward sister's experience of the stay of a patient, she was able to capture the flow of everyday practice which Benner's taxonomy is unable to do. Thus, MacLeod was able to explicate the everyday, background structure and pattern, unlock the ordinary processes and the temporal nature of nurses' *knowing in practice* more effectively than Benner. Despite the ordinariness of this practice, there is a complexity in it that MacLeod's approach unpicks. Everyday, moment-by-moment practices are shown to be intuitive, patient-centred and oriented towards multi-layered goals. The ward sisters' practices demonstrate an understanding of patients' past and current experiences and of the future possibilities; something also found by Street (1992). Like Tanner *et al.* (1993), MacLeod (1993) found that *knowing the patient* is central to nursing expertise. Three distinct processes characterise how MacLeod's (1990) ward sisters related, through their care, to their patients and to the ward. These processes of *noticing, understanding and acting* are

---

[1] By 'making of the data' we mean how the researcher makes an impact on the process and capturing of data through choice of approach, personal leanings, values, beliefs and how these impact the gathering, interpretation and analysis/synthesis of data.

inextricably bound in a non-sequential and non-linear way. It is the quality of these processes that seems to contribute to the complexity, goal-directedness and patient-centredness of the ward sisters' practices. Again, we note that just as practitioners rarely articulate Benner's (1984) six areas of practical knowledge, it is rare indeed to hear them name the intertwining processes described by MacLeod.

MacLeod found that when the ward sisters had acquired theoretical knowledge, it became contextualised by means of their practical knowing, thus creating new *knowing in practice*. Street (1992) also found that this mix of theoretical and practical knowledge resulted in a perceptual knowing which is time-related and context-specific. MacLeod reported that the ward sisters learned continuously from the people around them and more commonly, in the midst of practice, rather than separately reflecting on their practice. Thus becoming experienced is characterised as learning all the time and as changes in noticing, understanding and acting. MacLeod points out that *knowing in practice* can be developed from experience without reaching consciousness and this is what distinguishes her study from Benner's (1984), where experience is seen as occurring when preconceived (and, therefore, presumably conscious) notions are turned around. The problem with MacLeod's findings about how the ward sisters learned is that she relies completely on retrospective accounts of their practice over many years, thus accuracy around recall is called into question. Moreover, this type of expertise development would appear to rely heavily on chance.

Titchen (2001) studied expertise by developing an innovative methodological approach that used both hermeneutic phenomenology and phenomenological sociology to reveal the tacit knowledge of nurses. By learning from the studies above, Titchen sought to overcome methodological flaws, for example, by articulating her self-awareness as data gatherer and interpreter (see Titchen & Higgs, 2007). Also influenced by the methodologies pioneered by Benner (1994), MacLeod (1990) and others, Titchen found a way to enable nurses to surface taken-for-granted practices and non-spoken meanings to investigate expertise in patient-centred nursing and its development. She gathered data through participant observation, in-depth interviews, reflective conversations, storytelling, reflexive accounts and review of documentation. Analysis and interpretation, using approaches developed within the two phenomenological traditions, revealed the complexity of the practical know-how or professional craft knowledge of a nurse with expertise in patient-centredness. Participants were invited to check out the data for accuracy and to comment on, contribute to and critique the interpretations developed.

The study offers a theorised account of practical know-how (professional craft knowledge) through a conceptual framework of skilled companionship (see Figure 4.1). Within three domains of professional craft knowledge (the relationship domain, rationality-intuitive domain and facilitative use of self domain), it describes the attributes of, and processes and strategies used by, patient-centred nurses as they go about their everyday work. Professional artistry is discerned in the complex *interaction* and *balancing* of: the knowledges in the domains, in *managing the interplay* between intuitive and rational judgement and between theoretical knowledge and practical know-how (epistemology); who the nurse is as person

Box 3.2   The professional artistry of skilled companionship

Imbuing the skilled companionship domains with being a person demands professional artistry in the form of synchronicity, balance, attunement and interplay. At first sight, taking the aspects of being human into the nurse–patient relationship and realising the concepts of the relationship and rationality-intuitive domains within the relationship may seem simple and ordinary, but they are not. The artistry component of professional craft knowledge of the expert nurse enables emotional, physical, existential and sometimes spiritual *synchronicity*. Synchronicity is defined as the emotions and movements of the nurse, for example, occurring at the same time as those of the patient. The nurse paces her physical movement through space and time to be in tune with that of the patient and she displays emotions that are congruent with the ways that both she and the patient feel. The nurse and patient exist together for a period of time as a *unit* working, growing and being together for the duration of the patient's journey.

Synchronicity, in combination with reciprocity, may allow transcendence to occur through the symbolic act of physical forms of caring. Artistry is also embodied in the nurse's *attunement* to her patient as a person and to his symptoms, responses, physical functioning and body topology. The complex *balancing* of the rationality-intuitive and relationship domains and managing the fine *interplay* between intuition and rational thinking and between the use of theoretical knowledge and practical know-how also requires professional artistry. Professional artistry is displayed in the selection of relevant strategies for the particular patient and situation.

(ontology); therapeutic use of self; and the dance, as it were, *synchronising* all these elements (see Box 3.2). This framework is contextualised in a rich description of patient-centred nursing expertise. Later work has also identified the importance of rationality-intuitive interplay (e.g. Judd, 2005; Christensen & Hewitt-Taylor, 2006).

Titchen tested the framework against research literature and concluded that it is new and that it has advanced practical and theoretical understanding of how to be patient-centred. It elaborated processes (concepts) and strategies, identified in the literature in this section, and created new ones and new relationships. It was the first study to begin to describe the nature of professional artistry. Titchen argues that professional artistry is the hallmark of nursing expertise and proposes that skilled companionship is potentially transferable to other nursing settings and health professions. Later research has demonstrated this transferability (Titchen & McGinley, 2003; Brown & Scott, 2004; Manley *et al.*, 2005). Evidence in these studies suggests that patients and relatives value skilled companionship. Titchen (2004) also established that nurses can be helped to develop expertise through everyday practice through the support of a parallel critical companionship relationship.

In summary, this set of studies of expertise and its acquisition highlight the complexity and nuance of the expertise within ordinary, everyday practice. It suggests that expertise is more complex than first described by Benner (1984), in terms of the relationship between theoretical and practical knowledge. The acquisition of practical knowledge and how it becomes imbued with theoretical knowledge is far more complex than conventional experiential learning models suggest (cf. Kolb,

1984). Such models view experience as a time-unrelated and discrete event, rather than the elusive, time-related, contextualised and personalised nature of experience (MacLeod, 1990), as indicated by these studies. These inquiries also show that nurses learn from experience consciously and unconsciously in different ways and not just from instances where preconceived notions are turned around. It has also been highlighted that the time-related nature of practical knowledge and its complex relationships can be demonstrated in more helpful ways than a taxonomy. Finally, these studies show us the complex nature of studying expertise and its acquisition as a dynamic whole.

The lived experience of nursing

Twisting the kaleidoscope, the next pattern emerges from a set of studies about the lived experience of nursing from the perspective of nurses, using ethnographic, phenomenological and critical science approaches.

Appleton (1993) used a Husserlian phenomenological method with a reflective and intuitive approach. Six patients who considered that they had experienced the art of nursing consented to take part and the five nurses with whom they had had this experience were included. Appleton's dense description of her methodology and extensive use of jargon make her account rather inaccessible (at least to us!). Five metathemes were identified:

a. the way of *being there* in caring,
b. the way of *being with* in understanding caring,
c. the way of creating opportunities for fullness of being through caring,
d. a transcendent togetherness,
e. the context of caring.

The nurse's being there in caring centres on a humanistic perspective of the whole person within an entire life, a feeling of compassion for the person in need and personal involvement in helping through caring about the person. The dignity and worth of each human being is honoured which allows the nurse to be open to seeing each patient as unique. She concludes that her study addresses the inter-subjectivity and contextual nature of the art of nursing. Appleton also suggests that nurses synthesise diverse sources of knowledge and ways of knowing into the quality of caring which appears similar to MacLeod's (1990) finding that theoretical knowledge imbues *knowing in being*. Appleton's de-contextualised findings fail to offer detail of how nurses practise the art of nursing.

In an Australian study of predominantly experienced nurses, Lawler (1991) generated a theory in which the body and the person are seen as an integrated composite and in which part of nursing practice is seen as the facilitation of that integration. Grounded theory, ethnomethodology and a notion of disrupted social order provided the theoretical underpinnings. Lawler found that nurses learn to manage their own physiological and emotional responses to patients' bodies, thus making it possible for patients to manage also. They sometimes manage patients' bodies as objects – considered necessary to protect both themselves and patients against physical revulsion, or sexual connotations, but this objectification was done in a way that the patient as a person was not objectified or disembodied. Lawler discusses how nurses violate and negotiate normal social boundaries to touch areas of the body not normally accessible in public and how they attempt to delicately manage the social fragility of their work, particularly as the body is deeply inscribed with intimate meaning.

Conway (1996) used a grounded theory approach, combining observation, workshops and interviews to describe the knowledge used by nurses with expertise. Whilst Conway's study was informed by Benner's work, she concludes that there are four types of expertise, depending on the way of being or ontology of the individual and the organisational culture within which the nurse is practising. These types of expertise are described as technologist, traditionalist, specialist and humanistic existentialist in orientation. Practitioners operating within each of these worldviews use different types of knowledge. Technologists use anticipatory, diagnostic, technical and monitoring knowledge, whilst traditionalists, more concerned with survival, tend to use medical knowledge to get through the work. Specialists define their expertise in relation to technicalities associated with specific areas of nursing care. They use knowledge of assessment, diagnosis, are aware of the significance of quality of life for those they care for and display a transformative ability to extend their roles. Humanistic existentialists operate from a holistic practice perspective and use a range of knowledge, both theoretical and that associated with values and experience, underpinned by teaching from nursing and the social sciences. By showing that clinical expertise can operate in different ways, Conway pointed out the hitherto unarticulated place that values play in perceptions of expertise.

Practitioner-inquiry studies

Emerging more recently in the literature, the third pattern of studies comprises practitioners investigating their own expertise with the support of peers, facilitators and critical companions. The studies in this pattern are part of, or evolving from, the RCN EPP (Titchen & McGinley, 2003; Manley *et al.*, 2005; Hardy *et al.*, 2007). Our literature review did not reveal similar studies. Given that a description of the EPP methodology and attributes of expertise have been presented in Chapter 1 (see Figure 1.1), we only focus here on findings related to professional artistry and enabling the development of expertise through practitioner research.

Researching one's own practice, providing care based on rigorous knowledge of many types and giving a professional account of that practice are challenging activities for which many nurses need guidance and support. Based on that premise, Titchen and McGinley (2003) worked together to try out a new conceptual framework for blending all types of knowledge, that is, research knowledge, scholarly work, practical know-how and personal and local knowledges. It was proposed that this blending occurred through the professional artistry of a skilled companion (Titchen, 2001). From an analysis of Maeve's practice, they conclude that professional artistry enabled the blending of all types of knowledge that is essential for genuinely evidence-based, person-centred care and that it can be facilitated through critical companionship. Moreover, they propose that critical companionship, as described by Titchen (2004), is effective in enabling practitioners to gather, analyse and critique evidence from their own expert practice and to articulate this evidence to peers for critical scrutiny, learning and knowledge creation.

One of the research aims in the EPP (Manley *et al.*, 2005) was to uncover the nature of expertise in UK nursing. We set about achieving this aim by adopting a facilitation strategy based on an in-depth understanding, from the literature reviewed above, of how expertise is developed. The aim of this strategy was to help facilitators, critical companions and practitioners to understand the nature of expertise and how it can be revealed and presented to others for critical review. Therefore, the research team facilitated action-learning sets designed to prepare participants as practitioner-researchers, and critical companions as facilitators of practitioner research. Having gathered evidence of the participant's expertise, the participant and critical companion unpicked, dissected and explored in detail the *taken for granted* and *embodied knowing* within the nurse's practices, actions and thoughts and their consequences, impacts and outcomes. Together, and with peer participants and other critical companions in action learning, this evidence was not only deconstructed, but it was also reconstructed through using conceptual frameworks, chosen by the participants, to analyse and interpret their own evidence. Evidence and its reconstruction and synthesis were presented by the nurse participant in a portfolio for external critical review and accreditation by a panel.

A framework of expertise (see Figure 1.1), created by analysing the portfolios of evidence, offers a language for nurses to articulate and share with others that which constitutes their practice expertise. The framework indicates that professional artistry integrates and interplays the attributes of expertise (presented in Table 1.1). The study also sets out the practical know-how of enabling practitioner research. Thereby, it offers a unique framework for helping practitioners to inquire, critique and perhaps most importantly, continue to learn from the process of investigating their practice and ongoing development and articulation of their practice expertise. Thus, this study went further than previous investigations, in terms of enabling simultaneous articulation and development of expertise.

Our review of these three types of studies of nursing expertise suggests that the nub, essence, hallmark or pinnacle of expertise in any field of nursing practice consists of the capacity to meld, intertwine, link, interplay, synergise, synchronise and balance:

- theoretical knowledge, practical know-how and personal knowledges;
- noticing (picking up and recognising salient cues, patterns and issues), mature and practised understanding (theoretical, practical, intuitive/embodied) and acting (responsively, appropriately, mindfully and intuitively);
- intuitive and rational thinking/judgement (attunement/holistic perceptual grasp and conscious deliberation);
- theoretical and practical reasoning and perceptual grasp of distinctions and commonalities;
- seeing the parts and whole and moving between them;
- facilitating integration of body and the person;

- organisational and personal values;
- mature emotional intelligence;
- using self therapeutically (moral agency).

These different capacities are embodied and/or intuitive (precognitive) or they rely on ways of knowing that are cognitive, metacognitive (critical control of cognitions or thinking about thinking) and reflexive (awareness of self and impact on others). These capacities are at the heart of a newly emerging discourse about professional artistry. Therefore, we now make a final twist of the kaleidoscope to take a deeper look at the nature of professional artistry. Based on the idea that it is professional artistry that enables the practitioner to blend, synergise, balance and dance the different shards of glass or elements of expertise, we propose that artistry is the axis upon which our kaleidoscope of expertise turns.

Professional artistry

The hallmark of expertise

The literature we have reviewed in this chapter shows the complexity of what nurses with expertise do. However, very little of it shows how nurses combine this diversity and complexity creatively in each unique, engagement with patients, clients, families and colleagues. Over two decades ago, from his observations of professionals with expertise at work and building on John Dewey's pragmatic philosophy, Schon (1983) suggested that professionals mediate science in the messy world of practice through a kind of professional artistry that enables the use of genereralisable, propositional knowledge for the particularity of professional practice. Professional artistry is rarely referred to in the nursing research literature, rather the focus has been on investigating the art of nursing (e.g. Appleton, 1993) or nursing artistry which is primarily conceptualised as the helping, interpersonal relationship between the nurse and patient (e.g. LeVasseur, 1999). Professional artistry, whilst building on these conceptualisations goes beyond them as we show below. In the early literature, there was a tendency to polarise art from the use of science (see Darbyshire, 1999), although scholars, such as Carper (1978), who have had an interest in the epistemology of nursing practice have long since seen that nurses draw on scientific and aesthetic knowledges amongst others. More recently, it appears that nursing researchers are no longer separating art and science (e.g. Christensen & Hewitt-Taylor, 2006), and some scholars (e.g. LeVasseur, 1999) are seeing art and science in a creative synthesis which could be characterised, perhaps, as science is art and art is science. Nevertheless, the interplay of art and science and multiplicity of processes through which science, intuition and practical know-how is mediated into effective, practical, person-centred action is still largely ignored in the literature.

Influenced by Schon's notion of professional artistry, Titchen (2001), Titchen and Higgs (2001), McCormack and Titchen (2006) and Titchen *et al.* (2007) have undertaken empirical and scholarly research into professional practice including clinical reasoning, the development of professional expertise and the conduct of

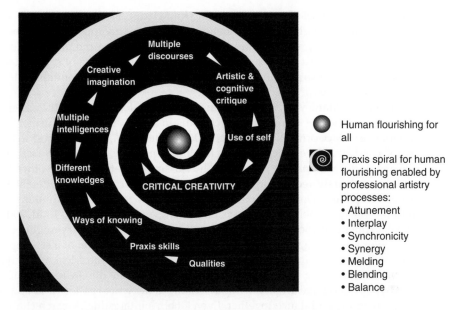

Figure 3.1 The dimensions and processes of professional artistry.

qualitative and practice development research to build up a picture of professional artistry in health care professional practice (see Figure 3.1). Extending beyond Schon's original conception, professional artistry is now seen as the artistry used by professionals to create unique responses to, and interventions for, others through *attuning, interplaying, synchronising, synergising, melding, blending* and *balancing* their:

- qualities (e.g. connoisseurship, discernment, appreciation, aesthetics),
- emotional, bodily, artistic and spiritual intelligences (capacity for, and quickness of, understanding or discernment),
- different kinds of knowledge (e.g. propositional, professional craft knowledge, personal),
- practice wisdom (possession of practice experience and knowledge together with the ability to use them critically, intuitively and practically),
- precognitive (embodied, intuitive), cognitive, metacognitive and reflexive ways of knowing,
- cognitive and artistic critique,
- creative imagination and expression,
- praxis (mindful doing with moral intent, illustrated in Figure 3.1 as a praxis spiral with the moral intent of human flourishing for receivers and givers of health care),
- use of multiple discourses (e.g. being able to move comfortably between language and meanings used by policy- and decision-makers and that used at the bedside),
- therapeutic/facilitative use of self.

Thus artistry is an act of production using knowledge, skill and technique and is distinct from, although it uses, aesthetics. Aesthetics is an appreciation of beauty, line, colour, texture and form and is necessary for creating the pleasing and enjoyable. In the context of nursing, aesthetics enables the giving of care that is not only effective but also pleasing to give and receive and which potentially enhances human flourishing for giver and receiver.

Building on Manley *et al.*'s (2005) finding that professional artistry appears to be generic across the 15 nursing specialisms included in the EPP, further investigations (e.g. McCormack & Titchen, 2006; Titchen *et al.*, 2007) suggest that professional artistry is generic, not only in clinical practice, but also in facilitation, research and development practices. The nursing literature, on the other hand, whilst increasingly recognising that nurses with expertise blend different types of knowledge (e.g. Donnelly, 2003) and that rational and intuitive thinking occur simultaneously in their clinical decision-making and practice (e.g. Judd, 2005), is not yet explicitly exploring the possibility that professional artistry might be even more complex, as suggested by Titchen *et al.* With the exception of a few sophisticated reflective accounts of practice (e.g. Johns, 2005) and empirical research (e.g. Gobbi, 2005), nursing research tends to focus on separate dimensions (colours or shards) of professional artistry, without looking at the whole pattern and how they blend, integrate and dance together. Even Gobbi's interesting research characterising nurses as both technical (hands on) and intellectual (using scientific knowledge) bricoleurs in the context of praxis does not seem to offer the sophistication of professional artistry, since the nurses are described as 'cobbling together' elements of knowledge from various disciplines and their own personal knowing repertoire to plan, design and evaluate patient care. In this book, we hope to shed light on how nurses with expertise are attuned to, and intentionally meld, blend, synthesise, synchronise, interplay and balance, rather than 'cobble together', the various dimensions of professional artistry.

Endless turning but resting for now

Within this chapter, we have explored the colourful patterns of what constitutes practice expertise through the metaphor of a kaleidoscope. This metaphor captures the many twists and turns a professional with expertise takes to find the right pattern for each particular situation and person. Whilst the literature is continuing to change as further work is articulated and presented, there is still little written about expertise as a dynamic whole. We pointed out that nursing research has tended to conceptualise the nurse with expertise in different ways, for example user and tester of theory through nursing interventions, decision-maker/ problem-solver, reflective practitioner, evidence-based practitioner or intuitive worker. These conceptions are limited because they focus on particular aspects of nursing care and not on the whole, so they miss the dynamic of professional artistry and the blending and melding of rationality and intuition with use of self.

This chapter has shown that particular research approaches can be used effectively to increase understanding of nursing expertise as a whole and, simultaneously within practitioner research, develop the expertise being studied. Practitioner research, conducted by nurses within a facilitative framework, also helps practitioners to articulate their expertise using language, values and meanings (i.e. discourses) that other professionals and policy-makers can understand (cf. Christensen & Hewitt-Taylor, 2006). Being able to do this increases opportunities for practitioners to influence health care for the benefit of patients and clients.

References

Adams, A., Pelletier, D., Duffield, C., Nagy, S., Crisp, J., Mitten-Lewis, S. & Murphy, J. (1997) Determining and discerning expert practice: a review of the literature. *Clinical Nurse Specialist* **11**(5), 217–222.

Appleton, C. (1993) The art of nursing: the experience of patients and nurses. *Journal of Advanced Nursing* **18**, 892–899.

Benner, P. (1984) *From Novice to Expert: Excellence and Power in Clinical Nursing Practice*. Addison-Wesley, London.

Benner, P. (1994) The tradition and skill of interpretive phenomenology in studying health, illness, and caring practices. In: *Interpretive Phenomenology: Embodiment, Caring, and Ethics in Health and Illness* (ed. P. Benner), pp. 99–127. Sage Publications, London.

Benner, P. & Tanner, C. (1987) How expert nurses use intuition. *American Journal of Nursing* **87**(1), 23–31.

Benner, P., Tanner, C. & Chesla, C. (1996) *Expertise in Nursing Practice. Caring, Clinical Judgement and Ethics*. Springer, New York.

Benner, P. & Wrubel, J. (1989) *The Primacy of Caring: Stress and Coping in Health and Illness*. Addison-Wesley, Wokingham.

Bonner, A. & Greenwood, J. (2006) The acquisition and exercise of nephrology nursing expertise: a grounded theory study. *Journal of Clinical Nursing* **15**, 480–489.

Brown, A. & Scott, G. (2004) Art and artistry in practice – a reflective account. In: *Delivering Cancer and Palliative Care Education* (ed. L. Foyle & J. Hostad), Vol. 1. Radcliffe Publishing, Oxford.

Carper, B.A. (1978) Fundamental patterns of knowing. *Advances in Nursing Science* **1**(1), 13–23.

Christensen, M. & Hewitt-Taylor, J. (2006) From expert to tasks, expert nursing practice redefined? *Journal of Clinical Nursing* **15**(12), 1531–1539.

Conway, J. (1996) *Nursing Expertise and Advanced Practice*. MarkAllen Publishing, Dinton.

Darbyshire, P. (1999) Nursing, art and science: revisiting the two cultures. *International Journal of Nursing Practice* **5**(3), 123–131.

Donnelly, G. (2003) Clinical expertise in advanced practice nursing: a Canadian perspective. *Nurse Education Today* **23**, 168–173.

Dreyfus, H.L. & Dreyfus, S.E. (1985) *Mind over Machine: The Power of Human Intuition and Expertise in the Era of the Computer*. Free Press, New York.

Gobbi, M. (2005) Nursing practice as bricoleur activity: a concept explored. *Nursing Inquiry* **12**(2), 117–125.

Hardy, S., Titchen, A. & Down, J. (2006a) *Authenticating Practice Development Principles through Inquiry-Based Learning as a Process for Transformation.* A symposium, NETNEP Conference, Developing Collaborative Practice in Health and Social Care Education, Vancouver, 14–16 May.

Hardy, S., Titchen, A. & Manley, K. (2007) Patient narratives in the investigation and development of nursing practice expertise: a potential for transformation. *Nursing Inquiry* **14**(1), 80–88.

Jenny, J. & Logan, J. (1992) Knowing the patient: one aspect of clinical knowledge. *IMAGE: Journal of Nursing Scholarship* **24**(4), 254–258.

Johns, C. (2005) Dwelling with Alison: a reflection on expertise. *Complementary Therapies in Clinical Practice* **11**, 37–44.

Judd, J. (2005) Strategies used by nurses for decision-making in the paediatric orthopaedic setting. *Journal of Orthopaedic Nursing* **9**, 166–171.

Kolb, D.A. (1984) *Experiential Learning: Experience as a Source of Learning and Development.* Prentice Hall, Englewood Cliffs.

Lawler, J. (1991) *Behind the Screens: Nursing, Somology, and the Problem of the Body.* Churchill Livingstone, London.

LeVasseur, J.J. (1999) Toward an understanding of art in nursing. *Advances in Nursing Science* **21**(4), 48–63.

MacLeod, M. (1990) *Experience in Everyday Nursing Practice: A Study of 'Experienced' Ward Sisters.* Doctoral Thesis, University of Edinburgh, Edinburgh.

Manley, K., Hardy, S., Titchen, A., Garbett, R. & McCormack, B. (2005) *Changing Patients' Worlds through Nursing Practice Expertise: A Research Report.* Royal College of Nursing, London.

Manley, K. & McCormack, B. (1997) *Exploring Expert Practice.* MSc Nursing Distance Learning Module, RCN Institute, London.

McCormack, B. & Titchen, A. (2006) Critical creativity: melding, exploding, blending. *Educational Action Research: An International Journal* **14**(2), 239–266.

Orme, L. & Maggs, C. (1993) Decision-making in clinical practice: how do expert nurses, midwives and health visitors make decisions? *Nurse Education Today* **13**, 270–276.

Purkis, M.E. & Bjornsdottir, K. (2006) Intelligent nursing: accounting for knowledge as action in practice. *Nursing Philosophy* **7**, 247–256.

Radwin, L.E. (1995) Knowing the patient: a process model for individualized interventions. *Nursing Research* **44**(6), 364–370.

Schon, D.A. (1983) *The Reflective Practitioner: How Professionals Think in Action.* Temple Smith, London.

Steele, S. & Fenton, M.V. (1988). Expert practice of clinical nurse specialists. *Clinical Nurse Specialist* **2**(1), 45–52.

Street, A. (1992) *Inside Nursing.* SUNY Press, New York.

Tanner, C.A., Benner, P., Chesla, C. & Gordon, D.R. (1993) The phenomenology of knowing the patient. *IMAGE: Journal of Nursing Scholarship* **25**(4), 273–280.

Titchen, A. (2000) *Professional Craft Knowledge in Patient-Centred Nursing and the Facilitation of Its Development.* D.Phil., University of Oxford, Ashdale, Oxford.

Titchen, A. (2001) Skilled companionship in professional practice. In: *Practice Knowledge and Expertise in the Health Professions* (eds J. Higgs & A. Titchen), pp. 69–79. Butterworth Heinemann, Oxford.

Titchen, A. (2004) Helping relationships for practice development: critical companion-ship. In: *Practice Development in Nursing* (eds B. McCormack, K. Manley & R. Gar-bett), pp. 148–174. Blackwell Publishing, Oxford.

Titchen, A. & Higgs, J. (2001) Towards professional artistry and creativity in practice. In *Professional Practice in Health, Education and the Creative Arts* (eds J. Higgs & A. Titchen), pp. 273–290. Blackwell Science, Oxford.

Titchen, A. & Higgs, J. (2007) Exploring interpretive and critical philosophies. In: *Being Critical and Creative in Qualitative Research* (eds. J. Higgs, A. Titchen, D. Horsfall & H.B. Armstrong), pp. 56–68. Hampden Press, Sydney.

Titchen, A., Higgs, J. & Horsfall, D. (2007) Research artistry: dancing the praxis spi-ral in critical-creative qualitative research. In: *Being Critical and Creative in Qualita-tive Research* (eds J. Higgs, A. Titchen, D. Horsfall & H.B. Armstrong), pp. 282–297. Hampden Press, Sydney.

Titchen, A. & McGinley, M. (2003) Facilitating practitioner-research through critical companionship. *NT Research* **8**(2), 115–131.

Section Two

Practitioner Expertise

4. Transformational Impact of the Expertise in Practice Project

Maeve McGinley

Introduction

I invite the reader to journey with me through my experience of the RCN's *Expertise in Practice Project* (EPP) (Manley *et al.*, 2005). As we travel, I aim to share a sense of my experience within the project, its impact on me as a nurse, what I gained from that experience and perhaps most importantly, how it continues to affect my current practice and that of others.

It has been a truly transformative journey, both personally and professionally. It has enabled me to look inside myself and it has awakened my understanding of what makes me an expert. Its effect has been such that it still informs how I facilitate learning (with my team and other practitioners) to transform their practice so that they too can deliver evidence-based and person-centred care.

The chapter comprises two sections. First, to fully appreciate what the impact and outcomes of participating in the EPP were for me personally and professionally, you need to have some sense of who I am and why I decided to join the project. Within the second section, I explore, in more detail, the impact the EPP journey still has on my current practice.

Section one: starting the journey

Great journeys of exploration and discovery usually have various stages. First, a preparatory stage, involving completing travel documents, employing an expert travel guide, reading travel guides and pouring over maps. The next stage might involve joining fellow travellers and their guides, moving on, learning new languages, experiencing new places, developing new skills, collecting souvenirs and recording experiences, completing a travel journal. The final stage involves returning home, sharing experiences with others and starting again a new beginning. My transformational journey was similar. First there was the application stage, then joining fellow participants and their critical companions, moving on into experiencing and learning a new language, frameworks, concepts and tools and gathering evidence and completing a portfolio of evidence.

Who am I?

I am a rich blend of characteristics, traits, knowledge, skills and experience, originating from both my personal and professional lives which come together to make me the person-centred expert practitioner that I am. I am married and living on the north-west coast of Ireland. I am a people-centred person who enjoys painting, gardening, music, holidays and fun. I am employed in a Community Health and Social Services Trust in Northern Ireland. My professional title is 'Clinical Nurse Specialist Bladder and Bowel Dysfunction'. The key elements of my professional role include specialist clinical practice, education, management and a range of regional activities. My academic and professional qualifications include a B.Sc. (Hons), R.G.N., Dip Nurse (Lond.), Dip H.E. Continence Care, Cert Health Services Management and District Nurse qualification. I have a number of publications (McGinley, 1984, 2001a, b). I was awarded the first Northern Ireland Nurse of the Year award. Locally, regionally and nationally, I have gained significant clinical credibility for my nursing expertise in the field of continence care.

I have had a passion for nursing since childhood and (due to significant episodes of illness during my career) I have gained invaluable insight into what it really feels like to be on the receiving end of nursing care and the importance of seeing situations through the patients' eyes. Not only am I a clinical nurse expert, but I am also enormously committed to delivering evidence-based, person-centred care.

Why then, when my clinical expertise was already recognised regionally and even nationally, did I feel that I wanted to put myself through this recognition of Expertise Project? There were a number of reasons and influencing factors that prompted me to do so.

Why the need to join the EPP?

First, I had been working as a clinical expert advisor, with an information technology student, developing software for an Expert Nursing System. He constantly challenged me to explain how I used different types of knowledge, how I came to decisions or made a diagnosis. I hoped the EPP would enable me, not only to understand, in significant depth, my expertise, but also to articulate expertise in such a way that others could understand and appreciate its true value, in terms of achieving health outcomes for patients and carers.

About the same time, I was aware that new professional career developments were taking place within nursing, such as the Consultant Nurse post, which might provide a new career opportunity for me. A core function of the Consultant Nurse's role is demonstrating clinical expertise (Manley, 2001). I hoped the EPP would help me understand the nature of my expertise, its strengths and weaknesses and provide me with strategies to address any weaknesses.

Second, I hoped the project might help me to compile a portfolio of evidence which demonstrated my clinical expertise. Although I already had a portfolio of evidence from the UKCC's Higher Level of Practice Project (UKCC, 1999), which demonstrated that I was working to a standard deemed by the UKCC[1] to be at 'a higher level' and that my practice was safe, it did not demonstrate or indeed illustrate the nature of my expertise in practice. What I needed was a body of evidence that I could use to provide practical illustrations of the value of my clinical expertise which I could use when bidding for additional resources or making an application for a Consultant Nurse post.

Third, I had no access to clinical supervision within my Trust, I felt that the opportunity to work closely with a critical companion might enable me to experience what clinical supervision was really like and further develop myself.

EPP project application

I had to complete an EPP application pack. I had to write a self-assessment against the attributes of expertise derived from a concept analysis (Manley & McCormack, 1997), outline my rationale for consideration as a potential 'expert'; identify and secure a critical companion for the duration of the project; get signed Trust Management support; and two references highlighting my attributes of expertise. These effectively were my 'travel documents'. I found compiling the nomination self-assessment particularly challenging. This may have been because I had not had any formal training or experience of structured reflection (Palmer *et al.*, 1994; Johns, 1996, 2001). Another reason for the difficulty was my unfamiliarity with the terms used to describe the attributes of expertise (RCN Institute, 2000).

Identifying and securing my critical companion also proved difficult. After much searching, thankfully, one of the EPP project team members, Brendan McCormack, kindly stepped in to act as my critical companion. Brendan's critical companionship and excellent facilitation of learning skills were key to the successful development in my knowledge, skills and understanding of expertise.

With travel documentation completed, my guide (critical companion) secured, I awaited final approval and a date to begin my journey. I used the waiting time to familiarise myself with the recommended project reading. Conscious of my lack of experience of structured reflection, I focused on that subject (Beckett, 1969; Freshwater, 1998; Johns, 1998). I also read up on the language of expertise, the terms used to describe the attributes and enabling factors (Manley and McCormack, 1997) and Titchen's (2000) conceptual frameworks. Relating Titchen's (2000) conceptual framework to my clinical practice and understanding the language she used when explaining them, at this stage, seemed like an impossibility.

Joining fellow EPP participants and moving on

As I joined my fellow travellers at our first action learning set (ALS) (McGill & Beaty, 1997), I felt excited, anxious and somewhat naïve. I was anxious due to my lack of experience in structured reflection and the realisation of its importance, within the project. I was further concerned that the knowledge of expertise and level of expert practice of ALS members would be much greater than mine. I

---

[1] Formerly the UKCC now known as the Nursing & Midwifery Council (NMC).

was naïve in my expectation that my critical companion, and/or the project team, would 'unpick' my expertise and gather the evidence to demonstrate it. I soon discovered that was my task with their support.

Action learning sets (ALS)

I found the ALS were an invaluable and most enriching experience. I felt able to check out my understanding of the project objectives, what I was required to do, what to expect of my critical companion, conceptual frameworks of skilled companionship (accompanying a patient/client on their illness/wellness journey) (see Figure 4.1) and critical companionship (Titchen, 2000) (refer to Figure 5.1) and many other key issues that I was concerned about. There were opportunities to discuss debate and critique my understanding of the expertise and reflection literature. I was able to observe and learn from the excellent questioning skills not only of the person leading the set, but also from the other set members. We developed a tool, in the form of a matrix, to help us, more easily understand Titchen's (2000) conceptual frameworks (see for example Table 4.1).

We used it at the end of each session, to reflect on the session. I could see, as we reflected, the various domains of knowledge and learning strategies that had been used and how they were actually used. This enabled me to get a real grasp and understanding of what I had been trying to read in terms of the frameworks and structured reflection (Titchen, 2000; Johns, 2001). I found that reflection, through action learning (McGill & Beaty, 1997), helped develop understanding of my knowledge use and in particular how effectively facilitation strategies can be used to develop learning. I felt the ALS were such a powerful way of learning and kept me so motivated that I decided I would, in the future, utilise that approach within my practice site.

Critical companionship meetings

Almost in parallel with the ALS activity, each nurse participant established regular meetings with his/her critical companion. These meetings, for me, felt like special guided tours.

My critical companion (Brendan) and I met via video conferencing. It proved a most efficient and effective method of meeting. We saved time and energy not having to drive long distances. It focused our minds and agenda, as meetings were strictly time limited. I could really concentrate on listening to and questioning Brendan as I had a video recording of the meetings and did not need to take notes. I used the recordings to reflect on the meetings which further enhanced my learning experience. As we travelled together, I experienced Brendan skilfully helping me to investigate my own practice, in terms of raising my consciousness of the nature of my professional knowledge base that informs my practice and how it is generated, and how I bring myself as a human being into my relationship with my patients. Reflecting on the video recordings, I could see when and how he skilfully used and balanced each of the critical companionship domains (relationship, rationality-intuitive, facilitative and use of self) as described by Titchen (2000) (refer again to Figure 5.1).

I gradually became more aware of the facilitation domain processes (consciousness raising, problematisation, self-reflection, critique) he was using to help me

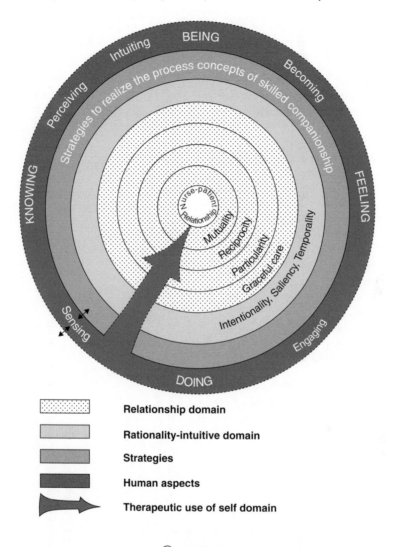

Figure 4.1 'Skilled companionship': a conceptual framework for patient-centred nursing. (© Angie Titchen (2000).)

examine my practice. He used, in particular, facilitation strategies, such as critical dialogue, feedback on performance, role modelling and high challenge/high support to do so. I felt I was working in a very helpful, negotiated partnership built on trust and mutual respect. Although I felt constantly tested, Brendan seemed to

Table 4.1 Critical companionship matrix

	Facilitation processes →	Consciousness raising	Problematisation	Self-reflection	Critique
Relationship processes	Mutuality Reciprocity Particularity Graceful care				
Rationality-intuitive processes	Intentionality Saliency Temporality				
Facilitation strategies	Articulation of craft knowledge Observing listening and questioning Feedback on performance High challenge, high support Critical dialogue Role modelling Use of creative imagination				
Facilitative use of self	Integrating self into the above				
Professional artistry	Attunement to and blending, melding, interplay, synchronisation, synthesis and balancing of any combination of processes (in *italic*) and strategies (in plain) to meet particular needs of individual practitioners in relation to their particular experiences, contexts and situations				

Source: Adapted from Titchen (2003).

be able to provide me with the right support, in the right measure (graceful care) when I needed to take my understanding to a new level.

During our initial meetings, we discussed, identified and agreed the aspects of my role (clinical practice, education, management and regional activities) from which I would source evidence to demonstrate my expertise. We went on to decide in detail, when and how I would gather 360° feedback and user narrative evidence required by the project. I constantly used Brendan as a resource against which to test my understanding of the literature I was reading. At one point, I found myself actually challenging Brendan about knowledge acquisition and use. I suddenly realised that to do so, my awareness of my knowledge base and its use must have measurably improved through the facilitation processes he used.

Evidence gathering, analysis, interpretation and evaluation

This next stage of my journey involved collecting evidence (souvenirs) and reflecting on experiences to put into my portfolio (travel journal). I selected activities from each of my role functions, to use as sources of evidence to demonstrate my expertise. For example, to demonstrate my expertise in clinical practice, I selected, with the patients' consent, a number of case studies and aspects of work I had done regionally, whilst providing specialist clinical advice to colleagues. These activities, along with the 360° feedback activity and user narrative, provided my main body of evidence.

Demonstrating my expertise from the evidence, however, required reflecting on and analysing each activity using the concepts and tools I had acquired through the project.

Qualitative 360° feedback

To obtain my 360° feedback evidence (refer to Chapter 13 for more information), I organised two 1-hour group interviews with two separate role sets. Each session was audio taped. The role sets for each group consisted of people (junior colleagues, peers, managers, educationalists), who had direct involvement with me in one or more of the work-based activities that I had selected for my evidence. Brendan carried out the interviews, basing his questions on ones I had drawn up. Selecting role set members forced me to examine all aspects of my expert role. Being the observer, rather than the interviewer, freed me to observe the group dynamics, non-verbal cues and learn from Brendan's skilled questioning techniques. Being present gave me ownership of the feedback.

Analysing the feedback was the greatest challenge I experienced in the project. It was at this point in my journey that I experienced what Freshwater (1998, p. 17) describes as 'a difficult phase of angst (the blackening)' before my transformation. Whilst the feedback was in itself extremely positive, the analysis really challenged my understanding and ability to use as a tool, Titchen's (2000) conceptual frameworks and to use a model of structured reflection (Johns, 1998). Initially, I felt positive about my knowledge, skills and expertise, yet, while analysing audio evidence, I began to doubt my expertise. I did not hear the role sets describe my expertise in the language that I was now so familiar with, in terms of describing the attributes and enabling factors of expertise. I had to unpick what they were saying to find suitable illustrations to demonstrate my expertise. This forced me to gain an even deeper understanding of the attributes and enabling factors. It also pushed me to come to grips with, in even greater depth, my understanding of skilled and critical companionship and how these concepts are parallel. I realised that most of the role sets had not actually observed me working directly with patients. So, understandably, they would have difficulty in providing examples to demonstrate attributes in that aspect of my role. This made me question my role as a skilled companion, and particularly, how I was going to evidence it. The user narrative together with the case studies would, I felt, adequately demonstrate my expertise in that aspect of my role.

I undertook a second stage analysis of the feedback using Titchen's (2001a, b) conceptual framework of critical companionship. This helped me identify my strengths and weaknesses in terms of my role. I found that in terms of critical companionship most of my knowledge domains were strong but I needed to strengthen my self-reflection and critique processes in my facilitation domain. Being able to compare how I worked with my team, with how Brendan worked with me and my analysis of my critical companionship domains all helped me realise that by improving my self-reflection and critique processes and by using facilitation strategies, such as critical dialogue, I could significantly enhance practitioners' learning. I also realised that I tended to decide what practitioners' needed in order to develop their expertise rather than finding out what they felt they needed.

Reflective piece

Using Johns's (1998) model of structured reflection on an incident within one of the sessions in the 360° feedback enabled me to begin to understand what made my clinical practice 'expert' compared to other practitioners. It raised my consciousness of the knowledge which Titchen (2000) argues is largely tacit and embedded in practice and of my precognitive way of knowing (see Chapter 12). I became aware of the types of knowledge (propositional, personal and professional craft knowledge) that I used and how I blended them in practice in an almost seamless way and even how I created new knowledge. I became very aware of my use of the three knowledge domains of person-centred care that Titchen (2000) described in the skilled companionship conceptual framework. I was able to evaluate the strengths and balance of each of my knowledge domains, when working with my patients. I could also see where my colleagues' skilled companionship domains required strengthening, for example, where they were not enabling a patient to share in decision-making about care, and how I could raise their consciousness, that whilst saying they engage in person-centred care, their actual care did not match what they said they did.

User narrative

The user narrative was gathered by Brendan, once ethical approval and consent from the user was obtained. Kate was mother and carer of my patient, Joseph, an 18-year-old boy with an undiagnosed neurodegenerative condition. (Kate and Joseph are pseudonyms.)

The narrative was a very powerful piece.

The narrative appeared to clearly indicate that, as a clinical practitioner, I demonstrated all the attributes of expertise and that I was also an effective skilled companion to others involved in this case. For example, Kate talked about how (until I came along) no one seemed to know why Joseph had so many infections, but that I was able to identify the probable cause. I knew what the appropriate course of action to take was and I applied a variety of knowledges to the situation, in order to make the most appropriate decisions (technical and aesthetic knowledge, demonstrating skilled know-how).

Using Titchen's (2001b) 'skilled companionship' model (refer to Figure 3.1) to analyse my expertise within this narrative, I clearly demonstrated expertise as a skilled companion to Joseph, Kate and other carers. My domains (relationship, rationality-intuitive, therapeutic use of self) appeared strong and well balanced. I seemed to effectively manage the fine interplay between my intuitive and rational judgment and between my theoretical and professional craft knowledge.

The practical strategies I adopted, to realise the process concepts within the domains, appeared to have been effective. For example the narrative highlighted how I was able to identify the key risk factors for Joseph through using my holistic knowledge and a scanner (saliency). I appeared to demonstrate graceful care with Joseph when Kate said:

> I feel comfortable with Maeve being in the house, I don't feel I have to put on a show for her, you know, and she knows all the different things that are going on. Maybe it's just Maeve herself, the person that she is, she just makes it easy to relax with her.

An illustration of when I used therapeutic use of self domain was given by Kate when she said:

> Maeve really listens to everything you say, and I find I know, like the hospital appointments, you know you're slotted into a certain time and I understand that, but I don't believe they listen to you. Maeve listens to everything you say and she thinks about it and she'd maybe come up with a few suggestions but she leaves it open, you know she leaves a lot open to us to decide.

The narrative made me very conscious of how users can distinguish between expert and non-expert practice. They may not have the language that I have learned about expertise but they have no problem in giving clear contextual examples to portray what they want to say. The narrative was both humbling and reassuring that I have been effective in achieving what I want to be, an expert skilled companion to my patient and his carers.

My professional title is 'specialist nurse' but this evidence demonstrated that I am, in fact, according to Conway (1998) a 'humanistic existentialist' expert nurse. I use a range of knowledge and operate from a holistic practice perspective.

Evidence portfolio

Having gathered evidence from a wide range of sources, I then had to amalgamate it, in a structured way, into a portfolio for formal review and accreditation.

Compiling and selecting material for inclusion in my portfolio, to demonstrate my expertise, brought me deep into my own subconscious and confronted me with the reality of how I and others perceive and understand expertise. It revealed to me the difference between my practice and that of other practitioners.

My reflective piece of evidence had provided an action plan, which I hoped to use to help work colleagues develop their expertise. Compiling the portfolio made me conscious of the new knowledge, skills and tools I was now using to examine my practice expertise and that of other practitioners. I realised that the language of expertise and the conceptual frameworks that I once found impossible to understand had become embedded in my knowledge and practice such that they were now a vital and integral part of my professional craft knowledge. My understanding of the attributes of expertise had developed so much that I no longer thought of them as separate entities to the conceptual model of skilled companionship. Rather, when I thought of 'knowing the patient' and 'moral agency' I linked them to Titchen's (2000) relationship domain, because I understood that to really know the patient I had to realise the concept processes within that domain. I was already beginning to evaluate my own and others' practice, using tools such as the attributes and then linking them to the conceptual framework. In doing so, I was identifying how I could develop and improve practice and, at the same time, showing an aspect of professional artistry, that is being aware that I was blending different types of knowledge in practice (metacognition – see Chapter 12).

Resting place: looking at the photo album

I reflected on my journey and produced an 'album of photos' (see Box 4.1) to show what its impact/effect has been on me professionally. Looking at these again now, I realise this is a snapshot of a higher level of consciousness I have gained from my experiential and developmental journey in relation to expert practice and its consequences, not only on myself, but on colleagues, patients and families and health care organisations.

Section two: a new beginning

Within this section of the chapter, I will talk more about how my journey continues, after the EPP ended, as I continue to share my travel log of experiences with others.

Work colleagues

During the EPP, I realised that the essence of my clinical expertise is my skilled companionship relationship with my patients and carers. I also have a responsibility, as an expert, to act as a critical companion to my team and other less-experienced practitioners. Before joining the EPP, I had become frustrated because some of my team's expertise did not seem to be developing as I thought it should. During the EPP, my evidence analysis (360° feedback, reflective piece), however,

Box 4.1   Photos/snapshot of the impact of my journey

- Increased awareness of the different types of knowledge I use in practice and how I use (blend) that knowledge to deliver evidence-based, person-centred care.
- Increased understanding as to how I generate new knowledge in and from practice.
- The ability to use new frameworks, concepts and tools to examine (deconstruct and reconstruct experiences) my own practice and that of others.
- An understanding of the differences between expert and non-expert practice and how that impacts on patients' and their carers' experiences.
- A growth in confidence and ability to articulate the nature and value of expertise to other practitioners and my organisation.
- Having the language needed to articulate my evidence of expertise to peers for scrutiny, knowledge creation and my organisation.
- Having evidence which demonstrates the value/benefits of expertise for patients and their carers.
- Having an action plan to enable me to help my nursing team develop their expertise.
- Having a clear understanding of the conceptual frameworks of skilled and critical companionship and their use as tools to examine one's practice and facilitate learning
- A very positive, powerful and personal learning experience within critical companionship.
- Recognition of responsibility as an expert practitioner to provide not only skilled companionship to patients and their carers, but also critical companionship to less-experienced practitioners who seek my help.
- Recognition of the need to develop, strengthen and use more effectively, my critical companionship, facilitation domain processes and strategies in order to develop practitioners expertise.
- Enhanced ability to critically self-reflect in a structured way and the realisation that guided reflection can be used as a means of seeking new and more effective ways to practice.
- Experience of how ALS and a critical companionship relationship can be very effective in supporting and facilitating learning.
- An insight into what it is that patients' and their carers' value in the delivery of expert practice. A realisation that they need and want to be respected, valued, listened to and involved in their care and decision-making.
- The recognition that given the government's pressure on health care organisations to ensure delivery of care is evidence based and clinically effective, my organisation needed to understand how developing practitioners' expertise, could help meet that political agenda.

uncovered problems in certain knowledge domains in myself and the team, which may have been limiting our ability to develop.

My critical companionship domains (relationship, rationality-intuitive, facilitative use of self) were found to be strong and well balanced, but certain concept processes (self-reflection, critique) within my facilitation domain were weak. The team's skilled companionship relationship domain was strong, but their rationality-intuitive domain (holistic practice, knowledge skilled know-how, saliency, reflective ability) was weak, resulting in an imbalance between their domains. This was most evident when they were discussing a problem case with me or a general physician (GP). They often had difficulty pulling out the salient points of a case. If challenged on their knowledge and reasoning, such as why they selected a particular course of action/treatment, they could not articulate their underpinning knowledge, give supporting arguments or provide evidence to support their decision. Their weaknesses tended to be in relation to conscious decision-making (intentionality); knowing what matters (saliency) and timing, anticipating and pacing (temporality). For skilled companions to be able to provide evidence-based, person-centred care their domains all need to be strong and well balanced (Titchen & McGinley, 2003). Team members seemed unaware of their knowledge base, how they used it and how to integrate new knowledge into their existing knowledge, such that it becomes part of their professional craft knowledge (knowledge acquired through professional experience). Given that evidence-based, person-centred care draws on holistic practice knowledge then my team needed to be aware of their own practice knowledge base if they were to be effective skilled companions to their patients.

The evidence analysis not just highlighted problems, but also revealed that by improving my own self-reflection and critique concept processes and using certain learning strategies (role modelling, articulating craft knowledge, critical dialogue, feedback), I could significantly enhance practitioners' facilitation of learning. As stated earlier, I discovered that I tended to decide what practitioners needed to develop their expertise, rather than finding out what they felt they needed.

I started sharing, very sensitively, my findings and action plan with the team. In partnership, we agreed to set up guided reflection sessions and provide role modelling opportunities. During the initial reflection sessions, the team identified their understanding of reflection and what reflective skills they had and where they needed to develop their knowledge and skills. Through reviewing and critiquing relevant literature and creating reflection opportunities in and on practice, I facilitated their learning. The team was invited to observe me working directly with patients (role modelling). An opportunity was created to allow them to question and critique my practice. I found the sessions, as Rolfe (1998) warns, challenging for myself but a great way to highlight to practitioners my craft knowledge and other types of knowledge and how I use them to provide expert care.

When the reflection sessions and the role-modelling opportunities were underway, I started to change the way I responded to the team when they sought my advice about problem cases. I stopped 'spoon feeding' them. Rather I began to challenge them to pull out the salient points of the case, justify/explain their reasoning and the knowledge they were using and to identify evidence to support their decisions. I challenged and supported them to articulate their craft knowledge, understand the knowledge they were drawing upon and to consciously identify any gaps in their knowledge plus how they might access knowledge to inform those gaps. Initially, I sensed increasing tension due to such a new way of working. Then gradually, I noticed that team members began to seek my advice in a different way. They began to use me as a resource to help them rather than just to provide answers. They became more confident, in articulating their knowledge, when discussing a problem case. They became assertive with other professionals when patients required any changes in treatment pathways. Increasingly, they were constructing and using their knowledge more effectively and so were more able to get the desired outcome for their patients. They appeared to be accessing and using more research evidence to broaden and deepen their knowledge base. Gradually, they appeared to be able to process new knowledge (research evidence) and integrate it into their practice.

As the expertise of individual team members has blossomed, so has their ability to develop expertise in other practitioners and to enable expert interventions to take place. A learning culture has really developed within the team, which Titchen and Binnie (1995) point out, enables personal and professional growth and fosters adaptability.

The organisation

At the time the EPP was drawing to a close, I felt I needed to raise awareness within my Health Care Trust, about my experience within the EPP. I wanted to articulate my new understanding of the nature of nursing 'expertise', that is how professional artistry brings everything together and how it can be evidenced. I wanted to share the importance and value of expertise in terms of delivering to patients and their carers, evidence-based, person-centred and clinically effective practice.

The government's clinical governance and clinical effectiveness agenda demands that health care provision be high quality, evidence-based, patient-centred and clinically effective (Rucroft-Malone *et al.*, 2002). I recognised that if my organisation was to meet that agenda, it needed to identify its expert practitioners, demonstrate that expert practice and to support the development of expertise to enable expert interventions to take place.

The Department of Health (1998) highlighted that within its clinical governance agenda the emphasis was on developing open and supportive frameworks to help organisations, teams and individuals reflect upon their performance and learn from their mistakes. One of the ways in which this could be done was through clinical supervision (RCN, 1998). In light of this, I sensed that I needed to influence the culture, within my organisation, in terms of the way in which it supported the development of clinical expertise, particularly, how clinical supervision was delivered. I felt that guided structured reflection was not utilised within the Trust's clinical supervision programme.

The first opportunity to share my experience of the EPP more widely presented itself when I attended an RCN 'Nurses as Political Leaders' conference. At the conference the attributes of a nurse leader were highlighted. I realised that they were a reflection of most of the attributes of an expert practitioner. This prompted me to share with delegates my experience in the EPP and new knowledge in relation to expertise. I realised from this experience that I could articulate expertise but most importantly that delegates understood what I was saying and were motivated by it. This gave me the confidence to begin to talk about the EPP to members of my Trust's Professional Nursing Forum (PNF). The PNF consisted of nurse managers, team leaders and some nurse specialists. I highlighted how I was now using the frameworks, concepts and tools to examine and develop my own team's expertise and how they could, more effectively, facilitate practitioners' learning. I began to question the type of clinical supervision being delivered in my organisation's Programme of Care.

When the project ended and I received confirmation that I had successfully demonstrated my expertise, I wrote an article for the Health Care Trust's News Journal, highlighting my experience in the project, how expertise can be demonstrated and how important expertise was in achieving positive health and social care outcomes for patients and their carers. About the same time, I met with the Director of Nursing and the Area Board's Chief Nurse to outline my learning resulting from the EPP and the benefits of the project to nursing on a wider front. I highlighted that learning from practice through reflection was an important mechanism for maintaining competency (Boud *et al.*, 1985) and patient-centred approaches (Titchen, 2000). I was invited to make a presentation on reflection to senior nurse managers. It prompted a very enthusiastic debate about the type of supervision being delivered within our Programme of Care, compared to the type of supervision that I was suggesting.

Following these discussions, an audit of clinical supervision was undertaken. Its findings confirmed my suspicions that the quality of delivery of supervision was very variable and did not appear to be impacting on developing practitioners practice in the way in which it had been intended. I was invited to meet with the Director of Nursing, the Programme Manager and Assistant Programme Managers to discuss the audit findings and what needed to be done to address problems identified. I highlighted the need to support Practice Development. I also recommended that a training programme on clinical supervision, based on the RCN Institute (2000) Programme, should be organised and implemented within the Trust, starting with nurse managers who were currently undertaking the supervision of staff. The programme could then be cascaded down through all the nursing staff. I recommended the RCN Institute (2000) Programme as it was based on the use of guided reflection within clinical supervision. A Practice Development-based post was created and filled. The Practice Development Officer, in response to the recommendations from our audit meeting, arranged the Clinical Supervision Development Programme. A facilitator, experienced in delivering the RCN Institute (2000) Programme, was brought in to run the programme, initially, for senior nurses, team leaders, allied health professional team leaders and specialist nurses. A strategy for taking forward supervision was developed and is currently being implemented.

Sensing that some nurse participants seemed unsure of how to implement, in particular, guided reflection, I offered to facilitate a learning set focused on clinical supervision. I felt that while the initial focus of the set would be how to use guided reflection within clinical supervision, it could eventually move on to offer set members who did not have supervision themselves, a group supervision facility. The learning sets are currently in operation and are being received positively in that they are enabling practitioners to implement the type of supervision that they agreed to deliver as a result of the training programme.

Since I undertook the EPP journey, a greater learning culture has been developing within my organisation. We are hopefully moving towards what Manley (2001) described as a transformational culture, in which staff empowerment and Practice Development are key characteristics. The changes in relation to how we are now delivering clinical supervision have the potential, not just to benefit patients and practitioners but also to contribute, effectively, to the organisation's objectives of developing more skilled, aware and articulate practitioners.

The patients

The user narrative evidence I gathered and analysed during the EPP demonstrated that whilst patients and carers want professionals to use their technical knowledge, they also want to be included where their views and values as a patient or carer are considered and facilitated into the process of care delivery and decision-making. This insight enabled me to develop my expertise and deliver care tailored uniquely for each patient. As my team's expertise developed, more patients and carers were receiving care which was increasingly evidence based and person centred. Similarly, the team began to develop the practice of other practitioners. Increasingly, patients and carers were receiving improved care delivery.

The impact of my experience in the EPP, in terms of improved care for patients, is illustrated through a project I initiated after the EPP ended. I had identified that males with benign prostatic hyperplasia (BPH; non-malignant enlargement of the prostate gland) were waiting at least 12–18 months for an assessment of their problem and even longer for treatment. Kuritzy (1998) indicates that the earlier BPH is detected and treated, decreases the chance for the patient to require surgical treatment. Prior to the project, I had highlighted the need to reduce the waiting time for assessment and treatment of this group of patients but with no success. When the EPP ended, I felt much more confident about articulating the needs of this client group to strategic commissioners. I was able to compile and present a robust business case to secure funding for 1 year to implement a pilot nurse led, community-based BPH assessment service. I recruited a nurse to implement the project. I used the critical companionship relationship with her, acting as her resource, challenging and supporting her on her journey through the pilot project. The project was independently evaluated. It was found to have more than achieved the project objectives. Patients were being seen at that BPH community clinic within 2 weeks of their referral and treated within 3 weeks, if treatment was required. Further, during the projects evaluation, patients reported feeling less anxious and able to ask questions when attending the clinic in their local health centre; it was more accessible locally; the information provided was adequate and easily understood. The quick access to assessment and treatment helped reduce not only the patient's worries but also those of carers.

The project was so successful that funding was secured to establish a permanent service. The significant improvement in the quality of service delivery, through this pilot project, was recognised at a regional level. We were awarded the top prize in the 2004 Health and Personal Social Services Quality Awards (Northern Ireland). The EPP empowered me to successfully undertake this initiative and helped me develop the knowledge and skills I needed to do so.

Myself (personal journey)

The experience of having a critical companion so enriched my thinking and learning during my experiential journey that I feared it would end as the project ended. As a direct result of my EPP experience, I felt so motivated to take action on so many work fronts I really needed someone to challenge and support me while I tried to create a culture of effectiveness within my team and my organisation. Brendan did continue to support me when I was preparing for the reflection presentation. He also acted as a resource to myself and my Director of Nursing working on bringing about a change in the Trust's delivery of clinical supervision. Further, he invited me to deliver a seminar, to Practice Development nurses, on the Skilled and Critical Companionship Frameworks (Titchen, 2000). I was also invited to one of Northern Ireland's university's to deliver a presentation to specialist nurse practitioners on my understanding and use of the Skilled and Critical Companionship Conceptual Frameworks within practice. The feedback from both of those seminars was so positive that it reaffirmed confidence in my ability to articulate my understanding of expertise and my knowledge use.

I was invited by the RCN Institute's EPP project coordinator to present my experience of the EPP in terms of personal impact and outcomes at a workshop at the RCN's Annual Congress 2002. I met Angie Titchen at the workshop. I discussed with her my need and desire to develop further my understanding of expertise, its development and in particular my professional knowledge base and how I could become a more effective critical companion. As a result of that discussion, Angie offered to act as my critical companion to help facilitate my continued learning journey. Brendan and Angie invited me to join them at a Practice Development colloquium meeting. This was an inspiring meeting that helped deepen my understanding of the theory underpinning Practice Development. It helped to maintain my motivation to bring about change within my organisation while facilitating my own professional learning. Working with Angie as my critical companion has enabled me to fulfil my critical companionship role and has culminated in a number of publications (Titchen & McGinley, 2003; Titchen & McGinley, 2004). It has also helped me to deepen my understanding of professional artistry in relation to drawing on my different knowledges, moving seamlessly between rational and intuitive ways of knowing and using practice skills to make each intervention with my patient and my colleague unique to their particular situations. My learning journey did not end as I had feared when the EPP ended. It continues even on to today.

Conclusion

In this chapter, I have walked with you through each stage of my EPP journey. As we travelled, I offered you a sense of my experiences within the project, its impact on me as a nurse, what I gained and how it has affected my current work. It has truly been a transformative journey for me personally and professionally. It has enabled me to look inside myself and awakened my understanding of what makes me an expert. Its effect has been such that it continues to enable me to facilitate learning and to transform others' practice such that they can deliver evidence-based and person-centred care. Further, its effect is reflected in the gradual transformation taking place in the culture of my organisation. Increasingly, the right context is being created, within the organisation, which enables expert interventions to take place. This can only help to ensure that the right treatment is given in the right away, for the right patient, at the right time and that it is delivered in ways that address the particular concerns and needs of the patient from his or her perspective.

Just like Jones *et al.* (1996), I have been on a stimulating and inquisitive journey which brought me through to a higher level of consciousness in relation to expertise. A journey through which, as a nurse, I was enabled to develop into the kind of person I want to be, fulfilling my therapeutic destiny and enabling those with whom I work to fulfil theirs.

This has been and is a journey I needed to do if I am to enable expertise to flourish.

To quote Thomas Beckett (1969):

> to be capable of helping others to become all they are capable of becoming we must first fulfil that commitment to ourselves.

Postscript

Since writing this chapter, Maeve has had to retire from nursing on health grounds. She is physically unable to nurse anymore, but through this chapter (and we anticipate further writing, if she is physically able), Maeve continues to share her nursing wisdom with others in a way that will inspire and enable a new generation of nursing expertise. Thank you Maeve.

References

Beckett, T. (1969) A candidate's reflection on the supervisory process. *Contemporary Psychoanalysis* **5**, 169–179.

Boud, D., Keogh, R., Walker, D. (1985) *Reflection: Turning Experience into Learning.* Kogan Page/Nichols Publishing, London.

Conway, J. (1998) Evolution of the species 'Expert Nurse'. An examination of the practical knowledge held by Expert Nurses. *Journal of Clinical Nursing* **7**, 75–82.

Department of Health (1998) *A First Class Service: Quality in the NHS.* Stationary Office, London.

Freshwater, D. (1998) The philosopher's stone. In: *Transforming Nurses through Reflective Practice* (eds C. Jones & D. Freshwater). Blackwell Science, Oxford.

Johns, C. (1996) Visualizing and realizing caring in practice through reflection. *Journal of Advanced Nursing* **23**, 1135–1143.

Johns, C. (1998) Opening the doors of perception. In: *Transforming Nurses through Reflective Practice* (eds C. Jones & D. Freshwater). Blackwell Science, Oxford.

Johns, C. (2001) Reflective practice: revealing the [he]art of caring. *International Journal of Nursing Practice* **7**, 237–245.

Jones, R., Blackwolf & Jones, G. (1996) *Earth Dance Drum*. Commune-E-Key Publishing, Salt Lake City.

Kuritzy, L. (1998) Current approaches to the management of BPH. *Clinical Geriatrics* **6**(12), 65–76.

Manley, K. (2001) *Consultant Nurse: Concept, Processes, Outcome*. Unpublished Doctoral Thesis. University of Manchester/RCN Institute, London.

Manley, K., Hardy, S., Titchen, A., Garbett, R. & McCormack, B. (2005) *Changing Patients' Worlds through Nursing Practice Expertise: Exploring Nursing Practice Expertise through Emancipatory Action Research and Fourth Generation Evaluation*. A Royal College of Nursing Research Report 1998–2004. RCN, London.

Manley, K. & McCormack, B. (1997) *Exploring Expert Practice Masters in Nursing Distance Learning Module*. RCN Institute, London.

McGill, I. & Beaty, L. (1997) *Action Learning*. Kogan Page, London.

McGinley, M. (1984) *History and Development of District Nursing in N. Ireland*. Unpublished B.Sc. (Hons) Thesis. University of Ulster, Coleraine.

McGinley, M. (2001a) Management of encopresis and the parents role. *Nursing Times Plus* **97**(22), 55–59.

McGinley, M. (2001b) *Wound Management Educational Resource Pack: Crest Guidelines*. N. Ireland CREST. CD-ROM.

Palmer, A., Burns, S. & Bulman, C. (1994) *The Growth of Professional Practitioners*. Blackwell Science, Oxford.

RCN (1998) *Guidance for Nurses on Clinical Governance*. RCN, London.

RCN Institute (2000) *Realising Clinical Effectiveness and Clinical Governance through Clinical Supervision*. RCN Institute, Radcliffe Press, Oxon.

Rolfe, G. (1998) Beyond expertise: reflective and reflexive nursing practice. In: *Transforming Nurses through Reflective Practice* (eds. C. Jones & D. Freshwater). Blackwell Science, Oxford.

Rucroft-Malone, J., Kitson, A., McCormack, B., Seers, K. & Titchen, A. (2002) Getting evidence into practice: ingredients for change. *Nursing Standard* **16**(37), 38–43.

Titchen, A. (2000) *Professional Craft Knowledge in Patient-Centred Nursing and the Facilitation of Its Development*. Kidlington Ashdale, Oxford.

Titchen, A. (2001a) Critical companionship: a conceptual framework for developing expertise. In *Practice Knowledge and Expertise in the Health Professions* (eds J. Higgs, & A. Titchen), pp. 80–90. Butterworth-Heinemann, Oxford.

Titchen, A. (2001b) Skilled companionship in professional practice. In *Practice Knowledge and Expertise in the Health Professions* (eds J. Higgs & A. Titchen), pp. 69–79. Butterworth-Heinemann, Oxford.

Titchen, A. (2003) Critical companionship: part 1. *Nursing Standard* **18**(9), 33–40.

Titchen, A. & Binnie, A. (1995) The art of clinical supervision. *Journal of Clinical Nursing* **4**(5), 327–334.

Titchen, A. & McGinley, M. (2003) Facilitating practitioner-research through critical companionship. *NT Research* **8**(2), 115–131.

Titchen, A. & McGinley, M. (2004) Blending self and professional practices in person centred care. In: *Developing Practice Knowledge for Health Professionals* (eds J. Higgs, B. Richardson & A. Abrandt). Dahlgren Elsevier, Oxford.

5. Working with Critical Companionship

Angela Brown and Karen Harrison

> Companion: a partner on a journey of discovery, someone who is reliable, an advocate, supporter who has genuine interest in development and growth.
> *Royal College of Nursing, 2000, p. 1*

In this chapter, the personal experiences of two critical companions Angela Brown and Karen Harrison will be presented. Angela and Karen met when they both volunteered to assist two practitioners on their journey of discovery to reveal their individual expertise. The two practitioners are Gill Scott (real name) and Susan Smith (pseudonym). Through participation in the Expertise in Practice Project (EPP), the Royal College of Nursing (RCN) Institute sought to contribute to what is known about expertise in practice and 'to test a conceptual framework for expertise' (Manley *et al.*, 2005, p. 3) by seeking volunteer nurses with expertise. To assist the practitioners to discover their expertise and assemble a portfolio of evidence to demonstrate it, they were invited to find a critical companion, as described by Titchen (2001). This chapter shares the experience of becoming a critical companion. Our journey is presented as a conversation between us, in which we have italicised, for clarity, the domains and processes of critical companionship.

What is a critical companion?

Angela: 'The first real exposure to the concept of critical companionship for me was the introductory reading provided by the RCN. I read the chapter on skilled companionship and then the one on critical companionship. I discovered that Titchen (2001) identifies critical companionship as a metaphor for a helping relationship. In our case, this relationship was about helping the nurses to become practitioner-researchers. This lulled me into a false sense of security because I thought I knew and understood about helping relationships from my years as a nurse and educator. Little did I know what lay ahead! A journey of discovery and pleasure for Gill Scott (the nurse with expertise who I was working with) and for me. We identified the experience "as one of the best and most fulfilling experiences of our careers" (Brown & Scott, 2004). Karen, can you remember your initial thoughts?'

Karen: 'Initially, the words critical and companion appeared contradictory; surely a companion would not be critical? As I read the work of Titchen (2001), I began to see that there wasn't the conflict within the concept that I originally thought. The notion of 'challenge and support' within a supervisory relationship was not new to me. With my mental health nursing background, I had worked for many years with clinical supervision (e.g. NHSME, 1993) which, in essence, is a form of companionship within a critical and supportive framework. Angela, tell me more about your early reaction to the critical companionship framework?'

Angela: 'I remember travelling to the first action learning set on the train and I had read the chapters provided, but not really looked at the conceptual framework of critical companionship as it is laid out in a series of concentric circles (see Figure 5.1). I remember being completely overwhelmed by its sophistication and complexity. I had always known that I am not really comfortable with representations of reality in this type of presentation, but this confirmed it. This identified the first learning opportunity for me, as I needed to get to grips with the process concepts if I was to assist Gill in this endeavour. My preferred orientation to new experiences is either to do it or seek comfort in the theory and so ...

'Critical companionship "reflects four theoretical perspectives" (Titchen, 2000a, p. 35). It is a conceptual framework, drawing on critical social theory, human existentialism, spirituality and phenomenology (Titchen, 2003). It is, therefore, not critical in the sense of criticising the work of the practitioner in an unconstructive way, but in the spirit of the critical social science concepts of Enlightenment; Empowerment and Emancipation (Royal College of Nursing, 2000, p. 1). I found Angie Titchen's (2000a) explanations of her influences for the development of this conceptual framework both familiar and reassuring – critical social theory (e.g. Freire, 1985), humanistic existentialism (e.g. Rogers, 1983), spirituality in the context of a non-religious framework (Campbell, 1984) referring to "symbolic acts of caring ... moderated love" (Titchen, 2000a, p. 36) and lived experience (phenomenology). Karen, can you remember how you felt about the critical companionship framework?'

Karen: 'I was late in joining the regional project group, other members having met at least twice before, so I relate to your sense of feeling overwhelmed, not only by the complexity of the framework and its diagrammatic representation, but also in needing to "get up to speed" with the others. Being a "visually orientated person", I found comfort in the very clear way the pictorial representation of the framework identified the three domains, i.e. the *relationship, rationality-intuitive* and *facilitation domains* and the dynamics within each. I entered this work, having read Titchen (2001), with the view that to enable Susan, the nurse I was working with, to articulate her expertise, it would be essential for her to make contact with her "self"; as someone of significance; someone constituted by relationships, meanings and memberships (Merleau-Ponty & Lefort, 1968). So this idea related, not only to person centredness, but also to a sense of valuing

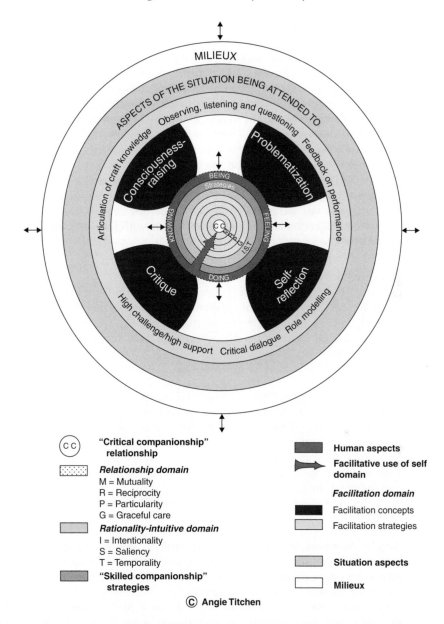

Figure 5.1 'Critical companionship': a conceptual framework for facilitating experiential learning. (© Angie Titchen (2000b).)

"self". I had a strong commitment to the work that lay before us and wanted to get the most out of this experience and help Susan to do so too. The action learning sets became an essential part of the project and enabled us to "dissect and analyse" the framework and translate the terms used within the domains into language we could understand. In a sense, Angela, as I am sure you would agree, we became critical companions to each other, within the peer group, offering challenge and support to one another. The sessions became increasingly useful in facilitating critical reflection and enabled me to prepare for the next session with Susan to embed my actions and also give me a sense of who I was as a (teacher) critical companion (Brookfield, 1995).'

Angela: 'You're so right, Karen, about the value of the action learning sets. I really appreciated them as one of the vehicles to help us, the critical companions, develop ourselves and our skill sets for facilitating practitioner-research. At the beginning, the action learning set provided us with the opportunity to explore the process concepts of critical companionship in a safe and stimulating group.'

The relationship domain

Closer examination of the critical companionship framework revealed that the relationship between the critical companion and the practitioner is at its heart (see Figure 5.1) and radiating from this relationship is the relationship domain. The *relationship domain* includes the four processes: *mutuality, reciprocity, particularity* and *graceful care*.

Titchen (2000a) defines these processes as:

Mutuality is working together of the critical companion and the nurse in a collegiate, partnership that is carefully negotiated (p. 37).

Particularity refers to the critical companion getting to know and understand the unique details and experience of the practitioner (p. 36).

Reciprocity is a mutual collaborative, educative, and empowering exchange of feelings, thoughts, knowledge, interpretations and actions between the companion and the practitioner (p. 37).

Graceful care is the support given to the practitioner by the critical companion (p. 37).

Angela: 'As the relationship between the critical companion and the practitioner is at the heart of the framework, I gave some detailed thought to how this relationship might differ from other "helping relationships". I was familiar with facilitator, mentor, educator, teacher and preceptor and so on; the list is long. When I joined the EPP, to help my understanding of the differences and similarities with other helping roles, I created two opportunities for peer discussion. At the same time as being a critical companion, I was a facilitator on the RCN Clinical Leadership Programme. I facilitated a workshop with a group of clinical leaders in a different city. We looked at helping relationships through a workshop activity. I then re-created this workshop at the 2002 Reflective Practice, Practice Development and Action Research Conference at the University of

Keele. These two activities helped me to clarify my thinking on critical companionship in the context of other helping roles. My conclusion is that it is all about the relationship; the relationship that develops is intimate and deliberate. My experience of critical companionship is that the relationship developed from a deliberate use of the critical companionship strategies and what emerged was a relationship that was to become enduring, mutually beneficial and rewarding. Therefore, the process becomes pivotal and reflects the humanistic existentialist influences: genuineness, unconditional positive regard and empathy (Rogers, 1983). Karen, how did you see the relationship domain?'

Karen: 'In parallel with the "person-centred approach" (Kitwood, 1997) that I adopt in my clinical work, as a guiding philosophy, I based my developing relationship with Susan with this same respect for her personhood. I do feel that at the heart of a person-centred approach is the regard held for the other and the relationship between the "helper" and the person we "help". I felt this underpinning personal philosophy was of significant worth in the project and indeed reflected the use of *particularity* – knowing the practitioner, as defined within the *relationship domain* (Titchen, 2001). Angela, can you explain how you approached *mutuality* or the partnership working that Titchen says is the most significant process in the framework and upon which everything else within it depends?'

Angela: 'The collegiality of our relationship was carefully negotiated through an agreed contract – *mutuality*. This established a working with relationship rather than a hierarchical or unequal relationship that can be seen in other more traditional helping roles. In hierarchical roles, the helper is often more knowledgeable/experienced than the learner in the particular clinical area. Within critical companionship, the helper is a more experienced facilitator accompanying a co-learner on an experiential learning journey (Titchen, 2003), but may not necessarily possess expertise in the same discipline. Gill worked in palliative care and I had no detailed knowledge of this type of clinical practice. This I found to be beneficial in the EPP as I was conscious of the possibility that if one knows something, it is easy to identify readily with the thing, without the required, deliberate exploration with the other person. I think this helps the individual to expose their expertise because they have to deconstruct their practice, rather than merely accepting it. Benner (1984) reminds us that nurses with expertise know more than they can say and through the use of clarifying questions the "treasures in jars of clay" are revealed (see Brown & Scott, in press). In creating my relationship with Gill, I used a deliberate strategy to get to know and understand her uniqueness, thus I was using the two process concepts or processes of particularity and *intentionality*. At my first meeting with Gill, we talked nursing, clarified values and beliefs and established what nursing meant to each of us. We shared our goals and aspirations for nursing, the project and ourselves. I was able through these discussions to begin the process of individualising the facilitation (*particularity*), choosing appropriate interventions and responses that recognised "where she was at". This first encounter established a relationship that was mutually trusting and respectful.'

97

Karen: 'I agree with you. Essential to any relationship is to care and to know one's self. Our own uniqueness and expression of caring is important within relationship development. Like yours Angela, the relationship with Susan began with a sharing of values, attitudes and beliefs about why we nurse – a values clarification (Edwards, 2001) and, as a result, a contract was developed and eventually documented. We agreed principles such as openness expressed through knowing, patience, interaction, courage, honesty, trust, humility and hope (Mayeroff, 1971). We both worked in mental health for older people, but in different specialities within this field, hers within functional mental health, and mine in dementia care. This enabled her to articulate fully her nursing and allowed me to explore and challenge practice, not with the eye of an expert in her field, but as an enquirer, an onlooker and a helper. We realised that we shared not only many aspirations and values for nursing, but also engaging in the process of championing for the client groups with which we worked. This notion of championing was driven by a sense of social and organisational ageism (and in my speciality – dementia "ism") and in a shared "passion" to nurse and to nurse well. The discussions were invigorating and restorative for both of us and were evident in the written records we each made.'

Angela: 'You know, Karen, it is really interesting that we had similar experiences and feelings. Did you give any thought about why you felt differently using this critical companionship approach?'

Karen: 'Like you, I sought other opportunities to explore (a) my values and beliefs about the nursing care I deliver and (b) the framework of critical companionship. In the first exploration, I held two focus groups: one for qualified nursing staff and the other for unqualified nursing staff, both working within mental health for older people. Using a values clarification activity (Manley, 2000), the articulation of the group members' individual values and beliefs were themed and clustered by each focus group to produce a statement of shared values and beliefs; the basis of which led to an underpinning philosophy statement for the service. It was both a relief and emancipatory to discover common ground. The second exploration capitalised on some local work that incorporated the framework of critical companionship in a post basic development programme for qualified nurses. The programme was jointly facilitated by a local university and the Trust's organisational development department. We presented this work at the ENB Mental Health Nursing Conference, Modernisation: Reforming mental health education and practice and investing in the future, Robinsons College, in 2001. Again, in common with you Angela, these activities helped me as a critical companion to embed the underlying principles of the framework into my existing educational, facilitation and supervisory roles.'

Angela: 'Karen, the fourth process concept in the *relationship domain*, *graceful care*, is, for me, one of the other differences from other helping roles. In her portfolio, Gill identified that:

The view that one does not become involved with patients is a long-established one'. The protective mechanisms nurses employ is well documented.
Menzies, 1960; Benoliel, 1982; Brown and Scott, in press

'I believe that this is also an inherent mechanism that I have carried from my own clinical practice into my education role, the need for boundary setting. However, in her portfolio, Gill said, "I was helped by Angela's warmth, acceptance, extraversion and her holistic thinking style", indicating that an emotional closeness developed between us. This is more than supportive. For me, it is the opportunity, as Titchen (2003, p. 33) identifies, to "bring together head, heart, body and spirit ... [within] person centred, evidence based practice". I found it interesting that the issue of boundary management was identified as an area not as well expressed in Gill's portfolio. As a result, we continued our discussions and deliberations long after the project ended and this resulted in a publication contributing to what is an important element that of boundary management within in a "helping relationship" (Scott & Brown, 2004). Karen, what's your experience of this?'

Karen: 'Critical Companionship calls for an intentional and authentic presence through which we both experienced wholeness and a single focus. I could not engage with Susan without giving of myself, so the relationship was more than just listening, being attentive or mirroring. Richards (1964) describes a transformation (in the helping relationship) where you both become a bigger whole. I felt this demonstrated a reciprocal *graceful care* of each other (which shows *reciprocity* and *graceful care* working together). Time at our meetings sped by and, after each session, there was a growing sense of bond and *reciprocity* in our articulation of our underpinning nursing philosophy.'

Angela: 'Well, Karen, we seem to be able to explain the *relationship domain*, however, we were, simultaneously, also in the *rationality – intuitive domain*!'

The rationality – intuitive domain

This domain includes three processes: *intentionality*, *saliency* and *temporality*.
Titchen (2000a) defines these processes as follows:

Intentionality is consciousness raising, self-awareness and thoughtfulness of critical companions (p. 37).

Saliency is the ability to know both consciously and intuitively what is important, what matters, what is of concern and significance from both the critical companion's and the practitioner's perspectives (p. 37).

Temporality is the critical companion's understanding of the importance of attending to the particulars of past, present and future time in helping a practitioner to learn (p. 38).

Angela: 'I remember the day I realised what *intentionality* really meant. I used to meet Gill at her place of work, an hour's drive from where I worked. The venue had been mutually agreed and at first I thought it was because it was easier for me to travel and park! Then one day driving to the meeting, I realised I was deliberately thinking about what I would say and do, regarding some outstanding issues that we had not being able to resolve. This was a defining moment for me in my critical companionship development as I had become more conscious and self-aware.'

Karen: 'I know what you mean Angela. For us, part of the contracting process identified that we would establish, at each meeting, what actions each would undertake outside each of the times we met. We did this intentionally (*intentionality*) because we found out that if either of us did not take our agreed actions to enable continued growth, moving forward was hindered.'

Angela: 'The other two processes in the *rationality – intuitive domain* are *temporality* (attending to time, timeliness, anticipating and pacing) and *saliency* (knowing what matters and acting on it). There was one particular point in the EPP when this became a critical process. Gill was reluctant to engage in the 360° feedback. This reluctance was completely contradictory to what I knew of her practice and reputation (*particularity*), so I waited for an appropriate cue, not so much in what she said, but in her body language, when we began to discuss 360° feedback. I knew this was essential to her development within the project, but more significantly I knew it was important to Gill (*saliency*). I thought about this and at first waited for her to feel ready to begin the process. After a while I felt I needed to probe a little more deeply into why there was this reluctance (temporality). Through the probing, she was able to recount a very painful experience of receiving negative feedback in the not so distant past and was, naturally, trying to protect herself from further hurt. Another of the illuminating moments, in our critical companionship journey, was resolution of this issue and the realisation of the potency of *temporality* and the critical part it played in such a personal and emotional journey of discovery. Moreover, there are often opportunities that we allow to pass by because we see them as too difficult or risky, but in this situation because of *particularity, intentionality, saliency* and *temporality*, I knew that the time was right to take the risk, using a strategy from the *facilitation domain* of critical companionship. This strategy of high challenge accompanied with high support is discussed in detail later in the chapter. Discussion about her reluctance to engage in 360° feedback brought Gill to a challenging realisation and the surfacing of one of the "treasures at the bottom of the jar", that is vulnerability and risk (Brown & Scott, in press).'

Karen: 'How interesting Angela. Susan prepared for the 360° feedback and identified participants, but was also reluctant to take the full and final steps to progress this feedback. As many nurses do, she disembodied her own needs and argued that she had insufficient time to commit to her own needs and development. Susan would often express that when her ward was busy, the only spare time she had to offer was her own clinical supervision, education and development time. She would often sacrifice this to meet the many and varied clinical and managerial demands that were made upon her. It is a trap to fall into and she was slipping down the slope. We also discussed her fear that someone would burst into the room and declare "impostor" and she would be "found out". Thereby, the process of a 360° review was potentially quite exposing for her.'

Angela: 'Oh Karen, I can readily identify with this feeling of being found out – it's known as an impostor syndrome or phenomenon (Clance & Imes, 1978) and is often associated with high achievers. I think that this analysis of the critical companionship framework has helped me to understand better this impostor feeling from a personal perspective. Rather than doubting my own performance as a facilitator and, just as Titchen and Manley (2007) say, by articulating my own professional craft knowledge (little gems), I have been able to increase my understanding of my everyday facilitation work and recognise and own my expertise and its impact on others. I can remember when I realised this change in myself. Do you remember, at the end of each action learning set, we used to close with a statement on our least and best experience of the session? I have notes from the set in April 2001 where I say, "[T]here is no least for me anymore, all best. Compared with the daunting process at the start, it has been so emancipating to be involved." The fear of being found out had gone away as I had realised my own expertise and impact. So what did you do to help Susan to overcome this fear?'

Karen: 'We took the view that we should consolidate her achievements to date by articulating her expertise and wait for the right time to gently push her forward over uncertain ground which again shows *intentionality*, *saliency* and *temporality* in action. We decided that she would capture more of her "expertise in action" in the form of narratives; these being "little gems" with clear currency and exchange in her articulation of her expertise.'

Angela: 'And so, Karen, this leads us to the deliberate strategies used to surface the expertise in the practice of Gill and Susan.'

The facilitation domain

The processes of the *facilitation domain* are *consciousness raising, problematisation, self-reflection* and *critique* (Titchen, 2003).

Titchen (2000a) defines these processes as follows:

Consciousness raising refers to enlightenment or bringing into the practitioner's consciousness the knowledge embedded in daily practice and the recognition of the nature of this knowledge (p. 38).

Problematisation is making problematic, practice currently seen by the practitioner as unproblematic (p. 38).

Self-reflection is a cyclical process in which practitioners critically reflect upon their own experiences, rational thinking and intuitions for learning and self and learning from, and improving on practice (p. 38).

Critique is a collaborative critical reflection upon a reconstructed experience and the situation in which it took place (p. 38).

By using these processes in a range of facilitation strategies, professional craft knowledge can be revealed. These strategies are:

- Observing, listening and questioning
- High challenge/high support
- Role-modeling
- Articulation of craft knowledge

- Feedback on performance
- Use of creative imagination and expression
- Critical dialogue

Angela: 'Using narratives (storytelling) is a particularly good way of surfacing the "gems" of practice or, in other words, identifying what is important (*saliency*). Hardy (1968, p. 5) reminds us:

we dream in narrative, daydream in narrative, remember, anticipate, hope, despair, believe, doubt, plan, revise, criticise, construct, gossip, learn, hate and love by narrative.

'This reminds me how important narrative is in all our lives and Gill and I have written about its important place in revealing expertise (see Brown & Scott, 2004).'

Karen: 'My experience supports that. Susan's narratives of her patients' stories and her nursing practice became some of the most moving literature I have read. One of the very real ways in which practitioners with expertise can demonstrate it and also influence the practice of those around them is in using narratives. One example was the use of a case study of empowerment. Susan had been working with a forensic client and the plan and resultant actions she used showed a high level of creative risk taking. The plan was developed through direct negotiation with the client, family members and professionals. The usual response of the nursing team would have been to have minimalised any risks to a point where the interventions and interactions with the client were stifling and non-therapeutic. Susan used her case narrative to demonstrate critical practice reflection in action (Schon, 1983) and a transition from ritualistic and routine practice, that is "thinking on your feet". Susan had found a vehicle to demonstrate her expertise to the rest of the nursing team. Through the medium of the narrative, she used her storytelling to demonstrate expertise and advanced practice.

'The person-centred relationships she developed with clients were a strong element but what was excitingly evident was her use of *saliency* in her risk assessment and management of some very complex situations. She described an intuitive knowing that was physically felt by her. This intuitive knowing we discussed at length, exploring the supporting literature, in particular that of Benner (1984) and Quine and Ullian (1978). We concluded that what she was possibly experiencing was the internalisation and sub-conscious simulation that Quine and Ullian (1978) identify. She showed how her nursing intervention(s) was based on empirical evidence which we felt was a demonstration of expertise. We also changed what was previously unconscious into conscious professional craft knowledge, I guess through the process that Titchen calls, *consciousness raising*. This was the kind of work we did together that resulted in *mutuality* becoming a reality in a relationship that was much more than a contractual one. Part of the journey we took was one of self-realisation and actualisation; she saw others (including me) as the "expert" and that she didn't belong with this enlightened band. Through the discussion, feedback, challenge and support, she was able to "see" what her colleagues saw in her practice. The moment when this happened was notably both powerful and empowering for her.'

Angela: 'I agree, Karen. *Articulation of professional craft knowledge* was at the heart of the EPP and appeared, to me, to be the whole purpose of the critical companionship within the project. Titchen (2000a,b) tells us that critical companions help this articulation by using storytelling, analysis and interpretation, interpreting and evaluating shared experiences and offering non-specific maxims. Once I had read this, I realised why I readily identified with this approach. My own personal preference for discovering the pertinent, relevant and implicit in any situation is through the use of stories and storytelling. Gill used narratives to reveal her expertise and together we analysed, interpreted, evaluated and made some attempts to describe what we saw. It became obvious, as we worked together, that she was very artistic and we used this quality to reveal her "treasures in jars of clay". Thus, by complementing her stories through *self-reflection*, art and poetry, Gill was able to identify the knowledge in her practice, become solution focused, more reflective and evaluative of her knowledge, skills and behaviours. As she revealed her expertise, we simultaneously engaged in *critical dialogue* to identify the evidence and theoretical underpinnings to the stories, reflections, poetry, art and feedback. The palliative care literature was well known to Gill so we sortied into other literature, known to me, to help her to surface her world view and identify her craft knowledge. The emerging portfolio became a rich picture of her expertise; "a metaphor of the artistry of nursing", as Gill said in her portfolio. She went on to say that "the evidence, including a collection of reflections, narratives and peer responses are metaphors of the individual acts of everyday nursing" (Brown & Scott, 2004, p. 108).

'When I examine what we did, I can see Titchen's framework in action. I think her framework brought what we did to life. I also think this framework is like any framework; it's there for us to reflect upon and test our own intuitive framework against in order to achieve personal and professional growth in facilitation. I also think that if we can make the framework more real for people, they will try some of the approaches.'

Karen: 'We too found that the use of narrative, whether that of the client, the family carer or the professional, can be a powerful learning tool. Whilst Susan did not participate in the panel presentation of her portfolio (the final stage of the EPP), she, nevertheless, went on to articulate her expertise and achieve a sense of actualisation, as described by Bishop and Scudder (1997). Thus, she recognised and honoured her skills, knowledge and abilities and knew that she was practising the art of nursing as described by Nightingale (1957).'

Angela: 'One of the other critical companionship evidence-gathering activities incorporated in the EPP was observation of the Gill's practice. As nurses we may think we are good at *observing, listening* and *questioning*. However, *observing, listening* and *questioning* about practice are not always easy. I remember being aware that the area of Gill's practice in palliative care was potentially problematic and this led me to consider very carefully what would be revealed. At an action learning set, another practitioner and critical companion said that they wondered about the purpose of observing practice. I responded by saying that I thought that observation of Gill's practice would "detract from the work we've done to date as I can now see the soul of her nursing". At the end of the discussion, we agreed that the purpose was to articulate expertise, but that there are other vehicles (Royal College of Nursing 2001).

'It is interesting though that I would never have questioned the use of observations of care in the RCN Clinical Leadership Programme that I was involved in at the time. I think it was because the observations of care were undertaken by the clinical leaders in partnership and then used to think about the patient experience. However, in the EPP, it was the practitioner who was observed. My revelation now is that whilst listening and questioning are powerful strategies to make what was hidden revealed, I missed the opportunity to deepen my questioning through observing her at work. I realise now that observing in a hospice was an issue for me and that by not reflecting upon my statement that observation could detract from the work done so far, I let myself off the hook. I remember feeling relieved that I did not have to observe in a palliative care setting.

'In retrospect, I think doing observation would have created an opportunity for me to expand my expertise as a critical companion. If I had observed her practice, we could have discussed, analysed and interpreted all the data she was collecting in the context of what I had seen and experienced with my senses, as well as heard. Although I was careful to provide *feedback on performance* (personal and through 360° feedback) and we discussed the outcomes of care, had I observed her practice, I may have had other questions to ask of each situation. For example, one particular story is prominent for me in that Gill described an intervention she had used that many would consider controversial (albeit evidenced based). Through an exploration of the actions, effects and strategies, she was able to identify her deliberateness in the approach with the patient, his family and the other health care providers. She captured this as part of her "reflexivity" and acknowledged that part of recognising expertise is to be aware of the challenges and being willing to be challenged by others (Scott, 2002). Had I observed her practice, I may have been able to ask her why this story was so different and also why the stories she had chosen to tell exemplified her expertise more than others.'

Karen: 'This reflects my experience of observation, Angela. I observed Susan undertaking group supervision sessions where she used her narratives to illustrate the power of "reflection in action". The potential impact this could have on improving the patients' experience of care within the unit was tangible. She enabled them to experience reflection as an awareness of their own context and of the influences of the environment and the community (within the ward) and raise their consciousness of the societal and ideological constraints on their previously taken for granted practice (Johns, 1996). This new awareness meant that they were able, collectively, to analyse ritualistic practices and consider a more rational–intuitive and person-centred approach.'

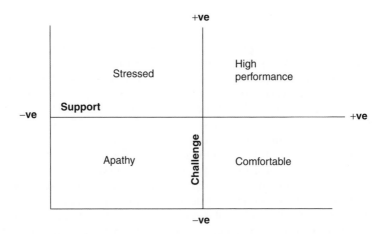

Figure 5.2 Challenge support matrix. (Adapted from Johns (1996). Reproduced with permission from Wiley-Blackwell and C. Johns.)

Angela: 'Karen, the strategy, *high challenge/high support* that we introduced earlier is, as you know, attributed to Johns (1996). I used this strategy in my interaction with Gill. Building on Johns's matrix, we devised and used the matrix in Figure 5.2 which was extremely useful in helping Gill to recognise where she was at the beginning of the project and where she was at the end. Gill identified that through high challenge/high support, she moved from stress to high performance based on wisdom and humility, as her words show':

What will keep a nurse so vulnerable that success and recognition of expertise is not corruptive and yet, suitably confident and determined to advance their cause? It is an awareness of both one's human frailty and growth potential; the willingness to experience both ends of the continuum and refuse mediocrity.

Scott, 2002, p. 21

Angela: 'So Karen we have used some of our experiences to illustrate the *facilitation domain* and we need to locate the framework within the overarching domain of the *facilitative use of self*.'

Facilitative use of self domain

Titchen (2000) describes the *facilitative use of self* as the overarching domain of critical companionship. Within it, the *relationship, rationality-intuitive* and *facilitation domains* are all used in their many forms and expressions, through the processes of professional artistry. These processes of blending, melding, synthesising, synchronising, interplaying and balancing the domains enable us to bring all of ourselves into the relationship with the person we are helping (Titchen, 2004).

Professional artistry

Angela: 'This idea of professional artistry is central in clinical practice as well. My recollection of Gill acknowledging her professional artistry is captured in the action learning set notes where I tell my colleagues that a process of self-actualisation has occurred for her. In discovering the essence of her nursing as spirituality, she had captured her individuality. She disclosed her discomfort about revealing her world view (i.e., a Christian world view which is rarely acknowledged within nursing journals and poorly understood by practitioners) to her colleagues. Role modelling critical companionship provided the opportunity for her to feel free to air this world view. She writes: "Angela was so supportive of me in articulating these thoughts, excited about their powerful influence in my life and the value of disseminating their principles more widely. Her respect for this personal disclosure and its potential was liberating, indeed an emancipatory research experience" (Brown & Scott in press). And for me, my expertise grew at the EPP review group meeting where Gill's submitted portfolio was reviewed. I was present at the meeting and was invited by the panel chair to say something about the experience of the process (as the critical companion)':

Working with her has been fabulous we hardly knew each other and found through these processes that I gained as much as I gave. Also, talking with like minded colleagues was just the best ever experience; there's not that quality time to talk through and around nursing. It's a powerful thing, to realise the gift of time to talk through developments and recognitions that celebrate the diversity of nursing. I have never discussed issues that underpinned my beliefs and values until this project, another important discussion makes you realise what underpins everything and manifests in all you do. And saliency, again you do not realise what you've got till you've had it.

RCN, 2002, p. 4

Karen: 'I agree, during our personal reflections within the action learning sets, it became clear to me that the journey taken by each critical companion and practitioner was very different; the journey for each went over very different terrain. Susan took a longer period of time to develop an ease with making personal reflections in identifying her expertise in any given situation and so I also observed that each expert's journey took varying amounts of time. Susan was able to articulate her professional artistry and made it to the "finishing line", in terms of producing a portfolio of evidence, but this was eventually outside the time scales of the project. However, the growth she experienced has allowed her a greater sense of worth and enabled her to feel comfortable in her advanced practice. I continued to meet with Susan, beyond the final completion of the EPP, still within a critical companion relationship to enable her to continue to develop and articulate her practice. Susan has since taken her place with other advanced practitioners and, through the journey she took, has progressed significantly within her career. Me? I too grew a lot as a result of the project and as a direct result of my role as critical companion, I found that I benefited "by proxy" and so now I am able to recognise and articulate my own professional artistry.'

Endings and potential

And so our critical companionship conversation must end, we hope that we have, through our conversation, provided some insight into the exciting process of critical companionship and, importantly, its usefulness in helping nurses and other health care professionals to reveal their professional craft knowledge and demonstrate their expertise. We believe that living the critical companionship framework is empowering for both practitioners and the critical companion and has positive outcomes for both. It enables a detailed examination of the underpinning dynamics of practice and facilitates the explicit description of professional interventions and actions that have thus far been difficult to articulate or illustrate. It is our contention that the process is as important as the outcome and that critical companionship is illuminating, liberating and transformational. We would encourage you to take a closer look at critical companionship and consider how you could use it in your practice.

Acknowledgements

We express our appreciation to Angie Titchen for her graceful care and professional artistry in the completion of this chapter; Gill Scott, thank you for the permission to use your name and excerpts from the portfolio and the opportunity to be involved in a memorable experience; Susan Smith, you know who you are, thank you. And last but not least, thanks to Roy Brown for his critical readership and companionship.

References

Benner, P. (1984) *From Novice to Expert, Excellence and Power in Clinical Nursing Practice*. Addison-Wesley, Menlo Park.

Benoliel, J.Q. (1982) *Death Education for the Health Professional*. McGraw Hill, London.

Bishop, A.H. & Scudder, J.R. (1997) Nursing as a practice rather than an art or a science. *Nursing Outlook* **45**, 82–85.

Brookfield, S.D. (1995) *Becoming a Critically Reflective Teacher*. Jossey-Bass Publishers, San Francisco.

Brown, A. & Scott, G. (2004) Art and artistry in practice – a reflective account. In: *Delivering Cancer and Palliative Care Education* (eds L. Foyle & J. Hostad), Vol. 1. Radcliffe Publishing, Oxford.

Brown, A. & Scott G. (in press) Treasures in jars of clay – working with critical companionship. In: *Illuminating the Diversity in Cancer and Palliative Care Education* (eds L. Foyle & J. Hostad). Radcliffe Publishing, Oxford.

Campbell, A.V. (1984) *Moderated Love. A Theology of Professional Care*. SPCK, London.

Clance, P.R. & Imes, S.A. (1978) *The Impostor Phenomena, Overcoming the Fear That Haunts Your Success*. Peachtree, Atlanta.

Edwards, S.D. (2001) *Philosophy of Nursing: An Introduction*. Palgrave, London.

Freire, P. (1985) *The Politics of Education; Culture, Power and Liberation*. MacMillan, Basingstoke.

Hardy, B. (1968) *The Collected Essays of Barbara Hardy*, Vol. 1. Harvester Press, Brighton.

Johns, C. (1996) Visualising and realising care in practice through guided reflection. *Journal of Advanced Nursing* **24**, 1135–1143.

Kitwood, T. (1997) *Dementia Reconsidered*. Open University Press, Milton Keynes.

Manley, K. (2000) Organisational culture and consultant nurse outcomes: part 1 organisational culture. *Nursing Standard* **14**(36), 34–38.

Manley, K., Hardy, S., Titchen, A., Garbett, R. & McCormack, B. (2005) *Changing Patients' Worlds through Nursing Practice Expertise, Exploring Nursing Practice through Emancipatory Action Research and Fourth Generation Evaluation*. RCN Institute, London.

Mayeroff, M. (1971) *On Caring*. Harper and Row, New York.

Menzies, I.E.P. (1960) A case study in the functioning of social systems as a defence against anxiety. *Human Relations* **13**, 95–121.

Merleau-Ponty, M. & Lefort, C. (eds) (1968) *The Visible and the Invisible*. Northwestern University Press, Evanston.

NHSME (1993) *Vision for the Future*. Department of Health, London.

Nightingale, F. (1957/1859) *Notes on Nursing*. Lippincott, Philadelphia.

Quine, W.V.O. & Ullian, J.S. (1978) *The Web of Belief*. Random House, New York.

Richards, M.C. (1964) *Centering*. Weleyan University Press, Connecticut.

Rogers, C. (1983) *Freedom to Learn for the 80s*. Charles E. Merrill, London.

Royal College of Nursing (2000) *Expertise in Practice Project Glossary*. RCN, London.

Royal College of Nursing (2001) *Expertise in Practice Project Action Learning Set Notes April*. RCN, London.

Royal College of Nursing (2002) *Expertise in Practice Project Review Group Report*. RCN, London.

Schon, D.A. (1983) *The Reflective Practitioner*. Avebury, Aldershot.

Scott, G. (2002) *Expertise in Practice Project Portfolio*. Unpublished.

Scott, G. & Brown, A. (2004) Boundary angst and negotiation in palliative care. *Spirituality and Health International* **5**(4).

Titchen, A. (2000a) *'Critical Companionship': A Conceptual Framework for Supporting Practice Development*. RCN Institute 2000 Short Course. Fostering an organisational culture of practice development. RCN Institute 2000, Oxford.

Titchen, A. (2000b) *Professional Craft Knowledge in Patient-Centered Nursing and the Facilitation of Its Development*. University of Oxford DPhil thesis, Ashdale Press, Oxford.

Titchen, A. (2001) Critical companionship: a conceptual framework for developing expertise. In: *Practice Knowledge and Expertise in the Health Professions* (eds J. Higgs & A. Titchen), pp. 80–90. Butterworth Heinemann, Oxford.

Titchen, A. (2003) Critical companionship: part 1. *Nursing Standard* **12**(18), 33–40.

Titchen, A. (2004) Helping relationships for practice development. Critical companionship. In: (eds B. McCormack, K. Manley & R. Garbett). *Practice Development in Nursing*. Blackwell Publishing, Oxford.

Titchen, A. (2007) *Revealing Hidden Rainbow Dancing: Professional Artistry and Practice Development*. Keynote address. 7th International Practice Development Conference 2007. Portraits, Panoramas and Palettes. Melbourne, Australia.

Titchen, A. & Manley, K. (2007) Facilitating research as shared action and transformation. In: *Being Critical and Creative in Qualitative Research* (eds J. Higgs, A. Titchen, Horsfall & H. Armstrong). Hampden Press, Sydney.

6. Critical Companionship – The Lived Experience

Alison Greggans and Margaret Conlon

Introduction

This chapter is about critical companionship. It articulates two people's combined views of experiencing critical companionship – from the facilitator's (Alison) and the practitioner's (Margaret) perspectives. The chapter reflects our experience of being involved in the Expertise in Practice Project (EPP) (Manley *et al.*, 2005), and the critique illustrates our interpretation of Angie's critical companionship framework (Titchen, 2000, 2003; Wright and Titchen, 2003), particularly the *relationship* and *facilitation domains*. Before we start, we would like to introduce ourselves.

Margaret

Prefers animals to people; loves watching little children; loves trees; ex-children's nurse, hated the uniform; found mental health; loved working in community. Experienced a real freedom to practise. Managed to find work that linked my passion for children with mental health. Worked with many *many* distressed and marginalised families and connected social and political beliefs with an energy for work. Alongside this was a drive for continual compensation for lack of school achievement so constant part-time studying was a way of being; many attempts to bring learning and practice together; frustrated by seeing potential for growth and change but unable to do anything; thought about pedalling water; met Alison; inspirational as a teacher; introduced me to action learning sets; felt growth; felt spirit; did EPP; laughed a lot; Alison gave me space to breathe; realised why I was tired; completed EPP; sensed difference from peers; found a new job; became more engaged in psychodynamic perspectives – a new channel; and now – and finally – a move to education! Transformative learning in action!

Alison

Loves anything Scottish (although English herself) and outdoorsy types of activities. Also loves trees and mountains and the weather. A bonus if you live in this part of the world. Currently pushing her own personal boundaries in terms of physical abilities – kayaking, mountaineering etc. I am pushing 50 and more determined than ever to live life. My mantra currently is 'feel the fear and do it anyway' … and I do – a lot! As an under confident learner (1976), I hated nurse training. Found ITU by default (couldn't get a job in midwifery) and suddenly the science started to make sense. I was able to join up the dots and fell in love with learning and helping others to do the same. Loafed around in ITU for about 16yrs (!) up and down the country. Was happy to stay in this loafing position but became bored. Got into education through working towards my degree at the RCN in 1990. Met Kim Manley – she was my tutor – introduced me to all sorts of information including philosophical aspects of knowledge and the freedom to think 'left field'. In life and in work, I encourage others to do the same. Now working in higher education (HE), I enjoy the challenge students bring from practice, helping them to think about their issues and the reasons why they keep going – or not in some instances. A wary writer – not a good confession for an academic – but have enjoyed writing this chapter with Margaret. We do laugh a lot. That's important in teamwork. Pretty scary having Angie as an editor to this chapter!

Our combined experiences provide the backdrop to our story. Writing our story for others to make sense of has been challenging. We grappled with how to present two voices which are distinct in both professional style and perspective. Although different, our individual styles have informed the debate and, by maintaining our individuality within the text, the respective relationships remain authentic.

My role as critical companion was to enable Margaret to surface her embedded know-how, *professional craft knowledge*, and articulate how this knowledge demonstrates her expertise in the care of children's and families' mental health. A shared working history, we believe, helped establish the critical companion/practitioner relationship, as we shared knowledge, values and perspectives about nursing, learning processes and about life – generally. This mutuality and a common professional identity were compounded within our experiences of action learning and facilitating education-based projects. We knew, or assumed, some of each other's practice idiosyncrasies, but what rapidly supported our ability to pay attention to the task at hand was having a shared respect for each other, as individuals and professionals. We both valued a willingness to take risks and an ability to keep it real.

To pull out evidence that was required for the portfolio, we reflected on three practice cases to break down what Margaret did. The analysis of these cases highlighted the particulars of Margaret's *professional craft*, and how she drew on her own expertise. This *craft knowledge* was demonstrated through her *felt* interpretations of practice, and at times was difficult for Margaret to spot and articulate.

As critical companion, I was using all of the framework's domains to facilitate Margaret's experiential learning, and reflect back the different types of knowledge Margaret was using in her own practice (ethical, empirical, aesthetic and self-knowledge – Carper, 1978). Intentionally using all these different knowledge/ evidence types supported Margaret to identify how effective she was in providing person-centred practices. As her facilitator, I too deliberately blended, intertwined and balanced different knowledge/evidence types to try and mirror effective person-centred and evidence-based facilitation. Titchen (2003) describes this *professional artistry* as an approach to help practitioners transform themselves and their practices to achieve patient-centred care. *Professional artistry* is shaped by who we are as individuals, the nature of the shared practice context and in this case, a collective professional history. Our story is therefore unique to us. Reflecting back, however, has enabled me to become more aware of my own *professional artistry* and understand how essential this self-knowledge is for being an effective facilitator in helping others become more person centred in their own learning.

In describing our experiences, we structure our thinking around four core components, which for us were crucial in enabling processes within the *relationship* and *facilitation* domain. These are:

1. reciprocation of power,
2. the degree of person centredness required within the facilitation process,
3. having an insider–outsider perspective,
4. the existence of high challenge.

These four elements structure the chapter, but first we provide a definition of what the *relationship* and *facilitation domain* are, as this may be helpful.

Defining the relationship and facilitation domains

The *relationship domain* emphasises the nature of the working relationship between the critical companion and the practitioner and is expressed in terms of its degree of *mutuality* (working together), *reciprocity* (giving and receiving), *particularity* (knowing and understanding the co-learner and the context of their care) and *graceful care* (use of all of self in the facilitation process).

The *facilitation domain* articulates the process of facilitation by the critical companion, and works with the *relationship domain* in action as well as all the others in the framework (see Figure 5.1). Facilitation through relationship involves activating, merging and prioritising *four* critical elements within the facilitation process:

1. **consciousness raising** – bringing to the fore tacit understanding about the nuances of everyday practice;
2. **problematisation** – through challenge and support, a process which enables reconsideration of deeply held beliefs about practice, and attempts to reframe assumptions about problems and practice-based issues so that solutions can be considered;

3. **self-reflection** – helping practitioners develop increasing self-awareness as to how their actions, behaviours and feelings impact on their own and others' practice, and moreover influence an understanding about practice experiences;
4. **critique** – the nature of the collaborative and analytical dialogue between the critical companion and practitioner regarding the practice-based culture, history, social context and politics.

The chapter combines a theoretical view of what happened through the experience of the critical companion and the expert practitioner. Margaret's reflections are embedded to illustrate the *felt* experience of engaging in the dynamic process of the critical companion/expert practitioner relationship.

Reciprocation of power

Titchen (2003) describes critical companionship as a 'metaphor and a conceptual framework'. We experienced it as a working philosophy of facilitating knowledge about *person-centred practices* through *shared learning* between the critical companion and the practitioner. Indeed these two features of the critical companion/practitioner relationship indicated to us how different this framework of facilitation felt from other facilitation experiences – which use for example experiential learning cycles (Kolb, 1984) reflective frameworks (for example Mezirow, 1981) and Heron's (1999) 'Facilitation Matrix'. The difference in using these frameworks from critical companionship is that the facilitator can adopt a more hierarchical position within the relationship, as well as a non-hierarchical one. Adopting the former position means that the facilitator may steer the direction of facilitation and take ownership of process which drive the rules of engagement towards a predetermined goal.

Heron (1999) advocates that facilitators deliberately weave different modes and styles of facilitation to achieve desired outcomes (hierarchical, cooperative, autonomous). The emphasis of person centeredness within critical companionship requires a high degree of inclusion, equality, transparency and authenticity between the critical companion and the practitioner. Hence reciprocation of power is dynamic and reflects where expertise is located – with the practitioner. In our experience of working together, critical companionship was characterised by openness which was not unusual for us. It didn't take us out of our 'role' as this familiar way of working had been built up over time. We had already established a shared understanding of the way we each worked, and we trusted each other's abilities to keep it 'safe' while being open to challenge. There was also no line of accountability between us which made the process feel more secure. Although still a risky course of action (having one's personal practice exposed to others always is), there was trust between us borne from a mutual respect of each other's roles and experiences.

Promoting openness was dependent on our *felt* equality in the relationship, which, in turn, enhanced the potential for utilising high challenge about Margaret's approach to, and the values which underpinned, her practice. This tacit agreement to 'go there' was unusual within other facilitative relationships Margaret had experienced, especially if the relationship between her and her facilitator was predicated on institutional power through the deliberate use of professional status. In these instances, it must have been difficult to be open, self-critical and feel free to speak out – indeed it may even be inappropriate if judgements about performance are being inferred. Critical companionship felt different for us, because the practitioner, as person, is the agent for change. Inherent in such person-centred approaches to facilitation is the degree of openness and trust. This openness can push boundaries in the relationship, especially if this is to be reciprocal. Unless this process is clearly negotiated at the start, consequences for working relationships can turn messy as the rules of engagement outside a facilitation context could become confused. Titchen advocates that within the *relationship domain*, the approach to facilitation adopted by the critical companion must demonstrate:

> a holistic, person centred, helping relationship in a health care context ... built on trust, high challenge/high support.
>
> *Titchen, 2003, p. 33*

Margaret's reflections indicate that this should not be taken on lightly, as demonstrated after one of our 'book chapter' discussions:

Whether it is group supervision/case exploration or individual discussion, many health colleagues will have experienced the sudden sensation of discussions becoming fraught. Opinions have clashed or worse, there is a suspicion that someone holds a belief that is quite different from your own. It is the sensation of someone carelessly or, unwittingly treading on a personal hot spot. Sometimes little or nothing is acknowledged openly but the tension is in the air. Sadly, personal values are only really visible when there is a sense of conflict. It feels as if your nerve endings are exposed for everyone to see but no one talks about it. I think we are all supposed to hold this professional cloak that is made of the same cloth, the same colour, feels the same way to wear.

According to researchers (Titchen, 2000, 2003; Wright and Titchen, 2003), the critical companion is a co-learner, democratic in attitude and uncensored in their critique of expressed professional performance by the practitioner. This is difficult to maintain if the critical companion's immediate concerns, as one's manager, suddenly become concerned with accountability and professional standards. Personal enlightenment may have to take a back seat as a more hierarchical rather than transformational approach may be required.

The fact that our relationship was not premised on any professional hierarchy felt freeing as it was egalitarian and unrestricted in its openness and partnership. This enhanced the potential for shared learning and was crucial for enabling a democratic and reciprocal process. This feature of the *facilitation domain* demonstrated to us how effective critique and self-reflection could be, when the facilitation relationship is truly self-governing.

Margaret's following reflections identify how the *relationship domain* advocated partnership working (*mutuality*) and how sharing of ourselves (*reciprocity*) supported each of us in our emerging understanding about the nature and specifics of Margaret's practices. As the critical companion, I was trying to use all aspects of myself, including my professional background, to understand what was going on and why. I put myself in the learning seat and attempted to understand Margaret's point of view in terms of her practice and the process of being facilitated. To do this, I used a variety of knowledge bases to my questions:

empirics – 'what are the pragmatics of your day-to-day work Margaret and what does this mean to the families and children?' 'What did you do next and on what basis were you making your judgements?'

aesthetics – 'how does talking about all this over and over again make you feel about your work and your experiences?' '[to myself] . . . Is she OK? . . . How did that last question make her feel? . . . What buttons am I pushing inadvertently? . . . Is she feeling safe? . . . Is she challenged enough? . . . Am I rushing her?'

ethics – 'am I alright to question you about this? [to myself] . . . I must make sure my questions are for her and not for me . . . as she is becoming more enlightened about the differences of her practice to others, what could be the outcome in terms of her place in the work setting?' 'Is she feeling supported?' 'Am I attending to what's going on?'

personal – 'I wonder how I am coming across as an absolute novice in this field?' 'Am I getting this? . . . What assumptions about Margaret am I making and am I remaining open to potentially conflicting agendas?'

To support Margaret in her learning 'journey' demanded, on my part, self-reflection, praxis, critical thinking, interpersonal skills and professional know-how. In so doing, I was using my own self as a professional to demonstrate *graceful care*:

I had experienced many other forms of supervision/mentorship/peer support but the experience of working with a critical companion was definitely different. Exhilarating and challenging, like lemon and lime zest shower gel. There's a dull resistance to being woken up but once you've started it, you wonder why you put if off for so long. As with many other busy health professionals, there was little time or opportunity to 'unpick' practice. Expertise stays at a very intuitive level and articulation of know-how is not encouraged. There is a level of constant doubt that is carried within you – especially as a fairly autonomous community practitioner. The doubting voice says 'am I doing any good' and 'did I make any difference?' Credibility and validity is really tested only when you are exposed. Testing was not the experience I was looking for – I knew that to develop and grow I needed time to reflect in a supportive and understanding environment.

Margaret's practice was unique in the culture in which she worked. This was depicted by the degree of autonomy displayed in the judgements made within complex cases. Her decisions were often on the spot, and she had no time to converse with others in her professional core group. If she had, she was not sure if these would have been accepted readily, despite the positive consequences of her actions for the clients she supported. There was a concern that the reflections on her practice would be similar to those she had experienced before, where she had felt exposed and tested and thereby stunted at times, in her growth as a professional. Within the critical companionship relationship, this concern was not realised. By allowing professional stories to slowly unravel, Margaret had space and time for reflection in an atmosphere of support. This enabled her to evaluate and critique her own practice and identify problems and issues for herself. It was here that the attribute, particular to Margaret's expertise, revealed itself – that of *being a maverick*.

The degree of person centredness required within the facilitation process

Ways of working (*one's professional craft*) are specific to each practitioner and are often embedded and difficult to identify oneself. This *craft knowledge* includes a fusion of various knowledge strands, for example, taught top-down and practice-based theories, experiential knowledge, empirical–rational and ethics. To really understand the practice situation and how expertise was located with Margaret's actions, I worked with her, observing and noting cues, checking, clarifying, questioning and probing. At times it was vital for me to parrot salient aspects of the story, so that Margaret could hear it 'back-to-front'. This helped us to draw a rich picture of practice and helped Margaret focus on the key elements of concern. McGill and Beaty (1992) refer to this as *attending* rather than listening and suggest that it demands using all of one's self to engage fully with what is being recalled. Through such engagement I could reassure myself that my interpretation was not open to bias or supposition, but rooted in Margaret's story and so grounded in her practice. This was enabled using a reflexive dialogue, which provided mutual learning and understanding.

Enabling such a dialogue is an example of how I was using my own professional artistry as a critical companion. I was aware of facilitating Margaret's understanding of the nature of *her* professional craft knowledge, and at the same time, her self-awareness of her own metacognitive thinking. In other words, I was thinking about my own thinking as a facilitator, of another's cognitive processes. This helped Margaret turn unconscious knowing into conscious reasoning. This was something I was continually trying to achieve with her, and the case studies – descriptive and empirically evidence-based accounts of Margaret's *professional craft* – helped us to focus on the salient aspects of her practice and reveal the *personal* nature of her own *professional artistry*. I attempted to draw out the *particularity* of Margaret's expertise by understanding and challenging why the phenomenon of her practice situation had been interpreted in the way it had. We used concept maps to enable salient issues within the stories and interviews to emerge.

Intuitive practice is embedded and wrapped in complex personal stories as well as professional knowledge and expertise. The extraction of this intuitive knowledge was not without its uncomfortable moments. We used concept maps to help us see connections and links that otherwise would not have existed. These concept maps grew densely and thickly over the page. As I commented in the portfolio, this method was very useful.

'As they (concept maps) unravelled across the page, my sense of fuzziness seems to slowly lift and be replaced instead with ordered strands that remarkably, make sense! The pleasure this produces is still tangible three weeks later as I realise that I am maintaining in clinical practice, a value system that I believe in and one that is predominantely respectful of the individuals I come across in the work setting'.

Through the concept maps and critical dialogue, new practice knowledge, or *professional craft knowledge*, was being revealed. Through this process, we raised personal theories pertinent to Margaret's practice and identified ways in which these theories had significance for her – significance in that it enabled growth and development. The *person* and the *professional* became interdependent, and at times inseparable. The critical dialogue I was attempting to promote, at times using Margaret's own personal stories about her professional craft, helped inform and bring to the surface the skills embedded in her practice, in particular, her aesthetic knowledge of the client, her rapid grasp on priorities and the ability to think outside the box. This fostered self-awareness and identified areas in her practice, *which for her* had real potential. This was also validated in the interviews with stakeholders and colleagues.

As an expert, it is vital to make one's practice-based theories accessible to others, to enable their own growth and development. As such, others' personal theories should make sense and be applicable in a variety of situations. Disseminating personal expertise becomes pooled 'know-how' for others to use (Benner *et al.*, 1996) and by reflecting in action, others can in turn validate these expert theories and assess their relevance in other situations. This is what Rolfe (1998) defines as Practitioner Centred Research (PCR). As the particulars of each practice case are so clearly described, it helps other practitioners judge the relevance and fit of PCR theory to their own practice setting; thus, the ability to implement and transfer PCR becomes far more apparent.

Critical companionship facilitates both the development and validation of inductively derived PCR knowledge. Being underpinned by phenomenology, critical companionship is concerned with extracting personal theories from the meanings and interpretations the practitioner reveals about their practice. This is clearly evidenced within both the *relationship* and *facilitation domains*. Meanings and significances about practice are highly subjective and pertinent to the practitioner's own specific experiences. As the facilitator, I enabled personal ownership of these emergent theories about Margaret's practice, so that her interpretation would impact on others' experiences and improve collective thinking and learning. Thus, enabling Margaret to articulate her craft and be explicit about her knowledge was only going to be part of her journey. Helping her to disseminate this new found practice knowledge to her colleagues, finding practice situations to test out these assumptions with her team, and, on the basis of this, enabling a cultural shift towards person-centred practices were still to be achieved. This, however, was not part of our remit with the EPP, but the way forward was nevertheless tangible.

As a critical companion, I was keen to maintain a level of challenge which was enabling Margaret to dissect her taken-for-granted actions and see them differently. I was at times astounded by the complexities embedded in Margaret's cases and, in a non-judgemental way, pushed for this view to be recognised. Through challenge, I applied a different lens for her to focus on, and so helped to reinterpret her well-known and recognisable introspections. As an outsider to Margaret's work situation and professional domain, this was relatively uncomplicated for me to do.

Unlike other supervised or facilitative practice-based sessions, unresolved tension was not a feature in a critical companion relationship. What was a more likely experience was creative tension and, at times, this felt fearless and limitless because of a feeling of safety that I could only attribute to the critical companion being an outsider. There was undoubtedly a positive and buzzing advantage to working with Alison as she became familiar with the specifics of my working know-how. There felt little lack of restraint or worry about the subtext. The knowledge that I could speak freely without fear of upsetting colleagues or worse, highlighting an ideology or deep-seated value that they did not hold, was extremely liberating. This feeling in itself surely supports the notion that the framework of critical companionship is founded on principles of emancipation and enablement. In previous supervision experiences, I have heard suggestions of not coping; or of being too involved, or of getting things out of proportion or of being told to 'concentrate only on what you can do, not on what you can't'. The need to conform and collude is greater than the need to explore the inner workings of intuitive practice (Johns, 2001). None of this was even hinted at as Alison permitted a relationship of mutual trust, alongside a permission to take risks and yet, remaining safe and contained. We had both invested in the journey of bringing deep knowledge to the surface for critical scrutiny because we were confident this would lead to the development of further creative thinking and emotional development. In the critical companionship framework, articulation of practice is seen as one of the products of the relationship – highly prized by some, but perhaps not by all!

As an *experienced* facilitator, I was able to facilitate this degree of introspection by deliberately challenging Margaret about her way of working. This was done to help her articulate the nature of the established work culture surrounding her practice, and relate this to how the politics, history and sociology of practice influenced her professional behaviours. Subsequently, I realised that what was occurring within the *facilitation domain* was something called *problematisation* in the critical companionship framework (see Figure 5.1), that is using support and challenge to reveal problems that have not previously been noticed. I was enabling Margaret to reconsider her deeply held assumptions about the newly surfaced problems within her cases.

This aspect of the facilitation process, initiated and supported through openness, attending, sharing and *graceful care*, enabled Margaret to reframe her problem of being seen as a *maverick* in practice, to someone who is seen as advocating patient-centred practices. Permission to '*go there*' in order to unpick this personal investment in her practice was not necessarily something we negotiated at the start, and in retrospect, should not have been taken for granted. As a facilitator of many students' experiences and someone who teaches advanced facilitation skills to clinical and educational colleagues, this has been an important learning point. It is now stressed to others that this willingness to receive such a high degree of challenge and introspection should not be assumed and should be continually checked out in the enabling process. Reciprocal respect should, therefore, be demonstrable in all facilitative relationships that deliberately use high challenge and support to *problematise* issues.

Having an insider–outsider perspective

Being comfortable with each other, stemmed largely from our prior experiences of working together, but also it came from my position as an 'outsider' looking in on Margaret's 'insider' practices. From this vantage point, I was in a privileged position to enable Margaret to hypothesise about the culture in which she worked and her contribution to it. If I had been a part of her culture (and so an insider), an objective view would have been more difficult to characterise, and it may not have felt real to Margaret. The difficulty as an outsider was to grasp fully the issues embedded in each case, while at the same time appreciate the layers of complexity located within Margaret's practice in terms of context and process.

As a critical companion, my role was to enable learning for both of us. Margaret's work domain, culture, practice-based issues (politics) and concerns, the nature of her expertise, for instance, all needed to be fully appreciated if connections, focus on feelings, relating old and new knowledge and transforming views of practice and ways of working could be enabled. I felt outside her sphere of practice and needed to get to grips with this very unfamiliar work-based context and the specialised knowledge and skills required of a practitioner working in this area. For Margaret, her learning was about her *professional artistry* or how she promoted person-centred practices for the children she worked with, and to some extent, their parents who were deemed to have mental health problems (in some cases). Not only did I have to quickly cover the bases of what her *professional craft knowledge* entailed, but she had to also adopt a process of inquiry which (a) related to an unfamiliar practice situation for her and (b) was challenging enough to promote critical thinking within this very able expert.

I was using my personal antennae to sense what was occurring so that an understanding from Margaret's point of view could be grasped. In other words, I was ensuring that my developing understanding of Margaret's practice was from her own unique interpretation of the phenomena of her work experiences. Challenge could then be applied appropriately. This was difficult as knowledge already acquired through previous experiences of working together could have blinded the facilitation processes. I needed to continually check in (e.g. Is this OK? How are you seeing this? Can you go into that a bit more?) and check out (e.g. How do you know? Can you be sure? Can I ask a ridiculous question? Explain to me. . . ?) to make sure the outsider view wasn't too far from Margaret's situational knowledge. In addition, such questions have the enormous advantage of enabling practitioners to articulate the taken-for-granted and surface their professional craft knowledge, often for the first time. Knowing about Margaret did not include the job or the work situation, but did include her beliefs, her working style and her interpretation of her profession. In short, I required a more holistic perspective to fully understand her as a whole person – who she was as an *individual* and a colleague. For Margaret, within her particular culture, the critical companion being an outsider was beneficial. But for me, this outside position was at times a struggle.

Alison's thirst for detail was immense – the detail, that Rolfe (1997) describes, as the 'swampy mess' that clinical practice whips up. This level of curiosity and inquisitiveness from someone who had not worked in mental health, seemed bewildering and rather perplexing. I struggled for a while in knowing whether to accept and trust the process or consider potential ulterior motives that could be driving her instead.

The felt authenticity behind the rather relentless enquiry, in retrospect, ultimately seduced me into allowing, what Johns (1997), cited in Titchen (2003), refers to as 'high challenge'. These 'challenges' encroached unnervingly on personal issues as well as professional. She recalls one point where I apparently told her to 'back off', but I have no memory of this. The sharpness of the process was evidently felt by Alison as well as by me.

The two spheres of professional and personal are of course entirely inseparable regardless of our professional demeanour. We joisted like toy soldiers threatening each other with swords, but all the time knowing we would never hurt one another.

Such security in a professional relationship is rare and freeing. Alison's facilitation style engendered aesthetic and timely challenges, which undoubtedly reflected her person-centred approach and facilitation style. Challenge though has to come from one who you respect, and who you believe is issuing their challenge for a meaningful and mutual benefit. The term 'high challenge' too easily invites well meaning, but less perceptive individuals to fire holes into well-placed armoury. The notion of 'high challenge' is that it has to be alongside 'high support' and that if the balance is weighted towards the challenge, the practitioner then perceives threat and is likely to respond defensively (Johns, 2001). I would be the first to acknowledge that my defence mechanisms were operating well – Alison knew also they were there and the ways in which they surfaced. She treated them gently and respectfully though and if something significant was inadvertently trod on, *reciprocity* and *mutuality* meant there was a capacity to let one another know.

The existence of high challenge

Permission to be person centred and challenge emerging perspectives was tacit in the agreement to participate in the EPP study, as it was realised from the outset that the exploration into personal practices would be significant. A theoretical grounding in Benner's work (1984, 1996) and familiarity with publications by authors such as Brookfield (1993), Sutton and Smith (1995) and Atkins and Ersser (2000) into advanced nursing practice equipped us both with a realisation that, for practitioners with expertise, it is normal to push boundaries, take risks and exhibit maverick practices. It is also essential for the expert to be taken out of their comfort zone, challenged to think differently and find new and better ways of achieving desired, patient-centred goals. Challenge does not mean to criticise negatively, rather it refers to using strategies that deliberately make the other think deeply in order to raise professional consciousness about practice. Challenge, therefore, enables the process by facilitating and deliberately provoking focus and intent.

It was helpful that trust between us had already been established, as this speeded up the principles of engagement and allowed focus and challenge to become part and parcel of our facilitative sessions. We did not have to establish safety or politeness necessarily. Respect for each other was already present and we both knew this. We knew unequivocally that judgements about practice behaviours would be made, but that these judgements would be used to inform strategies to enable Margaret to come to her own decisions about her practice and the salient elements within them. I was able to use my own *professional artistry* that is the blending of knowing when to intervene, pinpoint what seemed to matter in the dialogue and synthesise perspectives, as they emerged, to reflect back a coherent and tangible picture about Margaret's interpretation of practice events. As the sphere of professional practice was not shared, the challenge was done carefully and considerately, and in a manner that allowed Margaret to assert her view. I had to be aware of how the 'challenge' could have been construed and ensure that this did not impact on the process. Although comfortable with each other, we had to ensure that the challenge was appropriate and received in the spirit in which it was intended.

When challenging, and rather than be disadvantaged by the lack of knowledge about Margaret's context, the 'outsider' perspective enabled comments to be made about how she saw her practice as being ordinary or how difficult she presumed herself to be with others in the team; how she wasn't sure of the skill she brought to the team or what she offered, in terms of her individual style with the children and their families. All this was very much taken for granted by Margaret, but to me the practices were highly skilled. I was able to question the basis on which these assumptions were made, enquire as to the obvious in terms of organisational structures and management systems and organisational issues which had not been considered, and delve into the complexities of each practice case Margaret presented. These perspectives provoked the most searching of discussions as I could assume very little about her practice, apart from my prior knowledge of her ability as a practitioner and a thinker. Margaret comments:

> The early encounters with Alison left a slight sense of bewilderment. Other supervisors somehow want me to be like them and impose a level of their thinking rather than listen to my 'doing' . . . . Or even further, dig deeper to understand what was driving the 'doing'. I was conscious that in a way this allowed me to escape real critical examination and was on the one hand relieved by this (what might they find out?) but on the other hand, it left me uncertain and insecure – it is not very easy (or safe) being an agent of your own morality.

Challenge came in a variety of ways and any potential anxiety managed by our shared respect and prior knowledge of each other's ways of working. As an outsider, I had permission to ask almost daft questions which for Margaret was challenging in that she had to clearly explain the layers of practice – some of which were obvious – others were not so. Moreover, my constant inquiry promoted her to consider how these layers of practice integrated into a composite whole which could be accessed and understood by a potential novice. My appreciation of her expertise was helped by my own personal memories of nursing within adult intensive care units. Although a very different professional world of nursing in terms of clinical context, the espoused values and approaches she demonstrated chimed loud and clear with my own. This resonance of values and beliefs came about because we occupied familiar ground. This helped me to rapidly grasp the significance of the work and the risks Margaret took on behalf of her clients which in turn accentuated the clarity of the picture of her own expertise. How her espoused beliefs and values were translated in her practice provided opportunities for us to seek out the unique nature of this expertise and the consequence of this expertise were on those she comes into contact with – parents, children and colleagues alike.

> Alison was an insider in terms of some personal knowledge, but an outsider in terms of professional domains. I knew her as a lecturer when I was a student completing a postgraduate diploma. However, her professional life related to higher education and adult nursing, whilst mine related to mental health. Within my immediate professional world, she was, therefore, an outsider. There were times in our meetings when I can clearly recall an impending sense of apprehension about what I was saying. I had experienced it many times before, as the axe of judgement

> from another comes down on you and seems to cut off your tongue. I knew Alison held a quiet respect for what she described as my 'maverick practices' and I was aware of testing her limits of tolerance in a way that would not have felt possible if she held some kind of supervisory responsibility. I grew to trust her and attributed her lack of judgement to her outsiderness. It still amazes me – the axe never came – I was allowed to speak, and therefore explore, freely. I felt as if I could fly.

In the deliberate use of challenge, the facilitator must be mindful of how judgements can either impede or augment a facilitative process. If judgements are used in a way which imposes opinions and determines what is right or wrong, good or bad, they may censor the dialogue and silence the practitioner to the detriment of learning, transformation and inquiry. This can often be the case when the facilitator holds a position of power and status in the *relationship domain* and uses this positional status deliberately to their own advantage. If the judgment is used as a strategy for exploration, debate, consideration and validation, then the outcome can be positive in terms of another's growth, reflexivity, thoughtfulness and self-awareness.

Future challenges, tensions and possibilities – critical companionship and its fitness for health care in the next millennium

Demonstrating critical companionship requires significant understanding of the person who is being 'chummed' on their learning journey. The critical companion holds themselves up, not as an expert, a guide, a mentor or a co-counsellor, but as a mirror to enable someone to see themselves as others do and accompany them in their ability to accommodate this revelation. These facilitative skills are advanced, and exhibit the critical companion's *graceful care*. These skills are not to everyone's taste as they depict a preferred 'facilitative style' (Heron, 1999), the purpose of which could be inappropriate in some practice and educational situations.

As effective as it was for the purpose of the EPP, we assert that critical companionship is especially appropriate for use in practice cultures that value *reciprocity* and *mutuality* between professionals. It should be significantly adapted in clinical situations where professional hierarchies are apparent such as when models of clinical supervision espouse monitoring, assessment of performance and evidencing achievement of prescriptive outcomes of standard practices. For example, if the facilitation relationship is premised on hierarchy and authoritarianism, power and control, this could threaten the survival of the core principles underpinning the process of critical companionship within the *relationship domain*. Critical companionship therefore needs to be carefully, sensitively and incrementally introduced and attuned to the prevailing culture.

In our experience, hierarchical cultures are often the reality of many health practitioners and work-based settings. We recognise that the framework can be employed in different settings and practices to challenge hierarchical and autocratic organisations, but one needs to be mindful of the competing cost-conscious priorities which dictate measurable outcomes and quick fixes. The critical companionship framework could be used as leverage to deliberately extol and promote the increasing need for patient-centred practices which challenge top-down reductionistic directives.

Critical companionship cannot do this in isolation, but in the hands of skilled facilitators and practitioners, it can support the process of cultural change. By attending to the context and culture of practice, it is possible that critical companions as facilitators can enable patient-centred care to be evidenced through the implementation of facilitative processes (Kitson *et al.*, 1998).

We have to be realistic and balance clinician-based expectations with cost-efficient health care. The mantra for a flexible and adaptable work force is all well and good, but we believe that to implement critical companionship requires a real shift in mindset for the organisation, as the impact of real change could be far reaching. A gentle trickling of critical companionship in bureaucratic and tightly controlled organisations may offer opportunities for some joined up thinking.

In cultures which are not premised on learning and facilitation, conventional forms of 'supervision' are often top-down. In these situations, both players are often insiders of the same practice. Learning for the supervisor can therefore be limited as their expertise is assumed. Moreover, challenge of this expertise is not usually welcomed, and this level of knowledge can be used deliberately by the supervisor to drive the agenda for what is learned and achieved in a 'facilitative' context. The cost is the reduced ability to transform experiences into new creative learning. These key aims may be explained as being able to explore how the *self* intersects with *professional practice* in order to evidence *professional artistry* – the deliverables of which are *person-centred practices*. We argue that sustained critical companionship needs to be supported, resourced as a valuable person-centred philosophy. With careful consideration this framework can:

1. endorse and evidence patient-centred practices;
2. enable a shared vision of practice between facilitator and practitioner;
3. challenge how power can be used in positive and enabling ways;
4. advocate the *insider* and *outsider* perspective;
5. encourage deep learning which is significant for the individual and the organisation in which they work.

We emphasise that for successful critical companionship, clear and careful negotiation from the outset is vital. Personal and professional boundaries are defined by respective roles and responsibilities, which in turn are *significantly* influenced by practice cultures. The critical companion and the practitioner being facilitated need to be aware of how cultural norms of practice interface with facilitation processes and personal expectations. This will enable the extent to which the framework can be realised, negotiated and applied within a professional situation.

Postscripts

Alison: 'Candour, a willing spirit and an ability to keep it all real were crucial for us in this facilitation process, and in respect to the critical companionship relationship, a genuine curiosity to engage with the interpretations and meanings underpinning expert practice. However, for me, this had little to do with the framework, but rather who we were as individuals and our preferred working style – although to be fair, the framework does encourage this use of "all aspects of self" through the application of graceful care. My facilitation style I adopted at the time of the EPP was my normal default position. I was not consciously aware of how this default position mirrored attributes of a critical companion or indeed the framework in action. However, since the EPP (and reflecting back on this experience with Margaret), I am now far more aware of my own professional artistry in my practice. In terms of my own learning, I am making conscious efforts to apply this artistry, and in so doing, gaining a better understanding as to how I can use the critical companionship framework to greater effect.

'For us as co-researchers within the EPP, critical companionship had a shelf life within the bounded task of what we were charged to do. It was not an ongoing journey. It ended when the portfolio was completed, evidence extracted and Margaret's expertise articulated to the Panel. In the EPP, we had achieved our task. Margaret had researched her own practice, problematised internal and external obstacles and co-created new knowledge about her nursing expertise. But of course what had been done could not be undone and in many ways I was aware the journey for her had just begun, as had my exit strategy.

'And yes, we do laugh out loud when we meet and no we don't take ourselves too seriously!'

Margaret: 'There was no doubt that the influence of the critical companion experience was profound. I felt different and held a new level of confidence about my working practices. I know more now, about why I made certain decisions and what the root of some of these decisions was. The experience had offered a sense of validation. It was as if someone had polished the mirror so that it was gleaming bright.

'I struggled terribly though to articulate this new learning to my colleagues. I strongly doubted their interest and even felt a level of guilt about the time and energy I had invested in this and other similar projects. I wasn't sure they understood or made any sense of these quirky learning ventures of mine. I had made no visible difference to team functioning and this contributed to a sense of the "and so what" factor.

'This crisis of confidence seemed to produce a barrier with colleagues. I had experienced something like this before – it feels as if some of your neurones are exposed for everyone to see and yet nobody talks about it. I expected the sensation to pass so that I could then go on to articulate new knowledge and understanding to peers as was expected from the model (Titchen & McGinley, 2003). It didn't seem to pass though and my new learning remained internalised – there was a small sense of emancipation but it produced difference and distance. I somehow could not begin to articulate the experience.

'This was not something that Alison could help me with, as her "outsiderness" from the group prevented it. A key contradiction of embarking on critical companionship was that a core drive was to seek greater shared understanding and yet the dominant sense for me, as the process drove on, was of deeper difference and isolation. Perhaps the project had left too many questions; I was no longer sure that the role that was being prescribed was one that I wanted or one that I believed in. The EPP had also put me in touch with my tiredness – the intensity of the work and the constant exposure to emotional and social despair and deprivation was really quite overwhelming. I somehow could not get past this block and left the post 6 months later. There was no conscious connection to the EPP but one that I made retrospectively.

'I have though found new energy in higher education. The experiences and learning from the EPP are never far from my mind in one form or another. I hope now to contribute to a culture where others can safely question and explore their practice experiences, and be able to fly a little too.'

Acknowledgements

Thanks to Angie Titchen for her insightful additions and ongoing support in the development of this chapter. This helped focus our thinking and enabled our ability to express what we believe the essence of critical companionship is all about.

References

Atkins, S. & Ersser, S.J. (2000) Education for advanced nursing practice: an evolving framework. *International Journal of Nursing Studies* **37**, 523–533.

Benner, P. (1984) *From Novice to Expert Excellence and Power in Clinical Nursing*. Prentice Hall, London.

Benner, P., Tanner, C.A. & Chelsa, C.A. (1996) *Expertise in Nursing Practice. Caring, Clinical Judgement and Ethics*. Springer Publishing Company, New York.

Brookfield, S. (1993) On impostership, cultural suicide, and other dangers: How nurses learn critical thinking. *Journal of Continuing Education in Nursing* **24**(5), 197–205.

Carper, B. (1978) Fundamental patterns of knowing. *Advances in Nursing Science* **1**(1), 13–23.

Heron, J. (1999) *The Complete Facilitators Handbook*. Kogan Page, London.

Johns, C. (1997) *Becoming an Effective Practitioner through Guided Reflection*. Unpublished PhD Thesis, University of Luton cited in Titchen, (2003).

Johns, C. (2001) Depending on the intent and emphasis of the supervisor, clinical supervision can be a different experience. *Journal of Nursing Management* **9**(3), 139–145.

Kitson, A., Harvey, G. & McCormack, B. (1998) Enabling the implementation of evidence based practice: a conceptual framework. *Quality in Health Care* **7**, 149–158.

Kolb, D. (1984) *Experiential Learning: Experience as the Source of Learning and Development*. Prentice Hall, London.

Manley, K., Hardy, S., Titchen, A. & Garbett, R. (2005) *Changing patients' worlds through nursing practice. Exploring nursing practice expertise through emancipatory action research and fourth generation evaluation*. A Royal College of Nursing Research Report, RCN Institute, London.

McGill, I. & Beaty, L. (1992) *Action Learning: A Practitioner's Guide*. Kogan Page, London.

Mezirow, J. (1981) A critical theory of adult learning and education. *Adult Education Quarterly* **32**(1), 3–24.

Rolfe, G. (1997) Beyond expertise: theory practice and the reflexive practitioner. *Journal of Clinical Nursing* **6**(2), 93–97.

Rolfe, G. (1998) *Expanding Nursing Knowledge: Understanding and Researching Your Own Practice*. Butterworth Heinemann, Oxford.

Sutton, F. & Smith, C. (1995) Advanced Nursing Practice: new ideas and new perspectives. *Journal of Advanced Nursing* **21**, 1037–1043.

Titchen, A. (2000) *Professional Craft Knowledge in Patient-Centred Nursing and the Facilitation of Its Development*. DPhil Thesis, Ashdale Press, University of Oxford.

Titchen, A. (2003) Critical companionship, part 1. *Nursing Standard* **18**(9), 33–40.

Titchen, A. & McGinley, M. (2003) Facilitating practitioner research through critical companionship. *Nursing Times Research* **8**(2), 115–131.

Wright, J. & Titchen, A. (2003) Critical companionship, part 2: using the framework. *Nursing Standard* **18**(10), 33–38.

7. Expertise in Practice – Older People

Jonathan Webster

Chrysanthemum petals on a bedside locker.
You share your story with me,
your hopes and desires,
your anxieties and worries,
feelings of loss and hopelessness,
I listen, I hear, I see, I make sense of and understand.

A frost covers the ground outside your window,
I see a person who is recovering silhouetted against a steely grey sky,
but hear someone who is lost, fearful and worried.
We share your story with others, your hopes and desires,
your anxieties and worries, your wishes.
We plan no matter how difficult, we
listen to and question those who doubt,
we agree, negotiate and at times compromise.

Winter sunshine lights your room,
your hope is with those who understand,
they have heard your story and see you as a person,
they listen, they hear and act.

Introduction

The purpose of this chapter is to illustrate how expert, person-centred practice with older people is translated into care through the use of emancipatory practice development[1], by specifically drawing from a programme of practice

---

[1] 'Practice development is a continuous process of improvement towards increased effectiveness in patient centred care. This is brought about by enabling health care teams to develop their knowledge and skills and to transform the culture and context of care. It is enabled and supported by facilitators committed to systematic, rigorous continuous processes of emancipatory change that reflect the perspectives of service users and service providers' (Garbett & McCormack, 2002).

development that aimed to take forward person-centred assessment with older people within a district general hospital in England. Before doing this, however, it's important to start by defining what is meant by expert practice in older people's nursing in the context of contemporary health care.

Defining expertise in practice with older people

Expert care for older people has rightly attracted the attention it deserves through the raising of the profile of specialist gerontological nursing (McCormack & Ford, 1998; Ford & McCormack, 2000; Pritchard & Wright, 2001; RCN, 2004). Yet, clearly defining expertise with older people is both complex and challenging. Essential elements are the impact that expert gerontological nurses can have on both clinical outcomes in caring for older people (McCormack, 1998; Kydd, 2002; Lopez *et al.*, 2002; Forster, 2004; RCN, 2004) within the transformation and modernising of older people's services (Sturdy, 2004). More broadly publication of documents such as the National Service Framework for Older People (DH, 2001) and A New Ambition for Old Age (DH, 2006) in England and the Strategy for Older People in Wales (Welsh Assembly Government, 2003) as an illustration have raised the broader focus of the needs of older people within the context of health and social care policy and guidance. Other key elements that influence defining expertise in older people's nursing include a society that is changing, along with the needs of people accessing both statutory and non-statutory services. Across all services, there is a more ethnically diverse older population; people are living longer and are increasingly expressing their needs and aspirations particularly in relation to choice and individual control (DH, 2001; RCN, 2004).

The development of expertise in practice has been widely discussed and critically debated by different authors (Benner, 1984; Dreyfus & Dreyfus, 1986; Rolfe, 1998; Rolfe *et al.*, 2001; RCN, 2005). Expertise is seen to derive from a synthesis of both scientific and experiential knowledge (theoretical and practical) and through learning processes, particularly critical reflection – both 'in' and 'on' action (Schon, 1999). In her study into nursing expertise, Patricia Benner argued that tacit knowledge is the hallmark of expert practice; however, 'capturing' such descriptive accounts is difficult because the expert practitioner functions 'from a deep understanding of the total situation' (Benner, 1984). Identifying knowledge generated from practice through critical reflection and enquiry into practice can be viewed as a key element in enhancing practitioners' knowledge of their practice with older people and their supporters. Also, professional judgement, which can be subjective and unquantifiable, can be changed to an objective statement, grounded in knowledge gained from practice, which is illustrated in the following narrative:

I had been looking after John since his admission 3 days ago, on admission to my ward he was very frail and exhausted, he had previously suffered a stroke which had left him with a hemiplegia. His wife was worried about John being in hospital, since his admission I had spent time with her, getting to know them, what was important and what they planned for in the future. John's wife described to me how she had battled to get her husband home after his stroke as many professionals had told her that they wouldn't cope. However they were coping, life wasn't easy, however John and his wife had a routine that they liked, it worked well for them both. She described to me her anxiety whenever John had contact with hospital, just in case she was told that he wouldn't be able to go home.

I came on duty and knew something wasn't right. The nurse handing over John's care said that everything had been 'fine' and yes he did seem superficially 'fine', however he appeared less communicative, he seemed more vague, less himself. Before asking the medical team to assess I needed to make sure that I could describe what the problem was. I thought about what I needed to do, other patients I had cared for. I looked at his medication chart to see if there were any changes, I checked his vital signs, his temperature was slightly raised, it also appeared that he had been drinking less over the past 24 hours. In talking with John he told me that it felt uncomfortable to pass urine. I decided to check his urine and found traces of both blood and protein. I felt confident to say, these are the issues that I have identified, instead of something unquantifiable or nebulous such as something isn't right'. I felt confident too, to tell John's wife what we thought the problem was and to provide reassurance.

The care of older people within long-term settings is predominantly based on maintaining normal patterns of living as part of day-to-day activities. An approach to therapeutic care that is based on 'mechanistic' forms of decision-making is therefore inappropriate (RCN, 1998). Instead, nurses need to draw from factual knowledge that is deeply embedded in practice and yet is easily retrieved. Such tacit knowledge (i.e. difficult to explain or articulate) enables the expert nurse to engage in holistic decision-making and to avoid sole reliance on linear models (Benner, 1984) of understanding and conceptualisation. The expert nurse therefore bases decision-making not only on empirical evidence but also on professional craft knowledge (Titchen, 2000) that they are able to justify and articulate. However, what is less easily explained is how the expert nurse makes these decisions and how intuition is utilised (Rolfe, 1997).

Within the field of gerontological nursing, different authors have also described how expertise is reflected within their roles in working with older people and their supporters (Clegg & Mansfield, 2003; Webster, 2004; Manley *et al.*, 2008). According to Hardy *et al.* (2006), there is an international recognition of the role expertise has achieved in modern and effective health care systems; with evidence to support the claim that 'nursing expertise changes peoples' worlds, alongside workplace performance and organisational wide service developments (Manley *et al.*, 2005). Manley *et al.* (2005) further suggest that such nursing expertise is associated with specific characteristics expressed through 'professional artistry', which is recognised, by colleagues, patients and users. Recognition and possession of explicit expertise is therefore necessary within roles such as the consultant nurse who provides advice and guidance through the consultancy mechanism (Manley, 1997).

The Royal College of Nursing document, *The value and skills of nurses working with older people* (1993), describes what expert nurses offer older people (Box 7.1). These key components can be seen as being underpinned by *the attributes of expertise* (RCN, 2005) (Also refer to Box 1.2 and Figure 1.1). However, it has been identified that there are difficulties in clearly defining the attributes of specialist nursing practice in the care of older people within the context of core skills, the qualities needed to undertake specialist roles, perceptions of gerontological nursing and specialist versus generalist skills and knowledge (Oberski *et al.*, 1999; Kelly *et al.*, 2005; Reed *et al.*, 2007) needed to provide skilled, therapeutic care for older people and their supporters. Ford *et al.* (2004, p. 4) state:

> Studies of skilled practitioners clearly demonstrate that much knowledge is embedded in the actions of practitioners, but, when asked, they are unable to describe such knowledge, other than its technical aspects.

If this is truly the case in contemporary gerontological nursing, then expertise in the care of older people can be seen as being 'pigeon holed' into a set of taught technical skills with little or no value gained through experiential learning from practice with older people and their supporters that is readily articulated and described by the nurse. However, in making this argument, it is important to consider the significance of both technical and interpretative skills needed by nurses where ever the older person is being cared for (Webster & Hayes, 2008) to ensure good, consistent management. The National Service Framework for Older People (DH, 2001) identifies core elements of 'good management' within a hospital setting (Box 7.2) which should underpin both nursing and medical care/treatment. Training in which technical skills are taught is essential to ensure patient safety and competence in practice; however, training alone will not necessarily ensure the transfer of knowledge back into clinical care and work-based cultures in which experiential and theoretical knowledge are synthesised, the intended outcome being to improve the older person's experience of care. Emancipatory practice development can be seen as being key to enabling this to occur by 'liberating' both practice and practitioners by helping individuals and teams to break away from ways of working and clinical cultures that are not person centred, critically reflective or creative. This is discussed further and illustrated later in this chapter.

As previously discussed, defining expertise in the care of older people is as complex as it is multidimensional and multifaceted. Dewing (1994) cited by McCormack (2001) suggests that 'professional caring' is far more complex than 'providing nursing care' as it involves deep emotional involvement; self-awareness and the purposeful use of self; inter-subjectivity and aesthetic qualities, in which the self-aware, knowledgeable practitioner works with and in partnership with the older person and their supporters.

Workforce challenges

Having a skilled work force that has the core skills and ability to provide meaningful, therapeutic care to older people is central to providing quality-focused services. However, at times of financial pressures, less skilled, cheaper labour (RCN,

Box 7.1   The value and skills nurses working with older people

- Understanding the influences on care
  The Impact of ageism, the effects of class, gender, culture, ethnicity, religion and sexuality and how it might feel to be an older person or carer in today's society.
- Maintaining a positive approach
  Valuing the older person's life experiences and the meaning of those to the older person: focussing on what the older person can do, rather than on what he or she cannot do; building on the coping skills and strategies accumulated by the older person through life experiences; maintaining a perspective which includes the positive aspects of later life and adjusting to life changes and losses.
- Building and maintaining relationships
  Nurses' skills in communicating in sensory impairment, skills in subtle forms of communication such as body language, supporting skills, counselling skills, motivating and empowering skills, adjusting the pace of communication to the circumstances. Nurses' skills in therapeutic strategies such as group work, reminiscence and validation therapy are also valuable.
- Assessment
  Assessing an older person in health or illness is a highly skilled, highly complex process because of the interrelated factors of normal ageing – physical, psychological and social – and pathology. Assessing mental health needs in older age is particularly complex as is the nursing of older people who are behaving unusually, particularly when this is due to illness. Expert nurses recognise subtle changes in older people's health and can take action to help prevent deterioration.
- Intervention
  Expert nurses recognise that function may require more important than the effects of a particular disease. They also understand the effects of environment on an older person's health and functioning. Expert nurses have sound skills in rehabilitation and in working with other health care professionals in maximising the potential of the older person. Expert nurses can offer psychological support and therapeutic intervention for mental health needs. They act as key workers in professional networking. They are skilled in the care of older people who are dying, offering comfort, support and therapy both to the patient and their family. Expert nurses with older people are particularly skilled in planning discharge from hospital/transfer of care in maintaining their knowledge of local services.
- Developing expert specialist roles
  It has been demonstrated that patients who have access to specialist nurses are more knowledgeable, more proficient in self-care and more satisfied with the care they receive. These findings are clearly attributed to the nursing intervention. Following the appointment of specialist nurses, budget savings have been made because fewer patients have been admitted to hospital, lengths of stay have been reduced and there has been a reduction in the amount of wasted equipment. Specialist nurse appointments can also attract external funding.

Box 7.2   Core elements of good management within a hospital setting

> - Maintaining fluid balance
> - Pressure sore risk management
> - Acute confusion
> - Falls and immobility
> - Nutritional status and risk management
> - Continence risk management
> - Cognitive impairment
> - Rehabilitation potential
> - Depression
> - Infection control
> - Medicines management
> - Social circumstances
> - Family and carers' needs
> - How and where to access other specialist services
> - End of life care

2004) can be seen as being an alternative (from purely a financial perspective) to more skilled, expert nurses who provide, enable and lead care but cost more to employ. Assessing outcomes within the context of 'value for money' is a key indicator within current health care (RCN, 2004). However, measuring the cost-effectiveness of nursing is not easily achieved (Thomas & Bond, 1995). Balanced against this view is the need to consider future work force trends and the potential lack of availability of expert nurses as a result of an ageing workforce and greater global movement of nurses (Longley *et al.*, 2007). A lack of value placed on expertise is potentially compounded by nurses working in the field of gerontological nursing not being able to articulate or clearly demonstrate the difference that their involvement in care can make to the older person's experience of care and outcomes for therapeutic nursing and treatment within the context of organisational priorities.

In considering the future of advanced nursing roles, Policy + (2007) suggests that it is at least 5 years before the impact on patient outcomes and cost-effectiveness in advanced nursing roles such as those of the consultant nurse[2] can be identified and that decisions about role sustainability are reliable. This poses real challenges to nurses in such posts as frequently they are expected to demonstrate tangible outcomes very quickly leading to high impact changes that may or may not be sustainable. For practitioners working within the field of older people's nursing in 'expert' or 'advanced' roles such as that of the consultant nurse, this can be additionally challenging if they are working within services that may not have a specialist focus on older people's care and if there is no infrastructure

---

[2] Consultant nurses are cited because of the attention these 'new' (circa 2000) roles have attracted and because of the scope (covering four domains) of the role one core function/domain being expert practice.

to help them deliver on key organisational and national priorities of which there may be many. Similarly, support (through recognition of experiential and theoretical learning) is essential to help individuals to grow into such roles and not get 'stuck' at a certain level. When there is no clear support (personal and/or organisational), individuals may be 'pigeon holed' into carrying out activities that are easily identifiable and visible by others. Whilst these activities might be comfortable to them, i.e. familiar, they may not necessarily be appropriate for the advanced role as originally designed, which may in turn place the role at risk.

With the increase availability of post-registration gerontological graduate programmes, nurses and Allied Health Professionals have far greater opportunity of gaining a deeper level of theoretical knowledge and understanding of gerontological practice. However, it is debatable whether this alone (i.e. without experiential learning or an appropriate organisational culture) will enable change and development in practice settings. When there is immense pressure to deliver efficient services, at times of ongoing pressure as a result of financial and target imperatives (Webster, 2008), nurses working within perceived 'expert' roles can no longer assume that their position is 'safe' by right if they do not demonstrate clear outcomes and benefits to care within the broader organisational operational delivery agenda. Such political awareness and understanding of both the context of care and organisational drivers including astute awareness in 'organisational politics' (Redfern *et al.*, 2003) can be seen as being a core elements of expert practice in which the expert practitioner is able to work with, make sense of and influence the key clinical, operational and strategic drivers.

There are challenges in defining expertise in contemporary gerontological nursing, as expertise in the field of gerontological nursing doesn't sit within a neat, disease-specific box as it encompasses:

- many elements of essential, core nursing;
- specialist knowledge and understanding of the ageing process;
- holistic knowledge of the impact of ageing on the older person and their supporters;
- the development of caring, therapeutic relationships in which the person's desires and aspirations are kept central to care and ways of working.

Marr and Kershaw (1998) suggest that over the last three decades the management of care delivery has moved from task allocation to team nursing, patient allocation and primary nursing in which the desires of the person have taken precedence over the organisation. This is of particular relevance to older people's nursing and the influence that expert nurses in the field of gerontology can have in shaping how care is delivered and the importance placed on the centrality of the older person to care. Within England, the focus upon *The Productive Ward* (NHS Institute for Innovation and Improvement, 2007) can be seen as enabling nurses within a hospital setting to focus upon how they can use the time and resource available to care for patients more effectively. However, central to this is how innovation can grow, change and be sustained when there is immense financial pressure and ongoing major organisational change and restructuring. As such the expert nurse is vital not only in supporting and enabling others, but also by bringing a level of expertise and insight that others may not possess or have, so that implications and potential outcomes are clearly understood, recognised and acted upon.

Having developed a theoretical knowledge and understanding of gerontological nursing, the nurse whishing to develop expertise will then need to translate this theoretical knowledge into practice and the world of real-life clinical nursing. Reality can be 'messy' (Kelly *et al.*, 2005), 'murky' (Meyer, 2001) and 'challenging' (Webster, 2007), the ultimate aim being to improve the older person's experience of care through skilled, evidence-based, compassionate care in which the needs and desires of the person are kept central to all activity.

Perceptions of working with older people

Whilst the broad themes of expertise in nursing are relevant and appropriate to specialist care for older people (Rolfe, 1996; Rolfe & Fulbrook, 1998; RCN, 2005), there are clear challenges for the translation of such expertise into practice in a speciality that historically has been under-resourced and in some areas undervalued (Nolan, 1997). There still remains a view held by some that working with older people is of 'low status' (Kelly *et al.*, 2005) compared to other areas of specialist practice. Coupled with this is a broader view in which Meyer and Sturdy (2004) identify 'global challenges' in gerontological nursing.

Within health care, historically, it could be argued stereotypical images of working with older people have been reflected in the perceived level and type of care needed by them (frequently referred to and devalued as 'basic' nursing care) and the 'type' of nurse who chose to work in an 'elderly care' setting. However, the reality of specialist care for older people is that due to the complexity and diversity of needs that older people can have due to chronological ageing, nurses working within the field of gerontological practice need to be highly skilled and able to work and think creatively so that older people and their supporters experience care that is meaningful to them. This would therefore once again suggest that working with older people is far more complex than delivering just 'basic care' instead it is about essential, highly skilled nursing. In describing terminology that devalues older people, Crouch (1997) suggests that the effects of health care 'rationing' can lead to older people being perceived as an 'economic problem' in which language such as 'bed blockers' or 'delayed discharges' dehumanises the person and infers that because the person is old they are the 'problem' rather than the organisation and funding of services.

However crucially, it is important to influence the thinking and working of all staff ranging from those in executive positions to front line clinical staff who are either working in or commissioning services for older people. Supporting, developing and subsequently delivering expert practice should be seen as central to both practice and service delivery and not an added bonus that is desirable but not necessarily essential for efficient, quality-focused, person-centred services. However, key to this is ensuring that there is a clear and consistent focus on the needs of older people as key users of services, when the political health spotlight might be elsewhere.

Developing practice with older people

An emancipatory practice development journey

The context

As a newly appointed consultant nurse for older people in 2001, I was given the very broad brief of identifying the priorities for older people's nursing within the trust in which I was employed. The first 6 months of my appointment was spent working alongside staff in different clinical areas, communicating with and building a professional working relationship with different professionals and, importantly, working with and talking with older people and their supporters both within and outside of the trust. Getting 'under the skin' of practice and how the organisation provided services for older people enabled me to gain a real-life understanding of both how older people experienced care and the focus that older people's nursing had within the trust.

A recurrent theme that emerged from practice was how nurses 'see' people as they get older and perceptions of what it means to get old. This was highlighted in different ways ranging from observing and being part of practice with older people to discussions with staff both internal and external to the trust. Working in practice and alongside different teams, I experienced real-life clinical care and observed practices that recognised and valued the needs of older people and at other times less so. Although anecdotal, at times I felt that the 'patient' (the older person) had become disconnected from their past and who they were as a person – in essence the older person was seen by some nurses as being unidimensional, someone who was in hospital, was 'ill' and happened to be 'older'.

Working with older people and their supporters and different teams helped me identify key emerging themes from practice; specifically, how nursing assessments were carried out with older people and the value placed on the process of assessment as part of a continuum or 'journey'. Integral to this was how older people were seen as 'elderly patients' who were 'ill' or 'unable to cope at home' and seemed disconnected from their past and future. I was told by some nurses that 'individualised nursing care' was practiced and that 'we treat all patients as individuals'. However, based on observation and discussion, I was uncertain what this really meant and how it was embedded in the culture and reflected in day-to-day therapeutic working with older people. It seemed to me that finding out about the person, what was important to them and putting their desires and aspirations for the present and future at the centre of all activity needed to be more than 'caring' or 'empathy'. Based on an individual practitioner's own values and beliefs, it needed to be embedded in clinical care that underpinned expert therapeutic working with older people.

Enabling practice with older people

I recognised that from working with older people and clinical teams I was developing an understanding of practice and the context in which care was delivered. Recurrent themes were appearing and that priorities in practice were emerging centred around improving the older person's experience of care focused upon how nurses 'see' people as they get older along with the formal process of carrying out assessments with older people. As an experienced nurse, I recognised and valued the importance of the process of assessment (as an ongoing continuum) as it provides the foundations on which care is built and the cornerstone to planning and delivering person-centred care. I also recognised the level of expertise needed by nurses to carry out assessments that were meaningful and relevant by drawing from both technical and experiential knowledge. Benner (1984) clearly identifies that nursing knowledge in itself comes from a clear understanding of 'real' nursing and that knowledge forms an integral part of 'clinical expertise' and 'advanced practice'. This degree of understanding and insight is crucial as it recognises and values the skills of expert nurses and the positive impact that this can have on therapeutic care and working with older people and their supporters.

Importance of person-centred assessment

I recognised that the opportunity to carry out an assessment (that was not merely about ticking boxes) enabled the nurse to find out more about the person, what was important to them along with their immediate and long-term goals for care, this ensured that care was tailored to the person's needs and not what professionals thought was right. The plethora of literature relating to assessment identifies the place it has in underpinning professional practice. However, there is limited agreement about the parameters and objectives of assessment, how the practice of assessment is defined or the characteristics of good practice (Nolan & Caldock, 1996; Ford & McCormack, 1999). Increasingly, there is recognition that assessment of the needs of people as they get older are of paramount importance and that nurses along with other professionals play a vital part in this process (Meare & Bhowmick, 1995; Cohen, 2003). Underpinning person-centred assessment needs to be a philosophy of care that is embedded in person-centred practice. Ford and McCormack (2000) cite Kitwood and Bredin (1992), who identify that person-centred practice can be achieved if practitioners understand user needs, engage in positive work with the user; place central in all discussions/actions the desire to maintain/improve well-being. Person-centred assessment focuses on the needs as perceived by the person rather than those of the service provider or professional (Ford & McCormack, 2000); it focuses on the older person (and arguably those important to them) and not just nursing or health needs (Dewing & Pritchard, 2000).

In valuing the importance of the process of person-centred assessment, I was also pragmatic and recognised that in many clinical areas, staff were very busy and under pressure, the throughput of patients was immense and that the 'ideal' needed to be translated into what was 'workable' in the real world that is not always 'perfect' or 'ideal'. I was also aware that some staff and teams may not be prepared to consider developing new skills or challenging practices that they felt 'safe' and 'comfortable' with.

Helping to 'grow' expertise in practice

A key part of my role is in helping practitioners to challenge and question practice. I recognised that traditional methods of training and education did not always enable the translation of newly acquired skills and expertise back into traditional work-based cultures and that newly acquired empirical knowledge at times stayed at the door of the ward, particularly when the work-based culture did not support or nurture learning and the development of craft knowledge.

Practice development is central to enabling a work-based culture of innovation and development to grow and evolve and focused upon improving the person's experience of care. However, different approaches can lead to different outcomes. Manley and McCormack (2003, 2004) assert that there are two types of practice development, *technical* and *emancipatory*. Although there are similarities between both, by definition and purpose they are different. Technical practice development occurs as a consequence of practice compared to emancipatory practice development which is deliberate and intentional. Technical practice development can also be viewed as being driven from a 'top-down approach' that focuses upon technical skill and technical knowledge rather than a 'bottom-up approach' that aims to enable, transform and liberate both practice and practitioners. Emancipatory practice development and the empowerment of staff is focused upon developing a transformational culture (Manley, 2001) in which quality, positive changes to practice, leadership development and having a shared vision and the valuing of staff are core to how the team work. Manley (2001) further asserts that compared to technical approaches emancipatory practice development has two additional components:

- To enable practitioners to become empowered leading to the development of their individual and collective service.
- To foster the development of a transformational culture.

These additional components can be seen as needing to be underpinned by the seven emancipatory processes (RCN, 2006) that support skilled facilitation leading to the empowerment of practitioners (Box 7.3). A key challenge for practitioners involved with emancipatory practice development is the need to clearly understand the differences between emancipatory practice development compared to technical approaches, therefore informing their own critical intent through skilled facilitation and enablement.

Box 7.3 Seven emancipatory processes

There are seven emancipatory processes. Most are derived from the research methods of emancipatory action research (Grundy, 1982):
- Using self-reflection and fostering reflection in others
- Development of critical intent of individuals and groups
- Developing moral intent
- Working with values, beliefs and assumptions
- Focusing on the impact of the context on practice
- Seeing the possibilities
- Fostering widening participation and collaboration by all involved

Working with Albion Ward and Anne

Albion Ward is a busy, acute medical ward that provided care for older people within an integrated model of service delivery in a district general hospital. The senior nursing manager on Albion Ward agreed for her area to take part in the programme of emancipatory practice development that focused upon developing person-centred assessment with older people. The intention was not to introduce a new framework or tool for assessment but rather to help nurses within their team to review how they carried out assessments with older people, the focus being to enable greater person-centredness in assessment practices. The programme of practice development was made up of five distinct phases:

1. Working clinically with the team. I worked with the nursing team on Albion Ward on several occasions. This was not only to become familiar with the team but also to observe and be part of practice so that I could start to understand the clinical culture underpinning practice with older people.
2. Understanding the values and beliefs of staff related to working with older people and what they believed was important to carrying out assessments with older people. An anonymous values and beliefs questionnaire was developed which all nursing staff (registered and unregistered) were asked to complete.
3. Working with staff on a programme of practice development that focused upon the theory underpinning different areas of assessment and person-centred practice with older people. This approach finally brought both elements together to form person-centred assessment with older people. Coupled with this was the use of reflective exercises which (a) helped link the theory to practice regarding working with older people and (b) developed increased understanding and insight from practice.
4. Evaluation of development of practice by asking participants to share their story.
5. Evaluation of development by asking participants to describe how the programme had impacted on their practice and that of their teams after 3 months.

For the purpose of this chapter, I will focus upon phases three and four of the programme of practice development working with Anne (one of the participants) to demonstrate how expertise was created through emancipatory practice development.

Phase three

This phase provided the central time in which I met with participants and explored the themes related to assessment and person-centred practice with older people along with facilitating critical reflection. Our fortnightly, 2-hour sessions were divided into two parts:

- Exploring the theory underpinning the principles of assessment and person-centred practice with older people.
- Reflecting on personal learning based on reflective activities with specific themes.

This part of the programme lasted for about 20 weeks. At the first meeting of this phase, participants were encouraged to keep a reflective journal in which they could record observations, thoughts and reflections from the programme. It was also suggested that they would find using a formal framework to aid critical reflection of use, such as Gibbs's (1988) reflective cycle. A previous study that I had carried out identified the potential benefits of reflective writing in practice (Webster, 1999, 2002). I also recognised how reflective writing can help practitioners to translate their thoughts and observations from practice into tangible observations that both informed and generated understanding for the individual about their practice (Rich & Parker, 1995; Smith, 1995; Rolfe *et al.*, 2001).

Phase four
Consent was sought from participants before taking part in this phase. The intention of this phase being to identify how the process of practice development had influenced practice with older people by using:

- Didactic and reflective learning.
- The integration of skills and knowledge (both tacit and empirical) into practice.

Semi-structured interviews were carried out that aimed to identify how the process of learning (both didactic and reflective) had influenced their thinking and practice with older people. As part of this, participants were asked to create a picture to describe their views of the programme. This provided a focus for discussion as those taking part were asked to describe the picture. This level of creativity felt appropriate for this first evaluation as a key intention of the programme of practice development was focused on developing creativity in both professional practice with older people and thinking. Art-based activities can also be seen as encouraging individuals to express 'out there' what is normally 'hidden' or not expressed (Coulson & Stickley, 2002), greater emotional intelligence (Coats *et al.*, 2006) whilst learning both about oneself and the way in which we relate to patients and colleagues (Freshwater, 2004).

Anne's Story

Anne was a senior nurse on her ward and had worked within the speciality for a number of years. Working with her and nurses from Albion Ward, it became evident very early on in the practice development programme that they were unsure what to expect from the facilitating learning approach that I was taking with them as I explored their practice with older people. Initially, it seemed that some wanted me to 'teach' and weren't comfortable with being asked questions or encouraged to engage and reflect on their practice. I was conscious that at times I took on the key functions and activities of a practice developer (Garbett & McCormack, 2003), i.e. promoting and facilitating change, translation and communication, research into practice and education would overlap and merge with each other depending upon the theme being explored. These functions were reflected upon both collectively by the group and by individuals.

Phase three involved meeting with Anne and other participants over a 5-month period. These meetings became very interactive as the time enabled us to explore the key themes from the sessions. However, it also allowed for greater critical reflection based on the clinically based reflective exercises that she worked through between our meetings. I observed that as the sessions progressed, Anne became more confident and adept at critically reflecting upon her own practice and the clinical situations she was encountering on a day-to-day basis. The reflective exercises focused her thoughts on one area; however, she also spent time reflecting upon other situations she faced that were interrelated. Facilitation and critical questioning adapted strategies from critical companionship, and included mutuality, reciprocity, particularity and graceful care (Titchen, 2003). Anne was able to clearly articulate her own values and beliefs related to person-centred assessment with older people. Also, she was clearly challenging ways of working that were not person centred. Titchen and McGinley (2003) argue that both evidence-based and person-centred care draw from holistic professional practice knowledge, they suggest that skilled reflection enabled by critical companionship can enable this to occur. Within her team, Anne also described the strategies she was using to influence and enable others such as positive role modelling in which action was supported by articulation. Anne expressed the view that she had always tried to be a positive role model; however, she had not always been able to articulate why she was behaving in a certain way; she now felt increasingly confident to do so.

In describing how the programme of practice development had influenced her practice with older people, Anne drew a picture (Figure 7.1). Anne stated:

> I have got people out of their beds, on a journey, where they can see a door, and behind the door is sunshine, and then the door is open and there is sunshine, and there's happy faces and there's rainbows and bright colours.

Anne described how the programme of practice development had changed the way in which she worked with older people and their supporters and the profile of assessment within her own practice. She identified that at the start of the journey

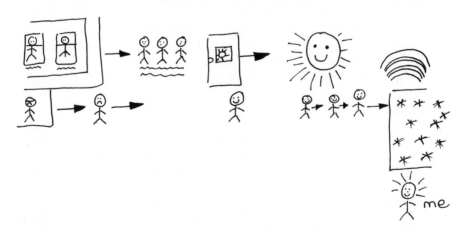

Figure 7.1 Anne's Picture

the colours used were 'grey' and 'dark'; however, now they were 'bright' and 'light'. She described how she now felt liberated and able to practice in different, more person-centred ways. The perceived barriers and blocks that she thought were present, that had previously stopped her practicing in the way she wanted to with older people, were not really there, but were 'merely excuses to stop us getting to know patients'. In describing how the programme of practice development had influenced her practice with older people, Anne stated:

> . . . its made me realise that everybody has a life, a past life and a future life, and it's made me realise that you need to get to know the person behind the illness to enable you to give better care that they want.

Anne described how she had used empirical knowledge and combined it with craft knowledge to inform how she worked with and cared for older people. Anne described a scenario that had occurred in practice:

> We had an older man on the ward who became very disturbed at night. He was unable to communicate his needs, however at night he would wander around the ward, going into people's lockers, he was generally very difficult to manage. The team were keen to have his sedation increased because the ward was so hectic, but I recognised how this would have affected him. I thought about what we had talked about and how it was important to find out about the person. I spoke to the man's daughter about what was happening at night, she informed me that during the war her father had been kept in solitary confinement, at home he always now slept with a light on by his bed. I ensured that this information was shared with the team, I also incorporated it into his care plan. As a result of leaving a light on by his bed he settled and slept well.

I recognised that increasingly Anne was articulating how the programme of practice development was helping her to develop her practice along with that of her team. She was applying knowledge gained through facilitation and critical reflection to her own practice with older people. She was also describing how she was using craft knowledge gained through facilitated critical reflection 'on' action to influence how she worked with and cared for older people and their supporters.

Parallel Journey

In reflecting upon my own role working with Anne and her team, I recognised that I had been on a parallel journey. Engagement was central to working with Anne and the team as without it collaboration in learning through practice development that focused upon empowering both the individual and 'collaborative' and enabling a transformational culture (Manley & McCormack, 2003) would not have taken place. Walsh *et al.* (2005) argue that engagement is central to any successful change; however, as such has been under theorised within the practice development literature. In exploring practice with older people on Albion Ward, facilitation had been key to the process of understanding, questioning, making sense of and developing practice with older people as I worked with Anne and her team.

Within the literature, there are multiple interpretations of what is meant by 'facilitation' and the role of the facilitator which ranges from a 'hands-on' approach to enabling change to more complex, multifaceted dimensions (Harvey *et al.*, 2002) in which it is about helping and enabling rather than persuading or telling (Aggergaard Larsen *et al.*, 2005). Harvey *et al.* (2002) further suggest that a key characteristic of skilled facilitation is that of not only affecting the context in which change is taking place, but also the ability to work with practitioners and in doing so make sense of the evidence being implemented. Furthermore, key to effect facilitation is the need to match the purpose, role and skills needed by the situation (Rycroft-Malone *et al.*, 2002) to the current context. Skilled facilitation can be seen as being core to practice development (Simmons, 2004) and effective working with both individuals and teams in the development of person-centred cultures of practice.

In facilitating the development of expertise in person-centred assessment with older people, at times Anne and I had travelled together, at other times along separate but parallel pathways as we explored and made sense ourselves of what we were learning within the context of our roles, culture underpinning practice with older people and teams in which we worked. At different times during the programme of practice development (that was ongoing), I had called upon (consciously and subconsciously) both technical and experiential knowledge that informed and underpinned how I worked and facilitated others. This called for both insight and understanding and the ability to make sense of and manage (if required) the many different variables that could occur during facilitation. At times this would take me away from my own 'comfort zone' and what I was familiar with and called for creativity through the use of both empirical and craft knowledge. I recognised that this intuitively lead to following different paths on occasions. However, I felt comfortable with diverting away from the planned route when necessitated by the situation. Underpinning this was joint learning with Anne and her team through critical reflection, this in turn subsequently informed my own actions that influenced how I worked with Anne and future teams as part of the same programme of practice development.

This can be seen as being clearly linked to the attributes of expertise (Box 7.2) as I synthesised different key attributes (and underpinning dimensions) of expertise such as 'holistic practice knowledge, saliency' and 'skilled know-how' into facilitation whilst working with Anne and her team. At the same time I was navigating my way around and working with broader organisational agendas along with many other sub-cultures. As a result of the insight and understanding gained through critical reflection, this informed how I worked and responded intuitively to different situations which subsequently informed my own learning and understanding as part of the programme of practice development. However, my journey was not purely about developing my own facilitation skills as a practice developer (although key), it was about making sense of a 'problem' that I had identified when I first came into my post in 2001 from which the programme of practice development had grown. Action research through its interrelated spirals based upon acting and observing, reflecting and developing a revised plan (Kemmis &

McTaggart, 1988) had enabled me to develop an understanding by working with Anne and by also being part of practice both as an 'insider' to the organisation and 'outsider' to the teams in which I was working.

Conclusion

This chapter opens by identifying the complexity of clearly defining expertise in the care of older people. Expertise in the care of older people does not fit into a neat box, similarly the context of nursing older people is infrequently neat and tidy because the real-life world of nursing and clinical practice can be 'messy', 'murky' and 'challenging'. Those in expert nursing roles do not work or function in isolation and as such can either capitalise or become vulnerable as a result of changing priorities within services or organisations. A reality may be that at times expertise may not be valued or seen as being of importance over more pressing requirements or agendas by individuals who do not see, understand or value the positive impact that expert nurses can make in delivering both the quality and strategic organisational agenda which are inter-linked. Therefore, the need to define clear measurable outcomes for both care and service delivery becomes an imperative along with the need to be able to clearly articulate and describe the impact of expert nursing at both micro and macro levels. The attributes of expertise can be seen as being a vital, conceptual resource to help nurses to articulate and make sense of how expertise is reflected within their roles which then in turn can be articulated and described to others.

Expertise cannot be described alone by tasks or technical activities as it is both multidimensional and multifaceted, requiring both theoretical and experiential knowledge that the expert nurse can use in a certain context and then translate and adapt to different situations. However, to achieve this, experts in clinical practice need support to develop both the skills and their understanding as expertise does not 'mystically' occur. Manley *et al.* (2008) in their cooperative inquiry into the leadership role of the consultant nurse working with older people identify the need to make explicit what is taken for granted. They also identify the need to support and make clear what is second nature and in turn the impact of expertise on older peoples' services. This highlights the importance of moving the notion of expertise in older people's nursing away from an ethereal concept to something that is measurable, visible and experienced by older people, their supporters and nurses working with older people in different settings.

Many nurses in expert roles in older people's nursing work across traditional interfaces and boundaries; therefore, the ability to synthesise knowledge and understanding through critical reasoning and then apply it to a different situation or context is key to expertise. Coupled with this is the need to be opportunistic and politically aware and to seize opportunities which will shape both local and national agendas. Expert knowledge (both theoretical and experiential) also needs to be fundamentally focused upon improving the older person's experience of care through empowering both practice and practitioners. This can be achieved by developing a greater understanding and insight into complex phenomena that can then be translated back into work-based cultures and environments through critical reasoning and skilled facilitation where older people and their supporters experience services or care.

Expertise is made up of the layers of empirical and craft knowledge gained from synthesising both types of knowledge that is underpinned by critical thinking and reasoning that influences how the expert nurse thinks, acts, articulates, enables others and clearly applies their knowledge to improve the older person's experience of care. Nurses working with older people need to be able to define and clearly articulate how expertise is reflected in their practice and the positive outcomes for care. For this to happen, organisations need also to support and enable expertise in practice to grow and flourish by creating and enabling, supportive, critically reflective cultures. Sustainable, expert person-centred care does not happen by accident, but through skilled facilitation that is underpinned by understanding the context of care, the values and beliefs of team members and a genuine belief to improve the older person's experience of care by enabling others and by transforming the culture of care.

Authors previously cited within this chapter have clearly identified the core elements of expertise in nursing and how it is clearly defined within contemporary health care. However, key to this is then how nurses apply this to their roles working with older people and their supporters, individuals, teams and the broader organisational situation/context. Reliance on describing the administration of technical tasks alone or the attainment of theoretical knowledge in isolation does not reflect expertise or the need for expert nursing. Similarly, technical approaches to developing practice will not ensure that expertise is translated and embedded into both clinical care and work-based cultures. The ultimate aim of expert nursing in the care of older people should be to improve the older person (and their supporters) experience of care through expert facilitation underpinned by a synthesis of both theoretical and experiential knowledge that is embedded in learning in and from practice. This can be seen as underpinning ways of working that keeps the older person central to all activity whilst facilitating a culture that transforms practitioners, teams and services and ultimately the older person's experience of expert, person-centred care.

Acknowledgements

My thanks to Loretta Bellman and Moira Whitlock for their help in writing this chapter.

References

Aggergaard Larsen, J., Maundrill, R., Morgan, J. & Mouland, L. (2005) Practice development facilitation: an integrated strategic and clinical approach. *Practice Development in Health Care* **4**(3), 142–149.

Benner, P. (1984) *From Novice to Expert*, pp. 2–5, 20–32. Addison Wesley, CA.

Clegg, A. & Mansfield, S. (2003) Nurse consultants and the care of older people: developing new role. *Nursing Older People* **15**(4), 14–16.

Coats, E., Dewing, J. & Titchen, A. (2006) *Opening Doors on Creativity: Resources to Awaken Creative Working. A Learning Resource.* Royal College of Nursing Institute, London.

Cohen, Z. (2003) The single assessment process: an opportunity for collaboration or a threat to the profession of occupational therapy? *British Journal of Occupational Therapy* **66**(5), 201–207.

Coulson, P. & Stickley, T. (2002) Finding a voice – artistic expression and practice development. *Practice Development in Health Care* **1**(2), 85–97.

Crouch, S. (1997) 'Bed blocking'. *Nursing Management* **4**(5), 24–25.

Dewing, J. (1994) Cited by McCormack, B. (2001) *Negotiating Partnerships with Older People – A Person Centred Approach*, p. 4. Ashgate, London.

Dewing, J. & Pritchard, E. (2000) *Nursing Assessment with Older People: A Person Centred Approach*, pp. 27–36, 52, 60, 62. RCN Institute, London.

DH (Department of Health) (2001) *The National Service Framework for Older People*, pp. 1, 30, 60. Stationery Office, London.

DH (Department of Health) (2006) *A New Ambition for Old Age, Next Steps in Implementing the National Service Framework for Older People*. Stationery Office, London.

Dreyfus, H.L. & Dreyfus, S.E. (1986) *Mind Over Machine: The Power of Human Intuition and Expertise in the Era of the Computer*. Free Press, New York.

Ford, P. & McCormack, B. (1999) The contribution of expert gerontological nursing. *Nursing Standard* **13**(25), 42–45.

Ford, P. & McCormack, B. (2000) Keeping the person in the centre of nursing. *Nursing Standard* **14**(46), 40–44.

Ford, P., Heath, H., McCormack, B. & Phair, L. (2004) *What a Difference a Nurse Makes*. Publication Code 000632. RCN, London.

Forster, S. (2004) In: *Nursing Older People: A Guide to Practice in Care Homes* (eds S. Carmody & S. Forster), pp. 1–11. Radcliffe, Oxford.

Freshwater, D. (2004) Emotional intelligence: developing emotionally literate training in mental health. *Mental Health Practice* **8**(4), 12–15.

Garbett, R. & McCormack, B. (2002) A concept analysis of practice development. *NT Research* **7**(2), 87–99.

Gibbs, G. (1988) *Learning by Doing: A Guide to Teaching and Learning Methods*. Further Education Unit, London.

Grundy, S. (1982) Three modes of action research. *Curriculum Perspectives* **2**(3), 23–34.

Hardy, S., Titchen, A., Manley, K. & McCormack, B. (2006) Redefining nursing expertise in the United Kingdom. *Nursing Science Quarterly* **19**(3), 260–264.

Harvey, G., Loftus-Hills, A., Rycroft-Malone, J., Titchen, A., Kitson, A., McCormack, B. & Seers, K. (2002) Getting evidence into practice: the role and function of facilitation. *Journal of Advanced Nursing* **37**(6), 577–588.

Kelly, T., Tolson, D., Schofield, I. & Booth, J. (2005) Describing gerontological nursing: an academic exercise or prerequisite for progress? *International Journal of Older People Nursing* **14**(3a), 12–23.

Kemmis, S. & McTaggart, R. (1988) *The Action Research Planner*, p 31. Deacon University Press, Victoria.

Kitwood, T. & Bredin, K. (1992) Towards a theory of dementia care: personhood and well-being. *Ageing and Society* **12**, 269–287.

Kydd, A. (2002) Focusing nursing care on the older person. *Nursing Times* **98**, 34–36.

Longley, M., Shaw, C. & Dolan, G. (2007) *Nursing: Towards 2015. A Report Commissioned by the Nursing and Midwifery Council.* NMC, London.

Lopez, M., Delmore, B., Ake, J., Kim, Y.R., Golden, G., Bier, J. & Fulmer, T. (2002) Implementing a geriatric resource model. *Journal of Nursing Administration* **32**, 577–585.

Manley, K. (1997) A conceptual framework for advanced practice: an action research project operationalizing an advanced practitioner/consultant nurse role. *Journal of Clinical Nursing* **6**, 179–190.

Manley, K. (2001) *Values Clarification Exercise. A Tool for Developing the RCN's Strategic Direction.* Royal College of Nursing, London.

Manley, K., Hardy, S., Titchen, A., Garbett, R. & McCormack, B. (2005) *Changing patients' worlds through nursing practice expertise. Exploring nursing practice expertise through emancipatory action research and fourth generation evaluation.* A Royal College of Nursing Report, 1998–2004, RCN, London.

Manley, K. & McCormack, B. (2003) Practice development: purpose, methodology, facilitation and evaluation. *Nursing in Critical Care* **8**(1), 22–29.

Manley, K. & McCormack, B. (2004) Practice development purpose, methodology, facilitation and evaluation. In: *Practice Development in Nursing* (eds B. McCormack, K. Manley & R. Garbett), pp. 35–40. Blackwell Publishing, Oxford.

Manley, K., Webster, J., Hayle, N., Hayes, N. & Minardi, H. (2008) Leadership role of consultant nurses working with older people: a co-operative enquiry. *Journal of Nursing Management* **16**, 147–158.

Marr, J. & Kershaw, B. (1998) *Caring for Older People – Developing Specialist Practice*, pp. 74–76. Arnold, London.

McCormack, B. (1998) Maximising life potential. *Elderly Care* **10**(3), 42–43.

McCormack, B. (2001) *Negotiating Partnerships with Older People – a Person-Centred Approach.* Ashgate, Basingstoke.

McCormack, B. & Ford, P. (1998) Nursing Older People, *Nursing Standard* **12**(24), 4–10.

Meyer, J. (2001) *Lay Participation in Care in a Hospital Setting*, pp. 1–9, 289, 311. Nursing Praxis International, Portsmouth.

Meare, J. & Bhowmick, B. (1995) Teamwork is the key to improving elderly assessments. *Care of the Elderly* **5**, 33–34.

Meyer, J. & Sturdy, D. (2004) Exploring the future of gerontological nursing outcomes. *International Journal of Older People Nursing* **13**(6b), 128–134.

NHS Institute for Innovation and Improvement (2007) Releasing Time to Care – The Productive Ward. Available from www.institute.nhs.uk/productiveward (accessed July 2008).

Nolan, M. (1997) Gerontological nursing: professional priority or eternal Cinderella? *Ageing and Society* **17**, 447–460.

Nolan, M. & Caldock, K. (1996) Assessment: identifying the barriers to good practice. *Health and Social Care in the Community* **4**(2), 77–85.

Oberski, I., Carter, D., Gray, M. & Ross, J. (1999) The community gerontological nurse: themes from a needs analysis. *Journal of Advanced Nursing* **29**(2), 454–462.

Policy + (2007) *Advanced Nursing Roles: Survival of the Fittest?* King's College London, London.

Pritchard, E. & Wright, J. (2001) Older people's specialist. *Nursing Older People* **13**(8), 33.

RCN (Royal College of Nursing) (1998) *Caring in Partnership: Older People and Nursing Staff Working towards the Future.* Publication code 002294, London.

RCN (Royal College of Nursing) (2004) *Caring in Partnership: Older People and Staff Working towards the Future*. Royal College of Nursing Publications, London.

RCN (Royal College of Nursing) (2005) *Changing patients' worlds through nursing practice expertise. Exploring nursing practice expertise through emancipatory action research and fourth generation evaluation*. A Royal College of Nursing Research Report, 1998–2004. RCN, London.

RCN (Royal College of Nursing) (2006) *Caring in Partnership: Two Years On*. Publication code 003102. RCN, London.

Redfern, S., Christian, S. & Norman, I. (2003) Evaluating change in healthcare practice: lessons from three studies. *Journal of Evaluation in Clinical Practice* **9**(2), 239–249.

Reed, J., Inglis, P., Cook, G., Clarke, C. & Cook, M. (2007) Specialist nurses for older people: implications from UK development sites. *Journal of Advanced Nursing* **58**(4), 368–376.

Rich, A. & Parker, D. (1995) Reflection and critical incident analysis. Ethical and normal implications of their use within nursing and midwifery education. *Journal of Advanced Nursing* **22**(4), 1302–1308.

Rolfe, G. (1996) *Closing the Theory Practice Gap*, pp. 17–18, 27, 134–137, 231, 232, 234. Butterworth Heinemann, London.

Rolfe, G. (1997) Science, abduction and the fuzzy nurse: an exploration of expertise. *Journal of Advanced Nursing* **15**(5), 1170–1075.

Rolfe, G. (1998) *Expanding Nursing Knowledge*, p. 32. Butterworth Heinemann, London.

Rolfe, G., Freshwater, D. & Jasper, M. (2001) *Critical Reflection for Nursing and the Helping Professions*, pp. 19, 40–74, 97, 128, 160. Palgrave, New York.

Rolfe, G. & Fulbrook, P. (1998) *Advanced Nursing Practice*. Butterworth Heineman, London.

Rycroft-Malone, J., Harvey, G., Kitson, A., McCormack, B., Seers, K. & Titchen, A. (2002) Getting evidence into practice: ingredients for change. *Nursing Standard* **16**(37), 38–43.

Schon, D. (1999) *The Reflective Practitioner. How Professionals Think in Action*, pp. 22–26, 50, 171–172. Avebury, Aldershol.

Simmons, M. (2004) 'Facilitation' of practice development: a concept analysis. *Practice Development in Health Care* **3**(1), 36–52.

Smith, C. (1995) Evaluating nursing care: reflections in practice. *Professional Nurse* **10**(11), 723–724.

Sturdy, D. (2004) Consultant Nurses: changing the future. *Age and Ageing* **33**, 327–328.

Thomas, L. & Bond, S. (1995) The effectiveness of nursing: a review. *Journal of Clinical Nursing* **4**, 143–151.

Titchen, A. (2000) *Professional Craft Knowledge in Patient-Centred Nursing and the Facilitation of Its Development*, pp. 111–149, 187. D.Phil. thesis, Linacre College, Oxford. Ashdale Press, Tackley, Oxfordshire.

Titchen, A. (2003) Critical companionship: part 1. *Nursing Standard* **18**(9), 33–40.

Titchen, A. & McGinley, M. (2003) Facilitating practitioner research through critical companionship. *NT Research* **8**(2), 115–131.

Walsh, K., Lawless, J., Moss, C. & Allbon, C. (2005) The development of an engagement tool for practice development. *Practice Development in Health Care* **4**(3), 124–130.

Webster, J. (1999) *Reflective Writing: A Study into the Process of Structured Reflection as a Tool for Individuals to Enhance and Develop Their Practice*. MSc dissertation, University of Portsmouth, UK.

Webster, J. (2002) Using reflective writing to gain a greater insight into practice. *Nursing Older People* **14**(9), 18–21.

Webster, J. (2004) Leading the switch to patient-centred care, *Professional Nurse* **20**(2), 20–21.

Webster, J. (2007) *Person-Centred Assessment with Older People. An Action Research Study to Explore Registered Nurses' Understanding of Person-Centred Assessment within a Framework of Emancipatory Practice Development.* PhD thesis, University of Portsmouth, UK.

Webster, J. (2008) Recognising, valuing and celebrating care for older people (Editorial). *Journal of Nursing Management* **16**, 97–98.

Webster, J. & Hayes, N. (2008) Specialists vs generalist care for older people. *Nursing Times* **104**(11), 12.

Welsh Assembly Government (2003) The strategy for older people in Wales. Available from http://wales.gov.uk/publications/circular/circulars03/NAFWC02003?lang=en (accessed January 2009).

8. The Role of the Consultant Nurse and Research in Articulating Expertise

Cheryl Crocker

Introduction

The consultant nurse role encompasses expertise in practice, education, consultancy, leadership and research. Research also includes service development and evaluation. It is therefore difficult to identify the exact level of engagement in research activity alone. In an evaluation study conducted by Guest *et al.* (2004), it was identified that the consultant role provided the credibility to develop services. There was evidence of a large number of initiatives which clearly involved research in some way. However, problems of evaluation and demonstrating impact were identified due to a lack of baseline data. Research tended to be longer term and as such there were few research outcomes cited (Guest *et al.*, 2004, p. 27). Overall, just over 48% of consultants stated they were engaged in research and development (Guest *et al.*, 2004, p. 24).

Demonstrating the nursing contribution to patient care and outcome is difficult. Spilsbury and Meyer (2001) demonstrated that available research is disparate and a range of methodologies have been used, which makes comparisons problematic. Their findings suggest evidence which reflects the positive impact of nursing care on patient outcome often fails to describe the structure and processes of care that contribute to what they call 'nursing-sensitive' outcomes (i.e. what nurses do). However, research invariably fails to address the 'invisible' (*sic*) aspects of nursing work (e.g. coordination of care, leadership and judgement). Moreover, the notion of expertise is not developed. Spilsbury and Meyer (2001) conclude that it may never be possible to define the nursing contribution to patient care, due to the ever-changing nature of nurses' work. Within this chapter, I aim to challenge that notion and report on the work completed as part of my doctorate research. The RCN Expertise in Practice report (Manley *et al.*, 2005) identified outcomes of expertise for participants, colleagues, organisations and patients. Research, I will show, is a tool that can be used to articulate expertise in practice.

This chapter provides an example where research has developed practice and, through the development of a nursing technology, provides a vehicle to develop and articulate expertise to others. I write this chapter from the perspective of a consultant nurse. Consultant nurses use additional expertise to develop and research actual practice and service provision with the intention of implementing findings en route.

Developing a nursing technology

Nurses adapt and change the sphere of their work in response to patient need, but rarely do they systematically monitor the process or impact of these changes. I aim to outline one such change to practice through a nursing technology. I will illustrate how expertise is key to the development of nursing technologies and I will introduce this through two concepts: (a) technology transferred and (b) technology transformed.

Nurse-led weaning was introduced by the consultant nurse in one Critical Care Unit in response to patient need. Weaning from mechanical ventilation was traditionally medically led. With six consultant intensivists, this was prone to be delivered inconsistently, in an ad hoc and uncoordinated manner. It was felt, as nurses were continually present at the patient bedside during these procedures, that they could initiate and lead weaning in a more systematic way. A review of the literature demonstrated that nurses have been using technology in the care of their patients but this was a double-edged sword. On the one hand, it could be used to reveal what nurses did and yet, on the other, it had the effect of masking their contribution (Sandelowski, 2000).

Through an ethnographic study, utilising participant observation and interviews, I collected over 250 h of field notes. I held a dual role, as consultant nurse and researcher, in my own area of work. As such I was able to describe in detail the culture of the unit and moreover describe my role as consultant nurse within the context of weaning from ventilation. This study was conducted over 6 months (full time) in one Critical Care Unit (comprised one high dependency and one intensive care unit). Twelve key informants were interviewed. These nurses were chosen because they were either involved in weaning patients or held key positions in the unit. Analysis of the interview data revealed four themes (Table 8.1).

Knowing the patient

Knowing the patient was inferred during interviews as essential to the delivery of patient-centred care. Observation of junior nurses practice revealed many nurses' knowing was framed in technological terms. These nurses assimilated information about their patients from a number of sources. One major source of information was the 24-h observation chart. This chart focused on physical data mostly generated from the available technology such as the ventilator and monitors. This had the effect of reducing patient care to a series of tasks with little attention paid to the psychological needs of the patient (Henderson, 1997).

Table 8.1 Themes of research

Theme	Sub-theme
Knowing the patient	Ways of knowing
	Continuity of care
	The role of the patient in weaning
The division of labour in weaning	Intra-occupational boundaries
	Inter-occupational boundaries
	The control of weaning
Nursing visibility	Nurses render themselves invisible
	Nurses are rendered invisible
	Making nursing visible 'doing the wash'
The nursing–technology relation	Definition of technology and weaning
	Weaning – a technology transferred
	Weaning – a technology transformed

In this sense, technology limited the extent to which nurses were able to get to know their patients. Knowing the patient is an important aspect of nursing (Tanner *et al.*, 1993; Ball & McElligott, 2002). Many studies have been conducted in order to define the exact meaning of knowing and attempts have been made to describe and analyse how this is realised in nursing (May, 1991; Jenny & Logan, 1992; May, 1992; Radwin, 1995, 1996; Henderson, 1997; Sandelowski, 1998; Luker *et al.*, 2000). In order to know a patient as an individual, a number of factors have been identified from the literature: mutual trust and rapport, a positive nurse–patient attitude and sustained patient contact (Henderson, 1997), the delivery of individual patient care (Radwin, 1996; Henderson, 1997), promoting the patient's own decisions and relinquish efforts to control the patient (Manley *et al.*, 2005) and continuity of care (Morse, 1991; Ball & McElligott, 2002). Knowing the patient is identified as an attribute of nursing expertise (Benner, 1984; Jenny & Logan, 1992; Radwin, 1996; Manley *et al.*, 2005).

In this study, patients were treated as passive recipients of care, yet their cooperation with weaning plans and strategies was essential. Nursing care practices served to limit patients' autonomy in weaning. Patients were expected to follow a weaning trajectory. This was identified as a predictable course of recovery with goals set by the medical or nursing staff, rather than the patient. This resulted in the patient assuming a passive role with little autonomy. Many of the nurses allocated to look after patients who were weaning were advanced beginners. The paradox is that whilst these patients have complex physical and psychological needs, they are not deemed to be critically ill and are more likely to be cared for by nurses who have not yet developed their nursing expertise. As a result of the study, these issues have been addressed. Continuity of care is emphasised and more experienced nurses are allocated to look after patients who are weaning. Patients are included in their weaning plan and both nurses and doctors accept that weaning trajectories are not linear.

The division of labour in weaning

The introduction of nurse-led weaning highlighted tensions inherent in boundary working. The transfer of technology to nurses resulted in a change in the content of nursing work which created tensions between nurses and between doctors and nurses.

In Allen's (1996) study, the organisation of work created tensions for nurses. Nurses found they did not have the time to spend doing what they perceived as tasks related to the core of their role (Allen, 1996). Nurses in her study stated at interview that they would control this by leaving doctor-devolved tasks until all nursing tasks had been completed. However, Allen (1996) observed that nurses continued to complete these tasks, regardless of their work pressures. In this (my) ethnographic study, nurses would leave weaning until other tasks had been completed; often, if they were too busy, weaning would either not progress or fail to commence. There are a number of reasons put forward for this. One is that the majority of nurses allocated to look after patients who were weaning were junior and therefore as advanced beginners they work to a schedule orientated to getting the (nursing) work done (Melia, 1987). Another explanation may lie with the complexity of weaning itself. Egerod (2003) found that the stages of weaning were difficult to identify leading to confusion regarding the onset of weaning.

Styles of decision-making adopted by junior nursing staff were a combination of what Stein (1967) described as the doctor–nurse 'game' and informal covert decision-making, as described by Porter (1991). However, this was not as unproblematic as previously described in the literature (Stein, 1967; Hughes, 1988; Stein *et al.*, 1990; Porter, 1991; Allen, 1997). Nurses also used an 'intra-occupational mediator', being the consultant nurse. This term has not been used in the literature before and was observed as an approach used usually by more senior nurses. This had the effect of giving the appearance that nurses were working in harmony with medical staff whilst at the same time influencing patient care. Nurses may have felt powerless. As identified by Allen (2001), nurses perceived position in health care hierarchy meant they felt they had little power to influence senior medical staff themselves, and therefore had to rely on an intra-occupational mediator (the consultant nurse). This approach can be explained by the authority and autonomy that the consultant nurse was perceived to possess (Manley *et al.*, 2005). This level of 'expertise', as described by Manley *et al.*, exuded a confidence that others recognised and responded to. Moreover, autonomy is recognised by a willingness to challenge whole teams and senior colleagues, if patient care is compromised (Manley *et al.*, 2005). In addition, the consultant nurse was the only nurse, with one or two exceptions, to use formal overt decision-making strategies. The consultant nurse challenged traditional ways of working, revealing a willingness to disturb status quo in order to achieve person-centred care. This could result in a difference of opinion with medical teams. As a result of the study, nurse-led weaning has been embraced and previous tensions between doctors and nurses have resolved. Nurses feel empowered and more confident. In introducing nurse-led weaning, the consultant nurse used her skilled know-how, enabling others through a willingness to share knowledge and skills (Manley *et al.*, 2005). There is evidence of team working rather than the professional groups working in silos.

Nursing visibility

Nurses rendered themselves 'invisible' in two ways. First, by their lack of participation in the ward round, and second, through the allocation of more junior nurses to patients who were weaning. The ward round was seen as the 'medical' round and as separate from nursing (Busby & Gilchrist, 1992). Both the bedside nurse and the shift coordinator were frequently absent from the round. When the shift coordinator was present, their role was limited to an information broker (Manias & Street, 2001), transcribing medical information to the next shift with minimal attention given to nursing care (Erkman & Segesten, 1995), or as Porter (1991) refers to as 'listening in on the side lines'. Nurses therefore missed the opportunity of using the ward round as a multi-professional team discussion and plan the care of a patient, which in turn enhances quality patient care (Thomas, 1989; Wright *et al.*, 1996; Felten *et al.*, 1997).

As a result of this study, I (as the consultant nurse) have changed how I use practice time. I accompany the team on the round, providing and articulating holistic practice knowledge, thus making more visible the nursing contribution to care and through a process of enabling others to participate through saliency and skilled know-how (refer again to Box 1.2 and Figure 1.1). As a result, nurses are much more visible and it has become custom and practice for nurses to participate. Nurses are able to articulate information about their patient to the medical teams, which enhances care.

Nurses attempted to make visible their contribution to care through 'the wash'. The 'wash' or 'bed bath' was seen as an important and essential part of routine aspects of nursing care. This study demonstrates that this routine was ritualised. Walsh and Ford (1989) define rituals as routine care tasks, performed without logic, whereas others have suggested a number of reasons why nurses engage in rituals. Wolf (1989) suggests this can be a therapeutic act, whilst Melia (1987) interpreted rituals as a way of getting the work done. Menzies (1970) suggested that decision-making can be stressful and rituals serve to limit decision-making releasing anxiety or tension. For nurses, the wash ritual offered a structure and helped organise their shift. Nurses no longer 'wash' at the same time as the ward round. Nurses coordinate their patient's care, and privacy and dignity are respected (an example of improved moral agency). In this way, nurses are now present at the time of the round and are better able to convey information about the patient to their medical colleagues.

Nursing–technology relation

Interviews and observation in practice revealed that nurses saw technology as machinery and equipment, which is congruent with the study by Barnard and Gerber (1999). However, nurses' view of the ventilator as a technology changed depending on the reason it was used. The ventilator has become a symbol of critical illness. Although nurses related to the ventilator in terms of equipment, it held a different meaning when weaning began. This is congruent with Sandelowski (2000), who stated that technologies are context dependent and this is reliant upon how they are used. Patients who were weaning were not considered critically ill. The ventilator was seen as a medical technology. This limited their role in the monitoring and recording of observations. Whilst nurses saw their role as monitoring and recording of observations, there was no need for them to develop further skills in dealing with the ventilator itself. Technological mastery has been identified as an essential component in the development of competence in critical care nursing practice (Ray, 1987; McConnell, 1990; Cooper, 1993; Walters, 1995; Locsin, 1998; Barnard & Gerber, 1999; Barnard, 2000; Little, 2000; Alasad, 2002; Wilkstrom & Larson, 2004). In this study, nurses did not master the technology but rather learned what Bevan (1998) described as 'superficial survival skills'.

Nurses' view of weaning was a reflection of the medical literature (Knebel, 1991; Mancebo, 1996; American College of Chest Physicians, the American Association for Respiratory Care and the American College of Critical Care Medicine, 2002). This view of weaning renders the patient as a passive recipient of care and serves to limit the nursing role. Nurses did not fully understand weaning in terms of the need to optimise and plan for weaning in advance of the patient being ready. There was little agreement about where weaning began and weaning finished.

Weaning: a technology transferred

Weaning was transferred from doctors to nurses. I define technology transferred to mean a task-focused approach to technology as 'equipment'. What appeared on the surface to be a relatively easy transfer of responsibility from doctor to nurse had not been the case. The transfer of a technology can also relate, as it does in this study, to different geographical places. There was a reluctance to transfer patients who were weaning to HDU and to use the non-invasive ventilators on ICU. Nurses saw weaning as a task devolved to them from the medical staff. Their role in weaning was limited by the technology. They focused on recording technology-generated data on to the 24-h observation chart. Barnard and Sandelowski describe the tensions that certain technologies present to nurses and suggest this is not the technology per se but the way nurses use and perceive them (Barnard & Sandelowski, 2001). Sandelowski suggests that technologies transferred are not simply the hardware components but also the values, norms and practices, and these may be in conflict with the receiving culture (Sandelowski, 2000). Receiving cultures, she suggests, may alter these technologies (Sandelowski, 2000). She goes on to state that nurses should determine which technologies are congruent with the values of nursing or as she puts it 'authentic tools of the trade' (Sandelowski, 1996, p. 13). The difficulty is in knowing what these are. I suggest one way of achieving this is to transform those (medical) technologies for nursing purposes, thus creating nursing technologies and it is here that nursing expertise is required.

Technology transferred

A definition

The transfer of technology refers to tasks, roles or use of equipment formally undertaken by one professional group that are devolved to another. This is commonly seen in the devolvement of tasks to nurses formally undertaken by doctors and referred to as an extension to nursing practice. This transfer does not include the devolvement of power or control of that technology. The transfer of technology may not always result in improvements to patient care/outcomes.

The transfer of technology often results in blurring of boundaries but it can also result in the creation of new roles specific to that technology as was suggested by nurses in this study (examples from nursing include clinical nurse specialists or advanced practice roles). In this ethnography, the transfer of technology served to limit the nursing role and as such the nursing contribution was marginalised.

Weaning: a technology transformed

There were examples when nurses interpreted technology not as a medical technology transferred to them, but used it to improve the care and therefore outcomes of patients who were weaning. I refer to this as a technology transformed. The literature does not clearly differentiate between a 'medical' technology transferred to nurses and a technology transformed by nurses. I therefore draw on a composite of literature to help interpret this concept. The following excerpt from this ethnography demonstrates how an expert nurse uses his skills and knowledge of weaning to enable him to assess patients and is an example of holistic nursing practice as described by Manley *et al.* (2005):

> You need to look at why patients are not weaning. It is not a case of just turning down the pressures you need to ask have they developed another hospital acquired infection? What is their fluid balance like? We know full well those patients who are long-term weaners get repeated infections. It's obvious if they are producing loads of sputum and they have a high temperature and you cannot wean. You need to look at other things like their fluid balance, if someone is exceptionally boggy (over hydrated), patients do accumulate fluid over a period of days so that is another reason why they do not wean. You need to look at the patient holistically.
>
> *Interview, P2*

His view was based on the need to see the patient holistically, using a systematic assessment in order to draw information about the patient's ability to wean. Furthermore, he saw weaning not just as following a protocol but in looking for and recognising patient cues, described as saliency by Manley *et al.* (2005) that would allow for an individual weaning plan to be made.

Alexander and Kroposki (2001) state in their description of a nursing technology that nurses require specialised knowledge of patients and their biophysical and psychological responses to ill health. What they fail to mention is the knowledge that constitutes 'knowing a patient'. This cannot be gained from biomedical data alone but requires the nurse to actually get to know the patient as an individual (Jenny & Logan, 1992; Radwin, 1996) and getting to know the patient requires expertise (Benner, 1984; Manley *et al.*, 2005). The provision of individualised and continuous care increases the probability of knowing the patient and is essential to successful weaning (Jenny & Logan, 1992).

A patient who had been on the unit for 20 days was demonstrating signs of altered mood. The next excerpt from field notes suggests the nurse was aware of the psychological needs of patients and the influence this had on weaning. The patient was withdrawn and anxious. His anxiety often resulted in an increase in respiratory rate and as such he would tire easily, thus weaning was often problematic:

> The night nurse was frustrated that the patient had not progressed in fact his weaning was deteriorating. There was a discussion about the patient's psychological status and it was decided to move the patient's bed so that he could see what was happening on the unit.
>
> *Field notes, ICU 9.0.04*

The next excerpt indicates how the nurse recognised patient cues and her ability to respond to them in a timely manner:

> I know from experience that when you come on to your shift and have handover about the patient, you start by looking at them from the baseline, by looking at the gases and look at the patient overall. You get a feeling what works and what doesn't. If it doesn't work you have a discussion with the intensivist or the nurse in charge. I think we are really good. We have initiated weaning and paid no attention to the doctors when it first came out (nurse-led weaning), so this is what we (nurses) do. We are quite eager not to sit on some body and wait for a certain time or wait for the doctors to come along.
>
> *Interview, P3*

In this example, the nurse does not wait for the doctor but is confident to initiate weaning, but recognises that there are a number of experts on which to call upon if a strategy did not work, then she would draw on the expertise of others in the team. Interestingly, she indicated she was eager to embrace nurse-led weaning by ignoring the medical staff when they were felt to interfere. This nurse indicated clearly that she needed to know her patient in order to plan weaning and this meant planning her work around the patient. Knowledge, experience and exposure were identified by Ball and McElligott (2002) as key nursing attributes to the recovery of critically ill patients and this related to the ability to identify patient cues:

> What works for one patient will not work for some one else and you need to get to know them, their personality has a lot to do with it, if they are anxious and you know what makes them anxious. You can see their pattern of respiration changing a lot of the time and the intervention you give, so you can plan your day and your daily tasks around them and support them.
>
> *Interview, P3*

The next excerpt is an account of my role as a consultant nurse. In my daily rounds of patients, I would review all patients who were weaning. The following patient has been on the unit a number of days and was therefore known to me. The patient was struggling to breathe but this was interpreted by the bedside nurse as a panic attack:

> I intervened by increasing the respiratory support for a patient who was breathless. The nurse had interpreted this as panicking but when I spoke to the patient she explained she had been unable to get her breath during the night and this frightened her. She was also anxious that she had not made progress, she was obviously tired and fed up.
>
> *Field notes, ICU 27.04.04*

In knowing the patient, I was able to pick up on the cues the patient was displaying and intervene. I was able to reassure her and ask her how she was feeling. I understood she was anxious and was able to use my expertise and experience to help the patient cope with her fear and frustration. I explained she had made progress but that weaning often meant going forwards and backwards and every patient's weaning was individual to them. We discussed her weaning plan and she appeared calm, her breathing was easier.

Alexander and Kroposki (2001) identify raw materials as patients and state they influence the technology used for the patient. This view does not take into account the nursing–technology relation and how this is affected by issues such as power, gender and the control of technology. The patient role is central in weaning. In this example, the patients were seen as an active partner in their care.

I observed one nurse who was very involved in the ward round. She actively engaged with the medical staff and her aim was to coordinate a medical procedure. This nurse recognised that the nurse's participation in the ward round was part of the nurse's role. It was important that the nurse was able to contribute in order to add to the medical knowledge about the patient. She was also proactive in finding out about the plan for the day in order that she could organise her activities accordingly. Field notes reveal that she planned her work around the patient, leaving her break until after the patient had been cared for and ensuring she did not miss the ward round:

> What we did is we went for a really quick wean and see if she can tolerate it. She had a tracheostomy so we gave her time to recover from that, after all it is a general anaesthetic. She just needed a bit of time, she was irritated by it (tracheostomy), she was coughing and coughing. We put her on CPAP, but that was a little too much for her. We did not want to push her, so we gave her some sedation to ease the cough. We gave her a little longer time and she did settle and she was more comfortable.
>
> *Interview, P8*

Important in weaning, according to Egerod (2003), is the need to experiment; at first, if one approach does not work then another is tried. The importance of recognising that each patient has an individual trajectory is demonstrated here:

I think a long day is a good thing because you know it is over a longer period of time and you can try different approaches to your weaning. Like the other month I went from the ventilator to low flow in a 12-hour shift which was fantastic. This was beneficial for the patient and I could tell within three hours that he was not going to be a slow wean. He was going to be quick and I would let him take the lead and I would support him gently and that was fantastic. He was a successful wean. Every patient is an individual.

Interview, P3

The role of the patient in this excerpt is not as a passive recipient of care but as a partner and the nurse demonstrated she worked with the patient in order to move his weaning on, she acted in a supporting role, monitoring and responding to his cues.

One nurse demonstrated how she was working proactively in order to expedite the weaning process. She used her skills as a nurse to assess and plan the care of her patient:

I am very interested in weaning myself and I really enjoy nurse-led weaning on the unit. I think it is very beneficial and I think when you come and you have a patient with so many problems, just looking at them visually, struggling to breathe. There are so many things that could be rectified to support them and that could be the underlying reason why they are unsuccessful. I like to sort that out. For example he (the patient) had no feed going and I started it again because yesterday he was vomiting and constipated and that is now resolved. I like to kick in with the nutrition and underlying support for him to get back to normal. If I could start looking at the weaning process and then to initiate it and you know contribute something to it. To start weaning his pressures or the level back down to whatever support he needs.

Interview, P3

This staff nurse demonstrates she was able to assess and plan the care of her patient on an individual basis. She knew him as a person and there had been some continuity of care. She actively enjoyed patients who were weaning. There was a sense of achievement if she managed to progress the care of her patient.

On occasions, as a consultant nurse, nurses would ask my opinion or ask for advice in order that weaning progressed. On other occasions, nurses felt at liberty to alter weaning plans in order that weaning was continuous and reflected the needs of the individual patient:

One of the respiratory physicians had written a weaning plan and the nursing staff ignored it. When I asked them why, they replied that the patient was doing well, so rather than take a step back by following the doctors plan they continued with their own plan.

Field notes, ICU 20.07.04

More frequently, I intervened in the patient's care when I recognised nurses needed help. On this occasion, I was approaching the patient's bed when I noticed the ventilator alarm:

> I noticed the ventilator alarm was reading apnoea, the nurse came over and said it had been happening a lot that morning. I was concerned but she did not appear to share this concern. I immediately changed the patient's mask, completed an assessment and explained what I was doing. I began to write a plan but the nurse felt the patient had only just arrived and therefore there was no need for a weaning plan yet. I explained weaning is not just about reducing the support sometimes it needs to go up as well and that was what I was doing. What was also important was the need to communicate this to ensure continuity of care.
>
> *Field notes, HDU 12. 08.04*

Planning for weaning is as important as actively weaning. Delays in weaning are experienced when nurses do not plan in advance. Although on this occasion the patient had just arrived, it was important to make a plan from the beginning for (non-invasive) ventilation. I was also able to see that the patient was mouth breathing and therefore a nasal mask meant the patient was not effectively ventilating. I changed the mask to a facemask.

The next extract from field notes is an example of my role as consultant nurse who is asked to review a patient in HDU. The nursing staff felt they were unable to progress the patient's weaning further:

> I am asked to visit a patient on the unit by a G grade who wants my advice on a patient they are finding difficult to wean. I visit the patient and the nurse at the bedside gives me a summary of the patient's medical problems. Whilst this is occurring I watch the patient. I notice how he is breathing, the rate, depth of the breath, use of accessory muscles, he looks a little sweaty but his pulse and blood pressure are OK. I speak to the patient and introduce myself, asking him 'how are you and how is your breathing to day?' Whilst I do this I place my hand on the patient in order to feel his temperature, I am also able to take his pulse, all the time though I touch him in a way as to say 'you are in safe hands, trust me'. He can answer me by mouthing sentences (he has a tracheostomy) but he does not appear breathless and can complete his sentence. He is fed up and appears anxious. After reading his medical notes and scanning the observation charts I listen to the patient's chest and examine the chest X-Ray. I complete a head-to-toe examination, noting his fluid balance over the last few days, I note he is oedematous (swollen). I scan his drug chart for drugs such as steroids, antibiotics (for course, strength and duration), diuretics (water tablets) and antidepressants etc. any information which builds a picture of this patient and how this will affect his weaning. I note he has pseudomonas (an infection) on his chest and this will inevitably increase the amount of sputum. He has been with us now for 12 days, the course of events lead me to believe his weaning will need to be gradual and he will require periods of rest. After I finish my physical

examination I return to talking with the patient. I ask him about how he is at home, what he hopes to achieve and how he feels his progress has been. It is obvious he had hoped to progress much quicker and is frustrated by the pace of weaning. I explain what the options are and suggest we devise a weaning plan together, the three of us, the patient, the bedside nurse and me. I negotiate goals, small periods of time off the ventilator with periods of rest, we plan one day at a time. The patient appears happy with this and after a chat about his family I leave. I return the next day to see he has met his goals and we repeat the process, this time increasing time off the ventilator. He appears happier today. Five days later the patient is off the ventilator and waiting to be discharged to the ward.

Field notes, HDU 13.08.04

This is an example of how a 'medical' technology transferred to nurses was transformed by the consultant nurse and used to improve patient outcomes (Chapter 3 identified this in the literature as a catalyst attribute). This excerpt demonstrates a number of characteristics of a technology transformed. The nurse is an expert and used her expertise and experience of weaning in order to assess and plan for weaning. An evaluation of previous weaning attempts was made. The patient is very much the focus of attention and involved in the assessment and planning stages. Goals are set that are patient focused and reviewed daily. The plan is individual and communication of that plan is an important factor to ensure that the consultant nurse includes the bedside nurse. Continuity is achieved as the consultant nurse reviews the patient on a daily basis. The consultant nurse takes responsibility for weaning, setting parameters for the bedside nurse and by providing informal teaching.

Definition of a nursing technology

A nursing technology can be defined as the delivery of proactive, patient-centred and individualised care, where care delivery centres on knowing the patient, drawing on nursing expertise with clearly defined lines of accountability, responsibility and autonomy. Nursing technologies are those developed by nurses in order to improve patient outcome. A nursing technology incorporates not only the object (equipment) but also the processes of care and knowledge associated with that technology. The definition of a nursing technology proposed by Alexander and Kroposki (2001) is limited. It assumes that everything nurses do is a nursing technology; however, as seen in this ethnography, technology can be transferred, and as Purnell (1998) has pointed out, not all technologies used by nurses are nursing technologies.

The characteristics of a technology transformed are listed in Figure 8.1. Nurses require knowledge, experience of and exposure to weaning. Experienced nurses work in a proactive manner providing close surveillance and immediately respond to patient cues and in this way are able to reduce the risk to patients. Weaning is nurse led, with patient-focused goals. Technology in this respect is an embodied approach to care, seen not as an adjunct to care, or as a means of bridging a gap between technology and care, but as a total process including the knowledge, skills and equipment that encompass the nursing care of the individual.

161

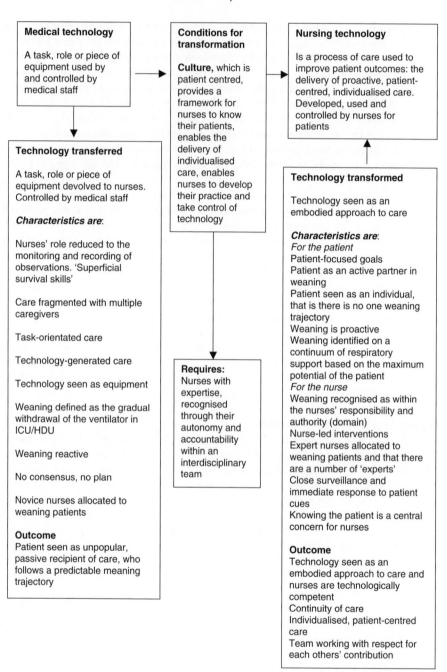

Figure 8.1 Defining concepts of technology transferred and technology transformed, their relationship and outcomes.

Weaning is planned when ventilation begins and is therefore proactive. Weaning is the nurses' responsibility. Nurses do not work in isolation but appreciate there are a number of experts in weaning to draw and learn from. They work as part of a cohesive team.

Conclusion

This chapter has demonstrated that expertise can be articulated to others through research. Research in this context has been *in* and *on* practice. The role of the consultant nurse has been made visible. The consultant nurse is a recognised expert in practice, but also uses research to develop and inform practice, not just their own, but for others. Outcomes from this research have revealed also how transforming care has the benefit of transforming technical, task, ritualistic care into patient-centred and negotiated interventions. The development of a nursing technology, as shown here, has meant that nurses examine their contribution to practice, articulate this to others and ultimately improve patient outcomes. Furthermore, nursing expertise has been demonstrated through the development of a nursing technology. This has been articulated through the example and differentiation between medical technology, technology transferred and a nursing technology that enabled transformation of practice.

References

Alasad, J. (2002) Managing technology in the intensive care unit: the nurses' experience. *International Journal of Nursing Studies* **39**, 407–413.

Alexander, J. & Kroposki, M. (2001) Using a management perspective to define and measure changes in nursing technology. *Journal of Advanced Nursing* **35**(5), 776–783.

Allen, D. (1996) *The Shape of General Nursing: The Division of Labour at Work*. PhD Thesis. The University of Nottingham, Nottingham.

Allen, D. (1997) The nursing – medical boundary: a negotiated order? *Sociology of Health and Illness* **19**(4), 498–520.

Allen, D. (2001) *The Changing Shape of Nursing Practice: The Role of Nurses in the Hospital Division of Labour*. Routledge, London.

American College of Chest Physicians, the American Association for Respiratory Care and the American College of Critical Care Medicine (Collective Task Force) (2002) Evidence-based guidelines for weaning and discontinuing ventilatory support. *Respiratory Care* **47**(1), 69–90.

Ball, C. & McElligott, M. (2002) Realising the potential of critical care nurses: an exploration of the factors that affect and comprise the nursing contribution to the recovery of critically ill patients. *London Standing Conference, London. WWW.ISCN. Co. UK* (report in full).

Barnard, A. (2000) Alteration of will as an experience of technology and nursing. *Journal of Advanced Nursing* **31**(5), 1136–1144.

Barnard, A. & Gerber, R. (1999) Understanding technology in contemporary surgical nursing: a phenomenographic examination. *Nursing Inquiry* **6**, 157–166.

Barnard, A. & Sandelowski, M. (2001) Technology and humane nursing care (ir)reconcilable differences or invented difference? *Journal of Advanced Nursing* **34**(3), 367–375.

Benner, P. (1984) *From Novice to Expert: Excellence and Power in Clinical Nursing Practice.* Addison-Wesley, London.

Bevan, M. (1998) Nursing in the dialysis unit: technological enframing and a declining art, or an imperative for caring. *Journal of Advanced Nursing* **27**(4), 730–736.

Busby, A. & Gilchrist, B. (1992) The role of the nurse in the medical ward round. *Journal of Advanced Nursing* **17**, 339–346.

Cooper, M.A. (1993) The intersection of technology and care in the ICU. *Advances in Nursing Science* **15**(3), 23–32.

Egerod, I. (2003) *Mechanical Ventilator Weaning in the Context of Critical Care Nursing: A Descriptive, Comparative Study of Nurse's Decisions and Interventions Related to Mechanical Ventilation Weaning.* PhD Thesis. University of Copenhagen.

Erkman, I. & Segesten, K. (1995) Deputed power of medical control: the hidden message in the ritual of oral shift reports. *Journal of Advanced Nursing* **22**(5), 1006–1011.

Felten, S., Cady, N., Metzler, M. & Burton, S. (1997) Implementation of collaborative practice through interdisciplinary rounds on a general surgery service. *Nursing Case Management* **2**, 122–126.

Guest, D., Peccei, R., Rosenthal, P., Redfern, S., Wilson-Barnett, J., Dewe, P., Coster, S., Evans, A. & Sudbury, A. (2004) *An Evaluation of the Impact of Nurse, Midwife and Health Visitor Consultants.* King's College, London.

Henderson, S. (1997) Knowing the patient and the impact on patient participation: a grounded theory study. *International Journal of Nursing Practice* **3**(2), 111–118.

Hughes, D. (1988) When nurse knows best: some aspects of the doctor–nurse interaction in a casualty department. *Sociology of Health and Illness* **10**, 1–22.

Jenny, J. & Logan, J. (1992) Knowing the patient: one aspect of clinical knowledge. *Image* **24**, 254–258.

Knebel, A. (1991) Weaning from mechanical ventilation: current controversies. *Heart & Lung* **20**, 321–334.

Little, C. (2000) Technological competence as a fundamental structure of learning in critical care nursing: a phenomenological study. *Journal of Clinical Nursing* **9**(3), 391–399.

Locsin, R. (1998) Technologic competence as caring in critical care nursing. *Holistic Nursing Practice* **12**(4), 50–56.

Luker, K., Austin, L., Caress, A. & Hallett, C. (2000) The importance of knowing the patient: community nurses' constructions of quality in providing palliative care. *Journal of Advanced Nursing* **31**(4), 775–782.

Mancebo, J. (1996) Weaning from mechanical ventilation. *The European Respiratory Journal* **9**, 1923–1931.

Manias, E. & Street, A. (2001) Nurse–doctor interactions during critical care ward rounds. *Journal of Clinical Nursing* **10**, 442–450.

Manley, K., Hardy, S., Tichen, A., Garbett, R. & McCormack, B. (2005) *Changing Patients' Worlds through Nursing Practice Expertise: Exploring Nursing Practice through Emancipatory and Fourth Generation Evaluation.* Royal College of Nursing, London.

May, C. (1991) Affective neutrality and involvement in nurse–patient relationships: perceptions of appropriate behaviour among nurses in acute medical and surgical wards. *Journal of Advanced Nursing* **16**, 552–558.

May, C. (1992) Nursing work, nurses' knowledge, and the subjectification of the patient. *Sociology of Health and Illness* **14**(4), 472–487.

McConnell, E. (1990) The impact of machines on the work of critical care nurses. *Critical Care Nursing Quarterly* **12**(4), 45–52.

Melia, K. (1987) *Learning and Working: The Occupational Socialization of Nurses*. Tavistock, London.

Menzies, I. (1970) *The Functioning of Social Systems as a Defence against Anxiety: A Report on the Study of the Nursing Service of a General Hospital*. Tavistock Institute of Human Relations, London.

Morse, J. (1991) Negotiating commitment and involvement in the nurse–patient relationship. *Journal of Advanced Nursing* **16**, 455–468.

Porter, S. (1991) A participant observation study of power relations between nurses and doctors in a general hospital. *Journal of American Nursing* **16**, 728–735.

Purnell, M. (1998) Who really makes the bed? Uncovering technologic dissonance in nursing. *Holistic Nursing Practice* **12**(4), 12–22.

Radwin, L. (1995) Knowing the patient: a process model for individualised interventions. *Nursing Research* **44**(6), 364–370.

Radwin, L. (1996) Knowing the patient: a review of research on an emerging concept. *Journal of Advanced Nursing* **23**(6), 1142–1146.

Ray, M.A. (1987) Technological caring: a new model in critical care. *Dimensions of Critical Care Nursing* **6**(3), 166–173.

Sandelowski, M. (1996) Tools of the trade: analysing technology as an object in nursing practice. *Scholarly Inquiry for Nursing Practice: An International Journal* **10**(1), 5–16.

Sandelowski, M. (1998) Looking to care or caring to look? Technology and the rise of spectacular nursing. *Holistic Nursing Practice* **12**(4), 1–11.

Sandelowski, M. (2000) *Devices and Desires: Gender, Technology and American Nursing*. University of North Carolina, Chapel Hill, NC.

Spilsbury, K. & Meyer, J. (2001) Defining the nursing contribution to patient outcome: lessons from a review of the literature examining nursing outcomes, skill mix and changing roles. *Journal of Clinical Nursing* **10**(1), 3–14.

Stein, L. (1967) The doctor–nurse game. *Archives of General Psychiatry* **16**, 699–703.

Tanner, C., Benner, C., Chesla, C. & Gordon, D. (1993) The phenomenology of knowing the patient. *Image Journal of Nursing Scholarship* **25**(4), 273–280.

Thomas, J. (1989) The changing role of the ICU nurse in medical rounds. *Canadian Critical Care Nursing Journal* **6**(1), 4–9.

Walsh, M. & Ford, P. (1989) *Nursing Rituals: Research and Rational Actions*. Heinemann Nursing, Oxford.

Walters, A. (1995) A heideggerian hermenutic study of the practices of critical care nurses. *Journal of Advanced Nursing* **21**(3), 492–497.

Wilkstrom, A. & Larson, U. (2004) Technology – an actor in the ICU: a study in workplace tradition. *Journal of Clinical Nursing* **13**(5), 555–561.

Wolf, Z.R. (1989) Uncovering the hidden work of nursing. *Nursing and Health Care* **10**, 462–467.

Wright, S., Bowkett, J. & Bray, K. (1996) Development in practice. The communication gap in the ICU – a possible solution. *Nursing in Critical Care* **1**, 241–244.

9. The Impact of Clinical Expertise on Patient Care in Rheumatology

Sarah Ryan

Introduction

Rheumatological conditions are both commonplace and diverse with as many as 200 different disorders (Symmons & Bankhead, 1994). Rheumatoid arthritis (RA) is a relatively common, chronic heterogeneous condition affecting 1–3% of the population in western countries with a 3:1 female preponderance (Hartzheim & Gross, 1998). It is the most frequent condition seen in nurse-led clinics. It is an autoimmune, inflammatory condition of the synovium which lines both the joints and tendon sheaths of the body. The inflammatory process results in pain, stiffness and fatigue. Systemic manifestations are common including weight loss and anaemia. The condition is characterised by unpredictability regarding the occurrence of symptoms, the efficacy of the treatment programme and the overall prognosis (Ryan *et al.*, 2003). Consequently, one of the objectives of treatment is to enable patients to cope with this unpredictability and to gain perceived control over the daily consequences of the condition. Other aims of treatment include reducing symptoms, suppressing the condition to prevent joint deformity and maintaining optimal physical, psychological and social function.

Treatment involves the use of drug therapy (to improve symptoms and reduce progression and deformity), exercise (to maintain muscle strength and mobility) and education to enable patients to develop self-management strategies to cope with the everyday symptoms. Living with RA has psychological and social consequences on mood, self-esteem, social relationships and work with patients twice as likely to experience depression than the general populations (Devins *et al.*, 1993; Dickens & Creed, 2001; Ryan *et al.*, 2003).

This chapter will explore how the attributes of nursing expertise, holistic practice knowledge, skilled know-how, knowing the patient, saliency and moral agency can be used within rheumatology nursing to improve health outcomes of patients.

Box 9.1   The elements of nursing (Wilson-Barnett, 1984)

- Understanding illness and treatment from the patient's perspective;
- Providing continuous psychological care during illness and critical events;
- Helping people cope with illness and critical events;
- Providing comfort;
- Coordinating treatment and other events affecting the patient.

Section 1: caring for patients with RA

In 1984, Wilson-Barnett described the key elements or functions of nursing which are as relevant today in caring for patients with RA as they were in the 1980s (refer to Box 9.1). If the nurse does not understand the illness from the patient's perspective, it is likely that care may be offered that has little relevance to the individual. Through applying the nursing attribute of 'knowing the patient', I am able to step inside the patient's world and obtain their perspective of the impact of their condition and what aspects are important to them. This is the first stage of an ongoing process of developing a therapeutic relationship with the patient. As the relationship based on trust and understanding develops, I will be able to promote the patient's involvement in decision-making. With the ultimate goal of the patient becoming an active participant in their own care, and being able to control aspects of their condition, for example using relaxation to help muscle tension and pain, the emotional consequences of a chronic illness need to be explored; if this is not addressed, the patient may continue to experience an array of feelings including anger, shock, grief and hostility. It is usual for the patient to experience low mood and heightened emotional reactions to any situation due to the physiological changes being experienced and the resultant impact on everyday activities. If these phenomena are not explained to the patient, they can often express feelings of guilt that they are not adjusting to the situation. If the emotional reaction to the condition has developed into clinical depression, this needs to be recognised with appropriate treatment offered if required.

Some nurses find it difficult working with patients whose conditions are not amenable to cure (Nolan & Nolan, 1995) and can experience feelings of helplessness or frustration when a patient is experiencing both physical and psychological symptoms. Through utilising the attribute of 'holistic practice knowledge', I use a range of knowledge and skills including cognitive behavioural techniques, physical exercises and work-based strategies to help the patient address the physical, psychological and social impact of their condition. Referral to other members of the team may also be appropriate including the occupational therapist to provide advice on aspects of hand function.

Helping patients manage their symptoms

Adopting a holistic, humanistic approach to care requires a change from the supportive role of 'doing for' the patient to a therapeutic approach, which necessitates enabling the patient to feel more in control. For instance, if the patient's main problem is reduced mobility, I need to employ saliency to help identify whether their is a sensory, affective or cognitive component (or a combination of all three) that is preventing the individual from trying to improve their mobility. For example, if the patient believes that exercise will increase their pain, they are not likely to engage in activity (cognitive component); if their mood is low, they may lack motivation to take an active role (affective component); and if they are not sleeping, this will increase their perception of pain when mobilising (sensory component). Consequently, the assessment will involve listening and responding to verbal cues as well as observing the patient's body language. If there is a large affective component, the patient will be withdrawn, offer little eye contact, express a lack of interest in everyday activities and display feelings of despondency regarding the future.

During the assessment process, utilising the attribute of 'knowing the patient' will enable the patient to describe their experiences to ensure that no cues are missed, which will be vital to informing the treatment plan. From this assessment, the treatment options, including graded exercise or cognitive behavioural therapy, exercise and relaxation, which has been shown to be beneficial in helping patients improve their activity levels (Burckhardt *et al.*, 1994; Seers, 1996), can be explained to the patient. Ultimately, the patient will choose the option that has meaning and relevance for their own situation. Deciding on an agreed management plan involves applying the attribute of moral agency; I provide the patient with information relevant to their situation and share my experience regarding how the problem identified could be addressed, for example using graded exercise to improve muscle strength and stamina. Although I express this option, I do not enforce this on the individual and I respect the individual's choice to address their problem from another angle such as participating in a yoga class. Therapeutic nursing has been defined as 'that practice where the nurse has made a positive difference to a patient or client's health state, and where he or she is aware of how and why this positive difference has occurred' (Powell, 1991).

Section 2: nurse-led clinics: added value to patient care

Once a diagnosis of RA has been confirmed, patients are often referred to a nurse-led clinic for the ongoing management of their care. The purpose and responsibilities of a nurse-led clinic are shown in Box 9.2.

Hill (1992) describes the role of the nurse in this context as essentially expressive in nature consisting of a combination of skills including:

- caring
- helping
- supporting
- teaching.

Wright (1991) supports this view adding that expressive skills are at the core of therapeutic nursing and include the ability to:

- be with the patient
- provide comfort
- provide education
- provide the emotional element of care.

Box 9.2 Purpose and responsibilities in a nurse-led clinic (Hill & Pollard, 2004; from Hill & Pollard, *Nurse Clinics: Chronic Disease Nursing*, Wiley-Blackwell)

- Managing the patient's condition;
- Identifying the patient's problems;
- Determining the patient's coping strategies;
- Appraising the patient's knowledge of the condition and its treatments;
- Establishing a care plan;
- Acting as a source of referral.

A case study will be used to illustrate the purpose of a nurse-led clinic.

Case study: Julie

Julie is a 38-year-old mother of two children, who was diagnosed with RA 3 months ago and is presently unable to work as a schoolteacher. She cannot understand why she feels so tired and so much pain. Her husband feels helpless to cope with the altered situation. Julie has recently been commenced on drug therapy for her condition and is finding it difficult to accept that it could be 4 months before the medication works. Julie has been referred by the rheumatologist to the nurse-led clinic to receive advice and support on managing her symptoms.

The nurse–patient consultation

One of the most important aspects in rheumatology nursing is the relationship that exists between the patient and the nurse. Using a framework such as Pendelton's model may provide a structure and help the nurse to optimise the consultation time available (see Box 9.3). I use Pendelton's model to help me to begin the

Box 9.3 Pendleton's (1994) seven functions for the consultation (from Pendleton *et al.*, *The New Consultation* (2003); by permission of Oxford University Press)

- To define the reason for the patient's attendance;
- To consider other problems;
- To consider an appropriate action with the patient for each problem;
- To achieve a shared understanding with the patient for each problem;
- To involve the patient in the management and to encourage acceptance of appropriate responsibility;
- To use time and resources appropriately;
- To establish or maintain a relationship with the patient, which helps to achieve the other tasks.

---

process of knowing the patient, as the model respects the patient's own perspective on the situation that has lead to the need to consult as well as involving the patient in the management of the problem.

Understanding the Lived Experience of RA

I need to provide time for Julie to share her experience, for example what it is like living with RA at that moment, and to listen to her concerns and anxieties. This involves the attribute of saliency. In that, as Julie describes what it is like to live with the RA on a daily basis, I can pick up cues and then clarify with Julie that I have perceived the problems she is experiencing accurately. Julie confirms that her main concern is the overwhelming fatigue that is with her for most of the day and a fear that she may not be able to carry on working. The use of open questions, an example of 'skilled know-how', enables Julie to share her experience (e.g. Can you tell me what the fatigue is like and what it is preventing you from doing? Can you tell me how you are feeling about the situation? What concerns do you have about yourself at the present?).

One of the main purposes of the initial consultation is for me to be able to relate to the individual and to enter their world and understand their needs, through applying the attribute of knowing the patient. I adopt a listening role and use clarification questions to ensure I have understood Julie's situation (e.g. so you feel that if you could manage the fatigue, this would help with your mood).

Providing meaning to Julie's experience

Julie wants to know why she is feeling so tired; using the attribute of moral agency, I explain that fatigue is one of the core symptoms of inflammation and that it would be unrealistic for Julie to be able to carry on engaging in all her activities when she has less energy. By providing meaning to Julie's daily experience, she is able to think about how she might address the identified problem, and consequently in the consultation, a goal is negotiated to plan the day balancing activity with rest periods enabling Julie to still feel that she is contributing to family roles. This also enhances Julie's sense of control, in that she can adopt a strategy to reduce the tiredness. Through knowing Julie, I can begin the process of increasing her perception of mastery over her condition.

At Julie's request, her husband is invited to the next consultation, so that he can contribute to the fatigue management, enabling the couple to be active participants in Julie's care. Julie perceives that this will reduce some of the helplessness that her husband has been displaying. Julie's husband identifies that he could ask his parents to babysit once a week enabling him to take Julie out so that they have time to enjoy each others' company.

Julie's other concern relates to her work, as a schoolteacher, as she is finding it difficult to reach the blackboard due to involvement of the gleno-humeral joint. An appointment with the disablement education advisor leads to a lower height blackboard being installed. I also discuss with Julie returning to work on less hours to help her manage her fatigue. Julie feels this would help her psychological status if she is able to contribute in her work role.

Interventions influential in developing a therapeutic relationship

These interventions reflect my own expertise and understanding from analysing and reflecting on, and in, my own practice about what are significant nursing interventions. I have used quotes from my PhD research to illustrate some of the interventions:

- *Obtaining genuine participation.* I find it is important to encourage the patient to participate in as many decisions as possible, as choosing from a range of options will heighten the patients perception of control. Patients who believe that they can influence their own condition report fewer physical problems and enhanced well-being (Newman, 1993).

> The nurse listened to me, everyone I had seen before said I must take up swimming but I don't like swimming and I don't see how it would help my pain. All I want to do is to be able to walk to the shops, and we talked about how I would start by walking part of the way and now I can go everyday and I am feeling so much better.
>
> *Dawn 46, RA 8 years*

- *Exploring lay beliefs.* The individual will bring their own lay beliefs and life experience to all situations. These are usually consistent over time and pertinent to the individual concerned (Donovan, 1991). I spend time establishing the patients' own beliefs about the purpose of treatment options; if rest is perceived as 'giving in', the patient is unlikely to engage in it but if the principles of pacing are explained and the benefit of rest experienced in terms of pain reduction, the patient may feel able to try and incorporate it into their daily routine.

> I wasn't exercising as I was afraid that the pain was damaging me knees once I know that I wasn't making things worse I found I enjoyed doing something to help myself.
>
> *Mark 45, RA 10 years*

- *Establishing realistic goals*: I know from experience that if a patient is trying to reach unrealistic goals, they will ultimately fail and understandably be demoralised. If a patient has had to reduce their leisure activities due to the pain, for example no longer participating in weekly badminton, it would be unrealistic whilst the condition is so active to continue with this activity but different exercises can be shown to the patient so that they can maintain their physical strength and still engage in physical activity.

> I thought that if I changed what I was doing I was giving in but when I spoke with the nurse she said I was expecting too much of myself now I go out for a meal once a week and I enjoy not having to cook so often.
>
> *Diane 55, RA 6 years*

- *Providing information specific to the individuals situation*. Donovan and Blake (2000) demonstrated that explaining to patients that their arthritis was mild when they were experiencing heightened symptoms did not have the desired affect of reassuring the patient. What I have found in my practice is that patients require validation of their problems (e.g. that pain is causing you a lot of problems at the moment and explanation provided within their own content). For example, I would state, 'I think the reason that the pain is causing you so much problem at the moment is that the new treatment we have just initiated has not had time to work; do you think this, or is there something else that you think is causing the pain?'

> Knowing that the fatigue is part of the condition makes it easier to manage, the nurse always seems to know just how big a problem it is.
>
> *Brenda 59, RA 9 years*

- *Involving significant others*. I always give the patient the option of including the family in the consultation.

> [H]e couldn't understand why I felt alright one day but had a lot of pain the next day, once the nurse explained that the pain could be variable he seemed to understand and help out more.
>
> *Jill 44, RA 12 years*

Evaluating practice

In order to explore the effectiveness of my practice, an independent researcher interviewed five patients with RA, whom I had reviewed in clinic on at least two occasions and asked the question: 'what is it like to be cared for by the nurse consultant?' (Ryan *et al.*, 2006b).

Two main themes were identified:

1. *Holistic person-centred care experienced and valued by the patient*.

> When the nurse consultant sees you in a consultation she thinking not just about you're physical problems, she thinks of other aspects of your life.
>
> *P3*

> I value my appointment with the nurse consultant, I know she will look at my joints, talk about my blood results and ask how my husband is.
>
> *P4*

2. *Feeling cared for.*

> She puts me at ease and looks after me and I know that when I see her I will
> come out better.
>
> *P2*

> She always seems very bothered about me, there's nothing I wouldn't talk to
> her about.
>
> *P3*

Developing a new model of care

Following the successful running of the nurse-led RA clinic, the rheumatology
team decided to introduce a new model of care for patients with fibromyalgia
based on the five attributes of nursing expertise that has been illustrated in the
case study about Julie.

Patients with fibromyalgia experience chronic widespread pain accompanied
by fatigue, stiffness and non-restorative sleep. A medical model of care has been
shown to have little to offer this patient group as analgesia is often ineffective
(Wolfe *et al.*, 1995), and although there is evidence to suggest that aerobic exercise
can be beneficial (Nicassio *et al.*, 1997), patients often have difficulty engaging in
activities due to the physical and psychological factors such as anxiety and depression that accompany the pain. I was given the specific remit of developing
a service for this patient group. The objectives of the new service are shown in
Box 9.4.

I arranged an open forum and invited all potential stakeholders including rep-
resentatives from the patient panel to attend to discuss the development and share
any anxieties. Some colleagues were sceptical about referring what they regarded
as 'complex patients' to a nurse perceiving that medical knowledge would be
required to manage patients with multiple needs. I invited colleagues to sit in
on consultations so that they could observe the bio-psychosocial approach being
used in the consultation. This proved useful not only in demonstrating the philosophy of the clinic but also in developing a closer working partnership with
colleagues. Through leading the change and having the organisational authority
to implement the new model, I was able to alter the culture of care for patients
with fibromyalgia. Manley (2002) identifies organisational authority as the single

Box 9.4 The objectives of a new model of care for patients with chronic musculoskeletal pain included

1. Improving the patient's physical, psychological and social functioning;
2. Reducing the fragmentation of the existing service and providing a clear pathway of care;
3. Reducing long waits to receive advice on symptom management;
4. Helping patients develop coping strategies to manage their pain.

most influential factor for achieving cultural change with regard to context. By remaining visible and demonstrating clinical expertise, I was able to gain credibility from the multidisciplinary team.

How the new model operates

I run two clinics a week with 30-min appointments. Referrals are taken from rheumatologists, rehabilitationists, orthopaedic surgeons, physiotherapists, general practitioners and nurses. The assessment and management of patients attending the pain clinic is based on the attributes of nursing expertise.

Firstly, saliency is employed to observe how the patient walks into the consulting room and it is noted whether the patient is very protective with their physical movements or has a very rigid body posture. Secondly, I ask the patient to tell me their story by taking me back to the time they first experienced any symptoms right up to the present-day impact of living with their condition. By using the attribute of knowing the patient, I am seeking to portray that it is the patient's expectations and experiences that I am interested in rather than my own interpretation of the situation.

I also ask the patient to share strategies that they may have used in the past to help with their pain and ask the patient to comment on their effectiveness. This utilises the attribute of skilled know-how by encouraging the patients to share their own knowledge and skills of their pain experience. It also provides me with the information as to what has been successful (or not) in the past in helping the patient to develop an element of control over their pain. It will also inform the discussion as to what options are open for the patient that will have meaning and relevance to their own unique situation. I can then, through the attribute of moral agency, provide information that will enhance the patient's ability to set realistic goals that we can monitor as a partnership and modify, if necessary. Through validation and explanation as to the patient's symptoms, I can start to embed new knowledge (thereby using the attribute of holistic practice knowledge). It is only by knowing the patient and hearing the patient's story that I can support the patient to take control of the situation (Box 9.5).

Box 9.5 Pain management strategies

1. Individual education and support;
2. Referral to a multidisciplinary pain management programme (as advocated by CSAG 2000) to focus on the development of behavioural coping strategies, for example pacing, relaxation, goal setting, developing a sleep routine, managing stress and anxiety;
3. Referral to other members of the multidisciplinary team where appropriate, for example occupational therapist;
4. Rationalisation of medicines;
5. Referral to a combined nurse consultant and liaison clinic to assess mood states that fall outside the nurse consultant's level of expertise;
6. Referral to voluntary organisations and community-based exercise programmes.

Box 9.6 Peer group members

- Two consultant rheumatologists;
- One manager;
- Two outpatient nurses;
- One inpatient ward sister;
- One consultant physiotherapist.

Evaluating the pain service

Two evaluations were carried out. First, an audit was performed to assess whether patients who attended the nurse-led pain service were still accessing other hospital specialities for the same pain problem. Second, a qualitative study was undertaken to explore perceived impact of the service from my peers.

An audit into the secondary care utilisation of 60 patients with fibromyalgia attending the nurse consultant led clinic (Ryan *et al.*, 2005) demonstrated that 53 patients reduced the number of different specialities being accessed 12–36 months after attending the nurse consultant-led clinic. Services patients were no longer accessing included rheumatology, imaging, orthopaedics, accident and emergency and gynaecology. The total number of secondary care appointments in all specialities fell from a median of 12 (range 1–76) to 2 (range 1–30).

To explore any perceived impact on the service following the appointment of a nurse consultant, seven peers (see Box 9.6) were interviewed by an independent nurse researcher. The peers were chosen by the nurse researcher from a role set of 12 on the basis that they had direct organisational involvement with the nurse consultant and represented a range of professions.

All peers were able to identify the role of the nurse consultant in developing a new culture that enabled a different model of care to be implemented for patients with fibromyalgia. Two examples from the interview data are included below:

Been excellent in actually developing a new model of how to manage these patients ... going away from the medical model ... where patients take ownership of these symptoms.

Rheumatologist 1

What has changed as a result of having a Nurse Consultant ... is the culture, so the culture perhaps um the hierarchical structure of doctors feeding down to nurses and allied health professionals has gone ... the role has almost given permission for other health professionals to see patients initially rather than being managed solely by the consultant.

Consultant physiotherapist

This new model of care is included in the Department of Health Musculoskeletal Service Framework to illustrate effective pain management (DH, 2006).

175

Section 3: the effectiveness of nursing interventions

Three randomised control studies have demonstrated the positive impact a rheumatology nurse can have on a patient's health status (Hill *et al.*, 1994, Tijhuis *et al.*, 2002; Ryan *et al.*, 2006a). These studies are described below:

1. Hill *et al.* (1994) demonstrated the value of a clinic run on nursing principles. This study was an evaluation of the effectiveness, safety and acceptability of a nurse practitioner (NP) in a rheumatology outpatient clinic. Seventy patients with RA were randomly allocated to either the NP clinic or a consultant rheumatologist clinic and seen on six occasions over 12 months. On study entry, the groups were well matched. At week 48, there was no significant difference between the two groups with both groups showing significant improvement in disease activity. However, the patients in the NP cohort showed additional improvements not mirrored in the consultant group. The improvement was in pain, morning stiffness, psychological status and satisfaction with care.

   One reason for this improvement could be that the NP had a longer consultation time of 30 min compared to 15 min. By having a longer consultation time, the NP can apply the attribute of 'knowing the patient' and understand the problems from the patient's perspective. This is valued by the patient and results in care that has meaning and relevance, which is more likely to have a positive impact on the patient's health status.

   One of the most noticeable aspects of the research was the marked difference in the referral patterns of the two practitioners, with the NP making greater use of other members of the multidisciplinary team, such as the physiotherapist. This is a more efficient use of resources as the patient can access preventative advice (e.g. minimising muscle wasting) at an early stage in their condition. The nurse was also shown to be a safe practitioner who was able to initiate and interpret clinical and laboratory data.

   Hill's work demonstrated that the nurse can add something extra to the management of patients with RA, and that extra is something that is valued by the patient.

2. Tijhuis *et al.* (2002) undertook an RCT regarding the effectiveness of nurse-led clinics. This study over 12 months was a six-centre study of 210 patients who had been experiencing increasing difficulty in performing activities of daily living over the previous 6 weeks. Patients were randomised into three equal groups, receiving care from either an outpatient team, a day patient team or one of six clinical nurse specialists (CNSs). Visits for care were not standardised and the average duration of care from the CNSs was 12 weeks, with a mean number of three visits. Inpatient and day patient care both comprised nine full treatment days. The primary outcome was functional status using the Health Assessment Questionnaire (Fries *et al.*, 1980). Results demonstrated significant

improvement in all three groups. By employing the attribute of moral agency, the CNS was able to provide specific, individualised information to the patient on how they could improve their physical function.

3. An RCT by Ryan *et al.* (2006a) examined the hypotheses that consultation with a CNS in a drug monitor clinic would have a measurable impact on the well-being of 71 patients with RA. Patients were randomised into two groups over a 3-year period. The intervention group was monitored by the CNS and an out-patient staff nurse reviewed the control group. Patients reviewed by the CNS reported a greater perception of being able to control their arthritis than those managed by the staff nurse using the Arthritis Impact Measurement scales (Meenan *et al.*, 1980).

By knowing the patient, the CNS was able to help patients cope with their symptoms through goal setting, pacing, addressing low-mood state and advocating exercise. It may be this attribute of nursing expertise-enabled patients to report a greater perception of control over their condition.

There was a higher dropout rate in the control group, which may reflect the role of the expert nurse in utilising the attribute of saliency. By focusing on patient-identified problems and providing care that has meaning from the patients' perspective rather than solely concentrating on the safety of their drug therapy. Ten patients from this study were interviewed by an independent researcher to explore ways of coping; the importance of nurse support in relation to enhancing positive control perceptions emerged as a clear theme in the intervention group (Hooper *et al.*, 2004).

Conclusion

This chapter has demonstrated how nursing expertise can be applied in a rheumatology setting. By providing care that has meaning and relevance from the patient's perspective, the individual can develop coping strategies to increase their perception of control over the daily symptoms of the condition, which include pain, fatigue and a reduction in activities. The five attributes of nursing expertise provide the nurse with a 'toolkit' which can be used to improve health outcome in patients with a rheumatological condition.

References

Burckhardt, C.S., Mannerkorpi, K., Hedenberg, L. & Bjelle, A. (1994) A randomised controlled clinical trail of education and physical training for women with fibromyalgia. *Journal of Rheumatology* **21**(4), 714–720.

Clinical Standards Advisory Group (2000) *Services for Patients with Pain.* Department of Health, London.

Department of Health (2006) *The Musculoskeletal Services Framework. A Joint Responsibility; Doing It Differently.* Department of Health, London.

Devins, G.M., Edworthy, S.M., Seland, T.P., Klein, G.M., Paul, L.C. & Mandin, H. (1993) Differences in illness intrusiveness across rheumatoid arthritis, end stage renal disease and multiple sclerosis. *Journal of Neurology and Mental Disorders* **181**, 377–381.

Dickens, C. & Creed, F. (2001). The burden of depression in patients with rheumatoid arthritis. *Rheumatology* **40**, 1327–1330.

Donovan, J. (1991) Patient education and the consultation: the importance of lay beliefs. *Annals of Rheumatic Disease* **50**(3), 418–421.

Donovan, J.L. & Blake, D.R. (2000) Qualitative study of interpretation of reassurance among patients attending rheumatology clinics: 'just a touch of arthritis, doctor?' *British Medical Journal* **320**, 541–544.

Fries, J.F., Spitz, P., Kraines, R.G. & Holman, H.R. (1980) Measurement of patient outcome in arthritis. *Arthritis and Rheumatism* **23**, 137–145.

Hartzheim, L.A. & Gross, G.L. (1998) Rheumatoid arthritis: a case study. *Nursing Clinics of North America* **33**(4), 595–602.

Hill, J. (1992) A nurse practitioner rheumatology clinic. *Nursing Standard* **7**(11), 35–37.

Hill, J. (1999) Patient education and adherence to drug therapy. In: *Drug Therapy in Rheumatology Nursing* (ed. S. Ryan). Whurr, London.

Hill, J. & Pollard, A. (2004) Nurse clinics: not just assessing patients joints. In: *Chronic Disease Nursing; A Rheumatology Example* (ed. S. Oliver). Whurr, London.

Hill, J., Bird, H.A., Harmer, R., Wright, V. & Lawton, C. (1994) An evaluation of the effectiveness, safety and acceptability of a nurse practitioner in a rheumatology outpatient clinic. *British Journal of Rheumatology* **33**, 283–288.

Hooper, H., Ryan, S. & Hassell, A. (2004) The role of social comparison in coping with rheumatoid arthritis – an interview study. *Musculoskeletal Care* **294**, 195–206.

Manley, K. (2002) Refining the consultant nurse framework: commentary on critique. *Nursing in critical Care* **7**(2), 84–87.

Meenan, R., Gertman, P. & Mason, J. (1980) Measuring health status in arthritis. *Arthritis and Rheumatism* **23**(2), 146–152.

Newman, S. (1993) Coping with rheumatoid arthritis. *Annals of the Rheumatic Diseases* **52**, 553–554.

Nicassio, P.M., Radojevic, V., Weisman, M.H., Schuman, C., Kim, J., Schoenfeld-Smith, K. & Krall, T. (1997) A comparison of behavioural and educational interventions for fibromyalgia. *Journal of Rheumatology* **24**(10), 2000–2007.

Nolan, M. & Nolan, J. (1995) Responding to the challenge of chronic illness. *British Journal of Nursing* **4**(3), 145–147.

Pendleton, P. (1994) *The Consultation: An Approach to Learning and Teaching.* Oxford University Press, Oxford.

Powell, J. (1991) Reflection and evaluation of experience pre-requests for therapeutic practice. In: *Nursing as Therapy* (eds R. MacMahon & A. Pearson). Chapman Hall, London.

Ryan, S., Dawes, P. & Kirwan, M. (2005) A retrospective audit of secondary health care utilisation of patients with fibromyalgia. *Rheumatology* **44**(S1), 375.

Ryan, S., Hassell, A., Dawes, P. & Kendall, S. (2003) Control perceptions in patients with rheumatoid arthritis: the impact of the medical consultation. *Rheumatology* **42**, 135–140.

Ryan, S., Hassell, A.B., Lewis, M. & Farrell, A. (2006a) Impact of a rheumatology expert nurse on the wellbeing of patients attending a drug monitor clinic. *Journal of Advanced Nursing* **53**(3), 277–286.

Ryan, S., Hassell, A., Thwaites, C., Manley, K. & Home, D. (2006b) Exploring the perceived role and impact of the nurse consultant. *Musculoskeletal Care* **4**(3), 167–173.

Seers, K. (1996) The patients' experiences of their chronic non-malignant pain. *Journal of Advanced Nursing* **24**(6), 1160–1168.

Symmons, D. & Bankhead, C. (1994) The incidence of rheumatoid arthritis in the United Kingdom: results from the Norfolk Register. *British Journal of Rheumatology* **33**, 735–739.

Tijhuis, G.T., Zwinderman, A.H., Hazes, J.M.W., Van Den Hout, W.B., Breedveld, F.C. & Vliet Vlieland, T.P. (2002) A randomised comparison of care provided by a clinical nurse specialist, an inpatient team, and a day patient team in rheumatoid arthritis. *Arthritis Care and Research* **45**, 280–286.

Wilson-Barnett, J. (1984) *Key Functions in Nursing: The Fourth Winifred Rapheal Memorial Lecture*. RCN, London.

Wolfe, F., Ross, K., Anderson, J., Russell, I.J. & Hebert, L. (1995) The prevalence and characteristics of fibromyalgia in the general population. *Arthritis Rheumatism* **38**, 19–28.

Wright, S. (1991) Facilitating therapeutic nursing and independent practice. In: *Nursing as Therapy* (eds R. MacMahon & A. Pearson). Chapman Hall, London.

10. Exploring the Relationship between Education Expertise and Nursing Practice

Nancy Jane Lee

Introduction

This chapter will use personal critical reflection to explore education expertise and its relationship to nursing practice. Expertise is a contestable concept, eluding precise definition or quantification. Its philosophical base has similarly been questioned (Selinger & Crease, 2006). Furthermore, professional practice expertise, such as that found in health and social care, is potentially controversial, with possibilities for professional vested interest, and control of access to knowledge (Fook *et al.*, 2000).

Initially, my reasons for even considering the relationship between education expertise and nursing practice will be explored. A professional doctorate programme will be outlined, being deliberately chosen as a case study for critical reflection, given its implied characteristic of research-based knowledge for application in the professional practice setting by the practitioner. In order to construct my critical reflection on education expertise, the following questions will be used:

- What is it that I think I am trying to do?
- How do I think it is done?
- How does the expertise relate to nursing practice?

The questions above do not represent 'evidence' in the sense of formal or empirical data, but personal and professional learning associated with subjective thought and experience. Experiential learning has been described by Weil and McGill (1992, p. 9) as 'the process that links education, work and personal development'. Having outlined the chapter's focus, the reasons for exploring education expertise are given below.

Rationale for exploring education expertise

Personal and professional interest in the nature of expertise has been prompted by three factors: professional experience, research relating to the nature of nursing expertise (Manley *et al.*, 2005), and the theory–practice gap in nursing. A consistent theme within the three factors identified is the inference that education and nursing practice are viewed as two separate halves of the whole nursing.

Practice colleagues occasionally tell me about 'the ivory towers' of academia or use the adage, 'those who can do and those who can't teach'. Sometimes, this is pleasant teasing and sometimes it is not. There is an implication that I am somehow out of the loop; that direct care delivery has precedence, is of more importance and has greater substance. The second factor prompting me to reflect on expertise relates to the wider contemporary literature concerning nursing expertise. This embraces clinical expertise, thus reinforcing the primacy of professional practice as the focus of nursing expertise. For example, Benner's (1984) progression from novice to expert relates clearly to the clinical nursing domain; a point identified by English (1993). Higgs and Titchen (2001) use the concept of graceful care to explore nursing expertise. Again, there is focus on the clinical domain, with patient attention, patient communication, recognition of patient individuality, along with self-knowledge and insight being seen as elements of graceful care.

Finally, the relationship or, as some would argue, the lack of a relationship, between education and nursing practice, can be found in the literature exploring the theory–practice gap in nursing. This has been described as the difference between the ideal state of nursing as espoused within educational preparation, and/or the practitioner's own values and beliefs about nursing practice, and the realities of professional practice. Maben *et al.* (2006) found that the much documented disparity between theory and the ideals of newly qualified nurses remained at odds with the pressures of service delivery in practice. Such disparity was also identified by Melia (1987), in relation to the occupational socialisation of student nurses. In essence, the students learnt nursing in the more powerful sphere of practice as opposed to the education environment. The three factors introduced above have prompted me to question my professional position in nursing and the nature, if any, of my associated education expertise. If not a practising nurse, then what is my relationship to and with nursing practice?

There are similarities here between nurse education and teacher education. Smith (2005), for example, explored student teacher perceptions of expertise in relation to their educators. It was found that the student teachers preferred professional development from a teacher educator who had recent professional practice experience. This was considered important to minimise the perceived contrast between the reality of teaching and the practice of teaching as presented by academic staff.

Furthermore, students associated their educators' expertise with subject knowledge, good knowledge of teaching principles, knowledge about child development and learning, research and development/awareness of research in the education field, self as teacher, respect for the student, role modelling and teamwork (Smith, 2005). Slick (1998) added the ability to bridge the gap between the espoused theory of teaching and the realities of professional life in the classroom. For example, in addition to external professional knowledge, an expert educator had access to a repertoire of knowledge and skill, which was difficult to articulate, and related to know-how and experience in the teaching setting. Colloquially, this could be described as 'trade secrets'.

Experts are considered to have a great command of knowledge in their subject area. However, according to Grunderman *et al.* (2001), command of the subject is not sufficient to be an expert or have expertise. It is further described as an ability to interpret knowledge creatively depending on the situation. The depth of knowledge combined with practical experience enables the expert to use salient knowledge tailored to reflect the individual situation at hand. An expert knows how and when to modify knowledge and skill depending on the context.

Implicit within Benner (1984) is the ability to progress through a process whereby practice, initially the slow, deliberate actions of the novice, progresses through advanced beginner, competence, proficiency, with a repertoire of knowledge and skills, to expert with the key skill of intuitive thinking. Fook *et al.* (2000) further distinguish between experiences as practice undertaken over and over again till it becomes routine. Expertise by contrast denotes innovative and creative thinking.

A *professional doctorate*

A focus for critical reflection

The previous discussion has illuminated my interest and education expertise and associated factors. A professional doctorate programme has been chosen as a focus for critical reflection and analysis of my thoughts about the nature of education expertise and its relationship with nursing practice. The ensuing discussion will demonstrate that the programme characteristics are intrinsically related to nursing practice, through its emphasis on the development and application of research strategies to generate knowledge and skill for use within the practice setting by the practitioner themselves.

Professional doctorates have proliferated in the UK in the 1990s and it has been suggested that their development in health and social care in England, in particular, is associated with service modernisation and adaptation (Ellis & Lee, 2005). The United Kingdom Council for Graduate Education describes professional doctorates as meeting:

> the specific needs of a professional group external to the University, and which develops the capability of individuals to work within a professional context.
> *United Kingdom Council for Graduate Education, 2002, p. 62.*

The professional doctorate programme I am associated with, the DProf (Health and Social Care), combines a doctoral level research element with facilitated modules. The modules address practitioner researcher knowledge and skill, critical reflection on professional ideas and values, critical reflection on the nature of professional practice and enhanced professional leadership for research in professional practice. The structure of the programme is outlined in Figure 10.1.

Students on the programme typically have senior roles in health and social care practice; clinical, educational, research based, managerial, or a combination. They

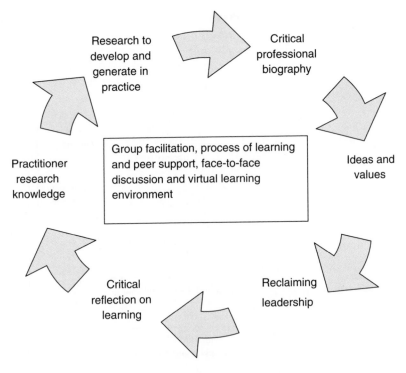

Figure 10.1 Outline of the professional doctorate, DProf (Health and Social Care).

may have consultant nurse or consultant therapist roles. Within the programme, there is emphasis on small group student discussion, personal development planning and peer learning. Face-to-face discussion and workshops are blended with the use of a virtual learning environment. The latter enables ongoing access to resources and support wherever there is an Internet connection.

Critical reflection on education expertise and nursing practice

Having briefly introduced the professional doctorate, there will now be exploration of the nature of education expertise through reflection on my role within the programme itself. As stated in the Introduction, the following questions provided a framework for reflection:

- What is it that I think I am trying to do?
- How do I think it is done?
- How does the expertise relate to nursing practice?

What is it that I think I am trying to do?

A pyramid of emerging education expertise is proposed as a result of critical reflection (Figure 10.2) and will be explored in detail here. Overall, I believe that

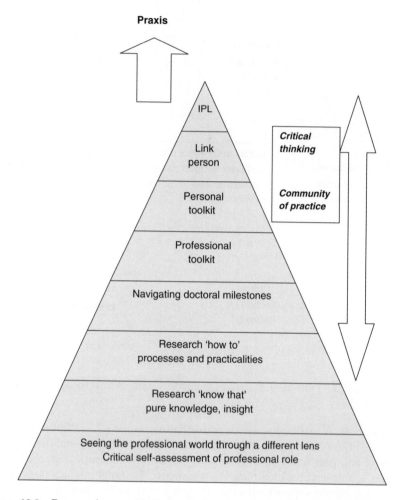

Figure 10.2 Proposed pyramid of education expertise within a professional doctorate programme.

enhancing students' curiosity and critical thinking about their professional practice, others' practice, the professional environment, its wider influencing factors and societal context, the experiences of the key actors in that practice, patients/clients/others, is the crux of any educational expertise I possess.

Within the professional doctorate, 'critical' is not concerned with pejorative or negative criticism. It is concerned with the ability to think through and question issues using a variety of perspectives, to use learning creatively, to develop and apply informed originality to professional practice. The ultimate would be the development of praxis, informed and committed action. This has been described as not only action based on thought and reflection, but also action based on principles of well-being, doing well and respecting others (Warelow, 1997; Glass, 2001).

Having given an overview of possible education expertise, the first theme emerging from my critical reflection relates to knowledge and its application and/or generation within professional practice. Doctoral study is considered to be the epitome of knowledge acquisition, demonstrating the ability to contribute original knowledge to a subject discipline based on creativity and independence of thought (Quality Assurance Agency/QAA, 2001).

However, despite the implied complexity and depth, there is little within my professional role that is concerned with didactic input, factual knowledge and information giving. Student learning instead involves a process, their learning process of enhancing and widening expertise pertinent to their sphere of professional practice. My role as facilitator is to enable an environment where the student professional can view the professional practice world from a different perspective. This involves challenging the students' comfort and assurance, in a constructive and positive sense within the boundaries of their professional expertise and then extending this further.

I view my role as engaging with the student in that process, embarking on the doctoral journey with the student, to consider what expertise is required from me and to help the student source expertise from others and importantly from within themselves. In summary, education expertise is associated with student engagement and facilitation of their own critical reflection. This is considered necessary to review and analyse the factors contributing to their professional practice and related research interests, and to assess their own learning needs in relation to professional practice and the development of research expertise within the practice setting.

Ideally, student analysis of the professional world will develop from their freedom to think and question, for example analysing their professional leadership or other roles, evaluating the wider professional context and the players within it, questioning their professional ideas or values, and enhancing knowledge/expertise to impact on practice through research strategies. The goal is reflection on the nature of knowledge, professional practice and evidence, using this as a foundation to develop practitioner research. In summary, my role is not concerned with accretion of professional knowledge per se as the students already have that by virtue of their own expertise within practice. Education expertise is associated with facilitating students' learning through questioning, critique and emerging creativity and interpretation.

Such knowledge is theoretical, possibly the term 'know that' is used to describe and differentiate it from other kinds of knowledge. In summary, my role is not to give knowledge in a one size fits all method; my role is to help tailor the process and movement through knowledge acquisition, appraisal, critique and confidence, depending on the student's individual need. This need itself is student identified and requires a partnership, using a process of analysis and reflection, to review key knowledge and skill and identify and plan for development.

Eikeland (2001) explores Aristotle's philosophy of theoretical knowledge. This is said to be concerned with truth and the pureness of knowledge for its own sake. It could relate to theory and factual knowledge or it could relate to philosophical appreciation. Though the above analysis is concerned with theoretical knowledge, there is also a pragmatic element concerned with 'how to'. Examples of 'how to' could include planning the research process for professional practice, how to engage with the practitioner researcher role. Other examples relating to research and nursing practice could be the practicalities of data collection, analysis and its management, management of change. In summary, how to engage with the practicalities of research in professional practice and strategies for leading research in professional practice are key to the student's learning.

According to Aristotle, practical knowledge or productive knowledge is concerned with the making of things, and knowing how to make things (Eikeland, 2001). In application to the professional doctorate, knowing how is concerned with how to make research in professional practice and how to develop doctoral level work that relates to professional practice.

In the pragmatic sense of knowing how to develop and apply research externally in professional practice as above, my expertise could also be used internally in the academic setting to navigate the key milestones in the doctoral process. Examples include periodic evaluation of the doctoral work completed to date, student self-evaluation and writing up. These are academic requirements and may be used as a quality assurance measure, to explore how the student is progressing, to identify research training and development issues and to ensure credibility, consistency and parity through peer review. Part of the education expertise involves knowing what is involved in the processes and helping the student navigate a pathway through them. In summary, education expertise involves acting as an interface between knowledge application in the professional setting and the academic requirements of doctoral study.

To date, the foundations of self-assessment and biography in the professional world, along with research know that and know-how, have been considered from the first to the fourth level of the pyramid in Figure 10.2. Further up the pyramid of educational expertise is the notion of a professional toolkit. Clearly, knowledge of research is not sufficient, in either education expertise or nursing practice. If it were, then the theory–practice gap would not exist. There are professional or interpersonal components which underpin practitioner research, for example leadership, change management, networking, motivation and communication. There may also be processes which hinder, for example, the tensions between the practitioner as researcher and the practitioner as professional, the challenges of undertaking research in the workplace, competing priorities, resistance to change, or too much change and uncertainty.

In the same way, a plumber has essential tools for the craft of the job, the student professional has a professional toolkit or repertoire of knowledge and skills that could be applied to their learning and research in the professional setting. Having the wrong professional tools or none at all could lead to dissonance in the practice setting, resistance to change, difficulty having shared ownership of research ideas and practice development.

Professional toolkit
The professional toolkit may require awareness of organisational culture. For example, 'Who needs to be directly involved in the research in practice; who are the

key people requiring awareness'? Leading research activities beyond investigation into tangible improvements in practice will require good leadership, motivation, stamina and change management. While students will have a repertoire of these skills in relation to their professional expertise, their application to research and practice at the same time is challenging. As Grunderman *et al.* (2001) suggest, expertise in one area, for example in the clinical field, does not necessarily imply expertise in other areas, for example people skills, leadership, research or administration.

The application of education expertise could relate to the development of the professional toolkit and ultimately to nursing practice, through elements of professional supervision, coaching and encouragement. There could be debriefing, significant event review, reflection for action and on action. The professional toolkit requires a wider impact than the local practice setting. It should relate to the dissemination of research and learning through conferences and the publication of papers, membership of professional networks or working groups. This could facilitate others' learning and promote collaboration. It must be acknowledged that these developments do not take place on an individual basis between the student professional and facilitator. Part of the development of education expertise, as stated earlier, involves the facilitation of an environment where students can equally share with their peers and engage in mutual learning and development.

As the professional toolkit relates to practice, thus the personal toolkit has application in relation to student motivation and enjoyment of learning within the professional doctorate experience. It also includes skills associated with critical thinking, analysis and reflection. While the previous elements of the pyramid are concerned with outcomes, professional and personal toolkits are concerned with processes and engagement within the experience itself. At a practical level, the personal toolkit could also be expressed as the balance of work life, home life and study life, ameliorating the competing tensions. For example, there is a double challenge for professional doctorate students. They are in the challenging situation of doctoral study, while simultaneously in the challenging situation of embedding, the ensuing knowledge and skill within professional practice.

To date, my critical reflection has explored knowledge and its processes along with toolkits for professional and personal maintenance. The term 'link person' is now used to refer to the resources and professional networks that students may access as part of their studies. While the student is grounded in practice expertise and local resources, there may be other professional associations, regional research networks, and other individuals who students can access to compare and contrast approaches and to establish presence and collaboration.

One aspect of my education expertise involves acting as a link person facilitating the sharing of information/networks and resources between students. This is a reciprocal process whereby receiving/distributing information between and with the students and myself builds a bank of expertise for the benefit of the students and also for my professional development. Part of education expertise involves having a broad view of health care and doctoral study strategies and using this as a resource. Part of the resource could involve the development of interprofessional learning (IPL), collaboration and understanding of roles.

When trying to respond to the question, 'What is it that I think I am trying to do?', critical reflection has enabled me to develop a pyramid (Figure 10.2) or model of possibilities that may apply to student development. The pyramid is transient, aspects of it will change, or there are elements that have not yet entered consciousness. Likewise, the components within the pyramid are not linear, there may be progression back and forth within the pyramid or more than one element will be worked on at any one time.

My perceptions of education expertise, the 'what' of education expertise have been explored. There are additional elements which influence the processes inherent within the pyramid itself. These will now be explored in relation to my second question, 'How is it done?'

The process of education expertise

How do I think it is done?

While the themes in Figure 10.2 summarise the proposed 'what' of education expertise, the arrows on the right-hand side of the pyramid demonstrate two critical processes evident at all levels within the pyramid. These are:

- critical thinking and questioning;
- communities of practice (Lave & Wenger, 1991).

Critical thinking

Educators exhort students to think and write critically, yet what does critical thinking entail? Clearly, a response given to me requires some expansion, 'I don't know how to explain it (critical thinking), but when I see it I know it . . .' Critical thinking involves looking at a subject through as many windows or from as many varied perspectives as possible. It may involve answering one question posed with another question, rather than offering an immediate answer.

For example, to respond to infection control targets on surgical wards by developing and applying the first immediate solution would be reactive and would not involve critical thinking. However, to ask questions about infection control, factors influencing the infection control target, its origins, reasons for its introduction, appraising evidence/knowledge relating to the target, using critical thinking to review the quality of evidence presented in the first place, would be possible components of critical thinking. Exploring the possible implications of the targets from the viewpoint of the multidisciplinary team, ancillary staff and patients, to ask about knowledge and skill, training needs, to ask questions about economics, evidence-based practice, and examples of good practice in other areas would be examples of critical thinking.

Within my education practice, developing and applying the principles above could involve small group discussion, one-to-one tutorials or discussion through the virtual learning environment. For example, students may want to discuss and question each other's professional practice and issues relating to the development and application of practice-based research. Mutual discussion and questions that are insightful and challenging, ultimately enhancing the development of practice ideas and sharing of knowledge and resources, is the desired outcome. In summary, the principles of critical thinking relate to development of that skill within the group and the ability to use it for the benefit of the group as a whole and the individuals' research areas within the group.

The above process is a simplistic representation of critical thinking in action, exploring the application of critical thinking within the student group and individuals. However, there is a myriad of other factors for me to internalise while trying to enhance a critical thinking environment. For example, I should be reflecting in action and evaluating the strengths and weaknesses of the group/individual processes involved. This may involve reviewing the dynamics and relationships within the group and the individuals themselves.

Critical questioning

Key questions in this internal dialogue could potentially relate to fairness and equity of participation in any group discussion, the quality of discussion and the student ease with the discussion. This is especially important and relates to the notion of criticality as constructive challenge and learning methods, rather than the direct assault of and individual's values and beliefs. There should be reflection on other issues that affect the morale of the group or individuals, for example, professional pressures, impending course deadlines, along with analysis of my own thoughts and feelings.

The balance between facilitating the external dialogue of critical questioning while maintaining a personal internal dialogue, relating to the strategies and processes involved, is challenging. Possible ethical tensions add an additional dimension. For example, as a group member, I can relate to and appreciate the students' professional situation.

In particular, some of the exciting challenges facing the student professionals have resonance with my own professional role. These tensions relate to the achievement of a balance between engaging with professional practice, while finding the time to reflect on practice, and used research and other strategies to enhance practice. However, as facilitator, there are other responsibilities in my role, which relate to fairness, equity and the development of an environment stimulating learning and curiosity. In summary, I am part of the learning group, while different by virtue of the role of facilitator.

Communities of practice

Lave and Wenger (1991) have developed and worked with the concept of communities of practice to explore the varied networks humans are involved with and from which learning and development emerge. Communities of practice involve members actively and have boundaries mutually understood and negotiated by the group. They act as a repertoire or database of resources and expertise that members of the community have developed over a period of time.

When I appraise the reflection on education expertise to date, then one major criticism is the implied one-way traffic inherent in the processes explored. Critics would rightly argue that my portrayal of education expertise suggests discussion from educator to student only. However, that is not the reality at all, or the implied nature of expertise. As stated earlier, the professional doctorate students are senior professional practitioners. Within the student community as a whole, some of the education expertise illuminated here already exists and can be shared and further developed through critical questioning, peer learning and discussion, and the elements of the pyramid in Figure 10.2. In addition, there are alternative elements of expertise which I do not possess, but which develops from the students' expertise. Alternatively, there may be other elements not yet identified. In essence, I do not know what I do not know about professional doctorates and student needs and wants. The student groups and I belong to a community of practice within the professional doctorate programme, whilst being members of other groups of professional or personal practice which may impact and feed into our learning within the professional doctorate.

A crucial element of my education expertise is to enhance the sharing of ideas, encourage peer learning and evaluation and foster the environment for that to happen. In essence, the aim is to develop a community of practice as espoused by Lave and Wenger (1991). For example, critical thinking could be developed from facilitation and discussion; it could develop from peer evaluation, peer presentation and assessment of learning, or the opportunity for informal discussion.

Within that, I include my own learning and development. There is an element of reciprocity. From the varied expertise available in the professional doctorate population and the wider academic and professional population as a whole, it is possible for us all to gain a broader picture of health and social care issues. This synergy is one aspect of the relationship between education expertise and nursing practice. The process of reciprocity relates to the provision of a learning environment or a community of practice in which research and development of professional practice can grow.

How does the expertise relate to nursing practice?

The final question within the critical reflection framework relates to education expertise and its relationship to nursing practice. While I do not contribute directly to the professional arena as a practising nurse, I can practise the skills and educational processes which indirectly inform and influence nursing through the practice of others. For example, previous discussion has identified the learning community, where I can help provide a space where student/practitioners can discuss and share development or practice-based research knowledge and skills. An exploratory study of professional doctorate student supervision needs indicates that such space is valued, a 'safe' place for reflection on professional practice (Lee, 2007). In addition, I can contribute towards and facilitate learning in relation to the pyramid in Figure 10.2. The application of learning contributes to advanced skills in creative thinking and enquiry about practice, in order to investigate or develop new approaches. Critical thinking and questioning are processes that students can apply to the nursing practice setting along with enhanced awareness of self and role in relation to practice. They are not academic skills to be used purely to complete theoretical work or to meet academic requirements.

My professional practice is no longer nursing practice. It is education practice for nursing practice, through the facilitation of processes, resources and support to enable others to undertake the practice-based research and development themselves. There is synergy with some of the elements of nursing practice expertise, enabling, facilitating, enhancement of individual skills, thinking about self in the context of practice. The components described above have resonance with those employed in direct patient/client care, good communication, empathy, forward planning, teamwork and role modelling.

Inherent within the student facilitator relationships of the professional doctorate are possibilities for reciprocity or the negotiation and exchange of professional elements. The exchange could take place between students and/or between the students and me. For example, know-how in relation to research processes, critical thinking, and resources to support doctoral study are exchanged for know-how about strategic developments in professional health and social care practice, analysis and appraisal of current issues. This is also demonstrable in the characteristics of the professional doctorate programme, which aims to make links between the means of developing knowledge and skill and the expertise to locate that within professional practice.

For example, the philosophy underpinning the programme focuses on research embedded in practice by the practitioner themselves, practitioner research. Education expertise can perhaps be better related to practice by virtue of the distance from that practice. For example, I am not of the same organisation as the practitioners, I do not share its culture, and I am not immersed in its values and direction. This gives me a broader view of the practice world rather than focused expertise and specialism. It also gives me a different relationship with the practice world. I am not bound to it by employment, or practice in that area.

While this is strength, it can also be perceived as a weakness. For example, my professional education has progressed along a continuum of diploma to doctoral studies. The progression has increasingly emphasised academic education as opposed to the maintenance of clinical dexterity. In summary, to maintain credibility within education, then I need to demonstrate competence in academic writing, appraisal and research participation. Sellers (2002) argued that nursing actively seeks and embraces academic characteristics in order to develop the approval and validation of more established academic disciplines.

Within the above argument, there is an implied dissonance which has legitimacy, the language and priorities of professional practice or those of education or academic practice. For example, the language of professional practice may be concerned with evidence-based practice, clinical outcomes and care pathways. The language of education may be concerned with curricula, research assessment and widening participation. How are links between education and practice to be maintained if we cannot mutually understand or speak the same language?

At the beginning of this chapter, there was some discussion of the theory–practice gap in nursing. Within this, it was suggested that there is disparity between the actual practice of nursing and that espoused from a theoretical and educational perspective. The discussion here has attempted to illuminate the possible components of education expertise and relationships to nursing practice by focusing on the skills of facilitation, critical thinking and creativity to enhance nursing practice. It has been suggested that the skills are key to the relationship between education and the professional doctorate students who are themselves working at levels of advanced practice and expertise.

Conclusion

Reflection on the everyday elements of my role has been an interesting and difficult process. However, exploring taken for granted activities has resulted in new perspectives relating to expertise and its place in education. The process of reflection has helped me identify strengths and weaknesses in my role, and to further explore the values and beliefs underpinning that role. This has also involved critical self-questioning. Given that expertise is difficult to express, not tangible, an automatic response in a given situation, can it be said to exist in my practice if I cannot illuminate it?

Discussion to date has attempted to explore the nature of education expertise and its relationship to nursing practice. During exploration, there has been emphasis on the personal nature of the reflection, rather than generalisations drawn from a range of empirical and other evidence. As such, the reflection is unique; another individual may give weighting to other components of education expertise based on their particular knowledge and experiences.

It must be acknowledged that not all of the associated components of education expertise lie in the hands of the academic. Clearly, there are other sources of learning for students, their own critical reflection and experiences, good role models and mentors from the professional group or within the students' workplace. Throughout there has been emphasis on the nature of education expertise as a process whereby the student is helped to identify and tailor learning and enquiry to their particular practice setting and research interests. As such, the independent nature of student learning and activity is characteristic of the higher levels of doctoral study, to develop creative and innovative approaches to professional practice through the development of research and knowledge.

A pyramid of expertise has been suggested, although this is not one directional or static. It is transient, and there may be additional elements to add to that pyramid as new experiences and knowledge are reflected upon and incorporated into my repertoire. Finally, critical reflection on education expertise has enabled me to find and articulate my own professional, educational voice and begin to explore it with clarity and purpose.

References

Benner, J. (1984) *From Novice to Expert: Excellence and Power in Clinical Nursing Practice.* Addison-Wesley, CA.

Eikeland, O. (2001) Action research as the hidden curriculum. Chapter 13. In: *Handbook of Action Research Participative Inquiry and Practice* (eds P. Reason & H. Bradbury). Sage, London.

Ellis, L.B. & Lee, N. (2005) The changing landscape of doctoral education: introducing the professional doctorate for nurses. *Nurse Education Today* **25**, 222–229.

English, I. (1993) Intuition as a function of the expert nurse: a critique of Benner's novice to expert model. *Journal of Advanced Nursing* **18**, 387–393.

Fook, J., Ryan, M. & Hawkins, L. (2000) *Professional Expertise: Practice, Theory and Education for Work in Uncertainty*. Whiting and Birch, London.

Glass, R.D. (2001) On Paulo Friere's philosophy of praxis and the foundations of liberal education. *Educational Researcher* **30**(2), 15–25.

Grunderman, R., Williamson, K., Fraley, R. & Steele, J. (2001) Expertise; implications for radiological education. *Academic Radiology* **8**(12), 1252–1256.

Higgs, J. & Titchen, A. (2001) *Practice Knowledge and Expertise in the Health Professions*. Butterworth-Heinnemann, London.

Lave, J. & Wenger, E. (1991) *Situated Learning: Legitimate Peripheral Participation*. Cambridge University Press, Cambridge.

Lee, N.J. (2007) *Enhancing the Quality of Research Supervision for Professional Doctorate Students Teaching and Learning Quality Improvement Scheme*. University of Salford, Salford.

Maben, J., Latter, S. & Macleod-Clark, J. (2006) The theory–practice gap: impact of professional-bureaucratic work conflict on newly-qualified nurses. *Journal of Advanced Nursing* **55**(4), 465–477.

Manley, K., Hardy, S., Titchen, A., Garbett, R. & McCormack, B. (2005) *Changing Patients' Worlds through Nursing Practice Expertise. Exploring Nursing Practice Expertise through Emancipatory Action Research and Fourth Generation Evaluation*. A Royal College of Nursing Research Report 1998–2004. RCN, London.

Melia, K.M. (1987) *Learning and Working: The Occupational Socialisation of Nurses*. Tavistock, London.

Quality Assurance Agency (2001) *Framework for Higher Education Qualifications*. Available from http://www.qaa.ac.uk (accessed March 2004).

Selinger, E. & Crease, R.P. (eds) (2006) *The Philosophy of Expertise*. Columbia University Press, New York.

Sellers, E.T. (2002) Images of a new sub-culture in the Australian university: perceptions of non-nurse academics of the discipline of nursing. *Higher Education* **43**, 157–172.

Slick, S.K. (1998) The university supervisor; a disenfranchised outsider. *Teaching and Teacher Education* **14**, 821–834.

Smith, K. (2005) Teacher educators' expertise; what do novice teachers and teacher educators say? *Teaching and Teacher Education* **21**(2), 177–192.

United Kingdom Council for Graduate Education (2002) *Professional doctorates*. UKCGE, Dudley.

Warelow, P.J. (1997) A nursing journey through discursive praxis. *Journal of Advanced Nursing* **26**, 1020–1027.

Weil, S.W. & McGill, I. (eds) (1992) *Making Sense of Experiential Learning, Diversity in Theory and Practice P9*. Open University Press, Buckingham.

11. Critical Creativity in the Development of Clinical Nurse Specialists' Practice

Liz Henderson

Introduction

The following poem was written by Susan during a PD programme for clinical nurse specialists (CNS). It is a creative reflection of a therapeutic encounter with John, a young man attending the bone marrow transplant clinic, and clearly illustrates the impact of nursing expertise:

> He shook . . .
> He looked uneasy, unsettled, unnerved
> He sweated
> He listened
> He questioned
> He heard
>
> Then he left, reassured, relaxed, at ease
> Smiling
> Understanding
> Nodding
> Pleased
> He shook . . . my hand

In exploring with Susan how she facilitated this transformation she replied:

> I relaxed. I very deliberately relaxed in front of him. I just spoke slowly and calmly and slowed the whole thing down, why I was here, what I could offer him, that I was here to support him in any way . . . by the end of the long session we'd identified all the things he was worried about, how he had coped in the

past and how he was preparing to cope with this... to cut a long story short he started to relax in front of me, you could just see the tension leaving him... such a change.

The attributes of expertise, identified on the RCN Expertise in Practice Project (RCN, 2003), are knowing the person, moral agency, saliency, skilled know-how and holistic practice knowledge. Facilitated critical dialogue with Susan around her narrative illustrated how she was drawing on holistic practice knowledge. She did this by establishing who John the person was. By focusing on what he really needed at that point in time, she responded very deliberately, skilfully and creatively, using all of self to engage with him in a way that was for his ultimate well-being. In this vignette, Susan's professional artistry is evident and bears all the hallmarks of nursing expertise.

This chapter presents a reflective account of the practice development (PD) programme in which Susan participated. The programme was aimed at enabling cancer and palliative care CNS to maximise the potential of their role and to recognise, appreciate and articulate their expertise in practice. The shared journey undertaken by the CNS participants and myself, as the facilitator of the programme, is outlined, providing an opportunity for gaining insight into the processes used and the impact of the development activities. It draws on and illustrates the work of McCormack and Titchen (2006), in their articulation of 'critical creativity' as a new world view for PD. Outcomes from the programme relate to three main areas: findings from CNS care stories, PD initiatives and elements of human flourishing evidenced by increased personal and professional effectiveness.

Critical creativity: a new paradigm for PD

The purpose of PD, as found in a concept analysis by Garbett and McCormack (2002), is to increase effectiveness in person-centred, evidence-based health care. This is brought about by skilled facilitators who work with health care teams to enable them to transform their workplace culture. These facilitators use systematic rigorous processes of emancipatory change that reflect the views of service users.

Manley and McCormack (2003) set out how this particular world view of PD, known as emancipatory PD, is underpinned by critical social science and informed particularly by Fay (1987). Active and critically reflective learning processes are used, aimed at enabling practitioners to become more self-aware, with increased insight into how their inherited dispositions and social influences place limits on how they view the world, influence their attitude to practice, as well as their relationships with others. The whole thrust therefore of emancipatory PD is to enable practitioners to become 'enlightened' about the nature of their situation, and 'empowered' to take action to overcome obstacles and bring about identified changes in self, practice, and the practice context. Critical social science is concerned that such action is self-generated, arising as a result of increased insight into the situation rather than from coercion or pressure from others. In so doing, practitioners become freed or 'emancipated' from forces or assumptions that previously constrained them and their practices.

Theories and sub-theories of critical social science

The activities and processes behind this 'enlightenment to emancipation' journey are set out by Fay (1987) in a complex scheme comprising eight practice theories and a total of 20 sub-theories. However, McCormack and Titchen (2006) critique Fay's (1987) theories of being critical, arguing that any meaningful explanation of how this complex scheme can be translated into actual practice is missing. Even sub-theory 10, which indicates 'how people are to carry out a social transformation', gives the impression that application of abstract theory to practice is a simple linear process, but as experience shows this is far from the case. Bringing about cultural or practice change is a challenging and hugely complex business. It necessitates the application of knowledge, skills and abilities, and requires a practical artistry which goes far beyond cognitive theoretical knowledge. McCormack and Titchen (2006) further point out that in Fay's (1987) scheme there is no recognition of moral or spiritual dimensions, which are often involved as people push out the boundaries to develop their practice.

McCormack and Titchen (2006) contend that engaging in such practical activity is a form of praxis (thoughtful, intentional doing with moral intent) in which practitioners identify the salient features of a given situation and, by drawing on all ways of knowing, consciously and deliberately attend to the particularities of the circumstance. In other words, they argue, practitioners need to employ a kind of creativity in order to be able to take in the whole situation and respond effectively. Repeated engagement in such creative activity enables practitioners to develop and refine their professional artistry (Titchen, 2000; Titchen & Higgs, 2001), without which their actions in practice would be routine, clumsy or inappropriate.

McCormack and Titchen (2006) therefore propose an augmentation to Fay's theory of 'transformative action' and in particular sub-theory 10, which identifies the need for a plan of action for social transformation. They argue that what is needed is a focus on the ways in which practice can be transformed through a critically creative engagement in practice. This augmentation, which highlights the need for holistic engagement in the situation, is termed creativity.

Critical creativity thus centres on three basic concepts, namely, praxis, professional artistry and human flourishing. Praxis is thoughtful intentional practice and includes the notion of moral intent which, from a critical social science perspective, involves social justice, democracy and equity. However, McCormack and Titchen (2006), from a critically creative world view, extend the concept of praxis to include human flourishing as the explicit moral intent and highlight the creativity of praxis articulated through action. From this angle, they suggest that praxis is achieved through creative thinking and critique *blended* with creative imagination and expression. The blending occurs through professional artistry, which according to Titchen (2000), Titchen and Higgs (2001) and Manley *et al.* (2005), is the hallmark of expertise. Hence, the person is actively drawing on all of their unique faculties and ways of being, to interpret the unfolding situation and, with skill and expertise, crafts a response that is uniquely her or his own, in order to enable all involved in the situation to flourish.

Person centredness is identified by a number of authors as key to human flourishing, linked as it is to a universal moral principle and belief about the

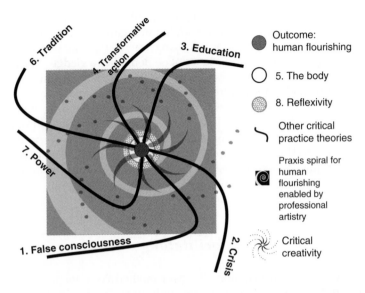

Figure 11.1 A theoretical framework for human flourishing located in the critical creativity world view. (*Source*: From Titchen & McCormack (2008) A methodological walk in the forest: critical creativity and human flourishing. In: *International Practice Development in Nursing and* Healthcare (eds K. Manley, B. McCormack & K. Walsh), pp. 59–83. Wiley-Blackwell, Oxford.)

intrinsic value of personhood (Binnie & Titchen, 1999; McCormack & Titchen, 2001; McCormack, 2004; Manley *et al.*, 2005). The means to achieve effective person-centred practice therefore is through creating the conditions which enable people to maximise their potential for growth (personally, interpersonally and professionally). Whilst endorsing what previously has been articulated in an emancipatory PD world view, critical creativity now moves beyond this in a 'yes-and' relationship, drawing attention to the need to *blend* criticality with creative imagination and expression for maximum growth and development. Thus, from a critically creative PD perspective, transforming the culture is brought about through practising in a manner consistent with the new understanding of praxis outlined above, with human flourishing viewed as both the 'means' and the 'end' of the PD work.

Titchen and McCormack (2007) therefore propose a new theoretical framework for human flourishing located within a critically creative world view (Figure 11.1). The praxis spiral arises as central with human flourishing located at the heart of the endeavour. Within what I would term 'creative praxis', the enabling processes are identified as blending, connecting, energising, reflecting, practising, learning and becoming. Critical creativity (like a gyroscope) then blends and melds the knowledge sources and unique ways of being, thinking, creatively imagining and doing, with human flourishing as the moral intent.

In synthesising the previous and newly emerging world view of PD, Titchen and McCormack (2007) have also begun to explore the relationship between Fay's eight critical theories and corresponding sub-theories locating them within a critically creative world view as illustrated in Figure 11.1. (Fay articulates the critical theories as a typology without showing any relationship between them.)

In recognition of the importance of embodied knowledge, which often precedes cognitive understanding, the critical theories of the body and reflexivity respectively surround the epicentre of the framework.

The framework thus offers new theoretical understanding of how practitioners can both transform themselves and enable transformation in others, by freeing themselves to value, draw on and *critique* all ways of being, becoming, knowing, thinking and doing, then to *blend* this (through professional artistry) with their own unique *creative imagination and expression,* in order to maximise both their own and others potential for growth and development.

Developing expertise as a facilitator

My interest in emancipatory PD as a methodology for individual growth and sustainable practice change began with attending the RCN PD School in 2000, increased while acting as critical companion (Titchen, 2000) on the Expertise in Practice Project (Manley *et al.,* 2005), and was further strengthened as a participant on a subsequent 2-year PD programme, facilitated by a leading UK expert. These experiences provided insight into PD methodology and an awareness of the underpinning critical social science.

With my interest stimulated, and seeing the relevance of facilitation to everyday practice, I undertook a facilitation e-learning course (website: http://www.campusone.ulster.ac.uk) and completed the RCN facilitation accreditation scheme. It was at this time I began to explore Fay (1987), and whilst fundamentally disagreeing with his atheistic stance, I appreciated the logic of the critical theories listed in his typology although I had difficulty assimilating and digesting them.

However, it was while going it alone and facilitating my first PD programme (with the support of a critical companion) that I started to develop as a facilitator and increasingly embraced creativity as a way of working as illustrated in this chapter. I drew on Fay's theories to try to inform and make sense of the experience. At the time of facilitating the CNS PD programme, critical creativity as a theoretical framework for PD had not been developed. However, this reflective chapter uses the framework to analyse and make explicit what I was doing at the time, and how I was developing expertise through active, reflexive engagement in facilitation practice.

The practice context

The practice context is a large teaching hospital in Northern Ireland, designated as part of the regional Cancer Centre. Medical and surgical cancer specialities exist with outpatient services, general inpatient wards, and an Oncology–Haematology Directorate. At the time of the programme, there were five Macmillan CNS palliative care in post, and five other cancer CNS posts. However, individual postholders seemed to have interpreted their roles in various ways, with one main exception. They all found they became so engulfed in clinical activity that other aspects of the role were hard to achieve. This echoes findings from a number of studies (e.g. Gibson & Bamford, 2001; Froggatt & Hoult, 2002; Skilbeck & Seymour, 2002).

Following discussion about this with the palliative care team leader, I agreed to facilitate a programme for the CNS. Working, at this time, as lead cancer nurse for the Trust, my role included line management responsibility for the identified CNS.

Methodology and design

This project was located within an emancipatory PD methodology. The underpinning philosophies, theories and narrative framework are reported in detail elsewhere (Henderson, 2004; McCormack & Henderson, 2007), but for purposes of this chapter, they are summarised within a critical creativity framework for human flourishing (Figure 11.2). It should be noted that the streamers of Figure 11.1 have been condensed into one streamer in Figure 11.2, labelled Fay (1987), with the other streamers now representing the array of influences brought to bear on the programme. This is entirely consistent with the way Titchen and McCormack (personal communication) see the framework being used.

The overall aim of the programme was to enable CNS to maximise their role potential through a programme of work-based and action learning. In order to

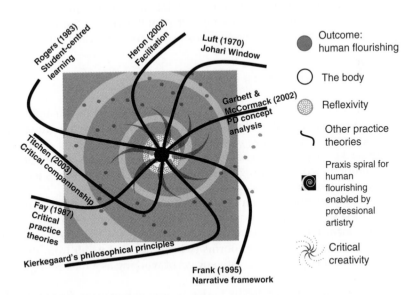

Figure 11.2 Underpinning theories and philosophies used in the PD programme, located in the critical creativity framework for human flourishing.

determine the effectiveness of the programme, two evaluation questions were agreed:

- How are CNS enabled to maximise their role potential?
- What is the impact of a programme of developmental activities on CNS and on their practice?

Programme of work

The programme, which ran over 2 years, was structured to enable learning around three ongoing action cycles, each commencing with a workshop on the topic, namely:

a. developing a shared *vision* for the project and the CNS role;
b. understanding the *culture and context* of care;
c. developing *leadership* to effect practice change.

We later added an 'emotional intelligence' workshop in response to emerging need, as understanding self in the context of the CNS role became an increasingly significant aspect of the programme. PD theory was also woven into the programme, with particular attention to understanding critical companionship (Titchen, 2003).

To provide a more explicit link to critical social science, the integrated development and data collection methods used during the programme are listed alongside Fay's critical theories (Table 11.1).

While this table illustrates the complex mesh of developmental processes used on the programme, it does not show the relationship between them. So in this way, it illustrates to some extent how a typology of theories (in this case, Fay's) fails to make transparent the links or relationship between the listed sub-theories.

The developmental journey

A brief overview of the programme journey is given to illustrate critical creativity in practice, with collective nouns used to describe the group experience, interspersed with my voice (as facilitator) in the first person. Pseudonyms are employed throughout the chapter. However, in acknowledgement of their poetic contribution, two of the programme participants' real names are used with their permission (Susan and Lesley).

My initial attention was on establishing conditions within the group that would enable the CNS to grow and develop, hence the attention on days 1 and 2 was around inclusion issues, laying the foundations for trusting positive relationships, and generating group norms (which included us all from the outset taking the risk of engaging in creative ways of working as a means of gleaning fresh perspectives).

A verse of a poem, written by Lesley, is used in two ways, first to show the type of chaos narrative initially heard and second to illustrate and frame our shared journey of learning.

Table 11.1   Fay's practice theories in use

Fay's practice theories	Integrated development and data collection methods used
1 False consciousness	• Making explicit values and beliefs (and using creative artwork to do so) • Using creative images and artwork to access preconscious understanding and to unlock barriers to verbal expression • Activity analysis to gain fresh insight into how CNS time was spent • Role clarification to gain others' feedback and perspective of the CNS role • Explicit references to the 'Blind and Unknown' quadrants of Johari Window (Luft, 1970) to enable insight
2 Crisis	• Developing a shared vision for the CNS role – to contrast espoused values and beliefs (vision of ideal CNS role) with the reality of everyday experience, thus creating tension • Monthly action learning sets enabled crisis (practice issues) to be presented and explored through facilitated questioning, active listening and critical dialogue • Situations of crisis that arose within the group were explored as the 'hidden' dynamics became manifest
3 Education	• Active reflective learning techniques – valuing experience as a basis for learning (structured reflection, critical dialogue, action learning) • Dealing with rather than avoiding crisis situations within the group as a deliberate learning strategy, to role model new ways of engaging, relating and acting • Culture workshop: learning about how we shape and in turn are shaped by the workplace culture • Cultural analysis • Leadership workshop • Emotional intelligence workshop and learning about self • Feedback from the stakeholder group to get fresh perspective • Narrating and analysing care stories and benchmarking, same against the attributes of expertise (Hardy *et al.*, 2002) as a means of generating new knowledge and developing professional artistry
4 Transformative action	• Developing fresh insights through critical reflection (about self, role, practice context) and taking responsibility for action

Table 11.1 (*Continued*)

Fay's practice theories	Integrated development and data collection methods used
	• Agreeing actions at each action learning set • Identification of work-based learning objectives (projects) • Taking action to alter time spent on various components of role
5 The Body	• Using creative movement to explore feelings then moving into reflexivity • Increasingly appreciating how the body is aware (e.g. experiencing a 'sinking feeling') then moving into reflexivity
6 Tradition	• Critical dialogue, use of creative images, and use of poetry to understand what parts of tradition in relation to the CNS role are worth keeping, what parts need changed • Confronting and challenging conventional (as opposed to autonomous) behaviours • Introducing care stories as a form of appreciative inquiry and exploring individuals' nursing expertise in the care given
7 Power	• Establishing a stakeholder steering group, with senior managers to take into account issues of power and authority • Engagement and critical dialogue to raise awareness of stakeholder perspectives and power bases across disciplines and at all levels • Observing, listening and questioning facilitation strategies to problematise power relationships in the workplace • Attention to process in order to establish nourishing conditions within the group for non-hierarchical, person-centred relationships to develop • Working with person-centred facilitation principles and raising consciousness about issues of power within the group
8 Reflexivity	• Thinking about and developing an awareness through workshops and critical reflection of 'being in context', and how this influences our thinking • Challenging our assumptions through critical dialogue • Identifying barriers and enablers in the workplace context and engaging in critical dialogue around difficulties encountered and how to overcome • Structured critical reflection within the group, identifying what prejudices or values may have influenced actions, developing the ability to look at things as other than they are (for transformative learning) • Regular reflection to evaluate progress made (using metaphor stimulated by creative images, or through the use of poetry) • Facilitator reflexivity in working with group

> Hustle, bustle, noise, clutter, spinning
> Out of control,
> Ideas, goals, plans, but no time to finish
> Does it have to be like this?
> Stop, take stock, think again.

'Hustle, bustle, noise, clutter: out of control'

The first line of this verse aptly describes the messy realities of practice and the CNS' feelings in the second line of being 'out of control'. Early stories presented through action learning clearly illustrated its impact. Presentations described ineffective teamwork, medical dominance, avoidance of conflict and denial. We could see how the pressures of the practice setting constantly impacts on us, albeit to varying degrees at different times, yet there was a sense of despair and of being resigned to the situation, since everything seemed to be subject to powers outside our control. These descriptions appear to provide illustrations of Fay's (1987) theories of crisis, tradition and power.

From a critical social science perspective, there was a need for participant enlightenment as to the ways in which their self-understandings were false. To reduce this 'false consciousness' (Fay, 1987), we engaged in high challenge (and support) during action learning with subsequent feedback and critical dialogue. To further raise awareness, concept maps of the presentations were created to feedback through visual impact of the type of disempowerment language heard. The aim was to reduce the 'blindness' and enable fresh insight that some action, no matter how small, could be taken to address the situation.

Ideas, goals, plans

Line 3 of the poem can be used to describe the next phase of the project, spanning 6 months, which were full of *ideas, goals, and plans* with three learning workshops taking place. The first, developing a shared vision for the CNS role, was to further engender a sense of crisis, by contrasting an alternate ideal for the role (Fay's sub-theory 3), with that experienced in practice. At a later evaluation, Dolores wrote, "I found the visioning very challenging, deep down I knew I wasn't meeting all the aspects of the role."

The next step made explicit the barriers to achieving the vision and the enabling factors to overcome these barriers. Subsequent to this day, we designed and undertook an activity analysis (Henderson, 2004) and role clarification exercise (Henderson, 2004) to check out our assumptions regarding how we spent our time and others' understanding of our role. Overall, people understood and valued the CNS clinical input but were less clear about the other sub-roles. In evaluation of this activity, Colette said, "[U]sing the questionnaire was a huge insight into how others perceive the role."

Nine months into the programme, we evaluated the progress to date at which participants reported their increasing use of reflective practice, facilitating others' learning, and role modelling person centredness. A detailed reflection of this activity linked to critical creativity is outlined in Box 11.1.

Box 11.1   Facilitator reflection linked with critical creativity; enhancing motivation

We had a really excellent morning, during which three of the group members presented issues around the purpose of the PD programme, their vision for the CNS role and how they had felt when initially joining the action learning set. Throughout all of this, there was a real sense of achievement and pride, and the energy in the room was really close and warm. On instinct, I knew I could work with that, knew it was right to just use that energy and through creativity intensify it, hence the exercise with postcards. I asked group members to select a postcard that symbolised their thoughts about where we were at as a group. It worked. There was a rich, intense and powerful feeling in the room and group members seemed to speak genuinely from the heart. We went off to lunch on a real high.

I felt energised, and really pleased at having done the right thing at the right time. I had experienced the use of visual images for the first time earlier in the week at a facilitators' group, and having learned from the experience I knew I could use it. I had previously studied Benson (2001) and Heron (2002) and had learnt that working in a creative way unlocks thoughts and enables, through metaphor, expression of ideas that otherwise would have remained unarticulated.

But it was my awareness of the camaraderie, companionship and warmth of feeling in the room that prompted my action. I wanted to intensify those feelings to stimulate further motivation for learning. I was using interpersonal empathy. I was very self-aware, present and attuned to the energies present in the room. I knew I felt good, and that they did too. On reflection, the verbal affirmations, the non-verbal smiles and good eye contact leading up to this would have given me information to draw on. However, at the moment of choosing to introduce the cards to enable evaluation, I was very consciously drawing on theoretical knowledge regarding creative group work, self-knowledge in relation to being able to enthuse others, knowledge of my colleagues and how they were feeling; then through intentional use of modulated voice, followed by energetic movement in kneeling down on the floor whilst quickly laying out the cards, I acted to test out my hypothesis.

The technique of altering the group dynamic is referred to by Heron (2002) as 'switching'. Heron (2002) suggests that switching promotes holistic learning, prevents alienation and sustains positive emotional arousal, and is a basic motivation for learning.

According to Benson (2001), psychological energy and feeling can be channelled by a symbol or image, transformed or integrated by it. Furthermore, the language of mental imagery and symbolism can help the analytical mind by enabling group members to connect and communicate with areas of themselves that may previously be hidden. Thus, the images on the postcards encouraged the CNS to observe possibilities, articulate these through metaphor, which in turn enabled their ideas to become more clearly defined.

This is an example of being critically creative. The postcard images were the tools used. But as facilitator, I was consciously drawing on and blending knowledge sources, whilst using my creative imagination, and engaging in creative expression with the intent of intensifying the conditions for human growth and flourishing (i.e. I was engaging in professional artistry).

But... does it have to be like this?

'But' then reality dawned. During the tenth action learning set, tension between two group members surfaced and was made manifest through silence. No one was willing to present an issue and it was apparent that something was going on within the group. I chose to challenge this and work with the silence. This provoked real anxiety in set members and some resentment. Twice in close succession, they tried to postpone dealing with the issue, the cultural avoidance–response surfacing. Tension in the group was extremely high. Line 4 of the poem asks *'does it have to be like this?'* I knew if we ignored this emerging problem, the growth of the group would be stunted, and what Johns (1992) refers to as 'the harmonious team façade' maintained.

At the height of tension, I suggested we stop and do a round of how individuals were feeling, in which emotions were identified as 'sad', 'helpless', 'confused', 'lonely', 'awkward' and 'distressed'. Opportunity was afforded for the issue to be addressed, but it became obvious that it was too difficult to speak out even in a safe environment. According to Belenky *et al.* (1986), silence or passivity is in itself an impoverished way of expression. To overcome this hurdle, I once again suggested we use visual images on postcards to depict our understanding of the situation, and to channel and transform the emotional energy from a destructive force to a productive exploration. This opened up through metaphor that there were interpersonal issues at the route of the problem, and how misunderstandings had escalated into conflict.

By drawing on group theory and paying attention to process, I was indicating to the group members that they had to take responsibility for themselves and help to negotiate their own solutions. What we were experiencing was the emotional pain of confrontation in dealing with, rather than avoiding the issues. What was unfolding here was in many ways an epitome of situations encountered by group members in the clinical situation and presented in early action learning sets. The pattern of confrontation avoidance and internalising feelings illustrates deeply ingrained cultural norms. From Fay's (1987) critical social science perspective, 'crisis' was occurring as a result of 'power' issues, brought into the open by my challenging 'traditional' behaviours. Articulating feelings helped to bring to consciousness 'embodied' knowledge, with the intent of moving us towards 'transformative action'. See Box 11.2.

We reviewed the process before leaving and reconnected as a group. A residential workshop on emotional intelligence took place the following month led by an external facilitator. At that, the two set members discovered why they had misunderstandings and engaged with each other in tentatively exploring it. This was a positive development in the pattern of interaction between team members.

'Spinning out of control'

In January, 1 year after the programme commenced, we presented our year's work to the advisory panel comprising stakeholders from senior management and multidisciplinary backgrounds. However, it soon became apparent that their understanding and expectations of a PD programme were totally different to ours. We tried to explain our learning journey and how we were growing and developing

Box 11.2 Facilitator reflection linked to critical creativity; painful growth

On this occasion, I was again drawing on many knowledge sources. Knowledge of the co-learners and reading what was going on identified that there was a problem. PD knowledge, facilitation theory, group theory and previous experience helped me to handle it, personal knowledge gave me the confidence to so act, whilst professional artistry helped mediate the theory into action and prompted the timing.

Johns (1995) asserts that to act ethically is a process of deliberation within the specific situation. In the midst of this situation, I had a conflict of values going on. I knew I was causing great anxiety, pain even to some of the set members. Yet I also believed that it was the right course of action for the overall benefit and growth of the group. So my intent was moral. However, the very fact that I was working in hierarchical mode and in control of the process meant that the responsibility for the group safety lay with me. This was quite a weighty realisation, but with an informed understanding and felt sense of commitment, I was quite prepared to work with the issue for ultimate benefit.

In terms of personal knowledge, I was very self-aware in the midst of the situation. By remaining calm, composed and present, and by interpreting what was happening, I was aiming to give the group confidence that the process was being attended to. This is another example of praxis enabled by professional artistry within a critical creativity world view, but this time in the midst of a painful situation, yet one that resulted in growth for us all.

as a result, but it appeared they were interested only in 'technical' outcomes (as is the norm in health service), perhaps illustrative of Fay's (1987) theory of tradition. At our subsequent action learning set, we engaged in a group reflection about this. As facilitator, I tried to highlight the many political perspectives we needed to be cognisant off and asked participants, '[W]hy did we have an advisory group?' The response from Angela represented a major challenge:

> You suggested it Liz, ultimately that is the crux of this whole entire experience, we have come to this completely naïve and we have gone along with what has come up as it came up and . . . and I just feel on top of what we already do we've just set ourselves . . . I mean we do this day and daily, but we're just talking about it in a different language now and we've allowed people like [advisory group members] make us feel almost inadequate . . . ?

As facilitator, I was aware of a sinking feeling inside, things seemed to be *spinning out of control* but I knew I had to 'hear' the story, even though it was hard to hear. See Box 11.3.

I listened, praised the honesty and attempted to explore the issues with the group, but when another set member who held a different perspective became vulnerable, I interjected by describing a time when I was a participant on another PD programme. I described not only the pain of the journey, but also the learning and growth that ensued. My intentions at the time were to provide a holding place amid the pain and offer hope and encouragement by bringing possibility into view, perhaps an illustration of Titchen's (2003) graceful care. In Fay's terms,

Box 11.3 Facilitator reflection located in the critical creativity world view

> My immediate awareness of a sinking feeling illustrates the interwoven nature of embodied knowledge. Holding my own turbulent emotions of disappointment, hurt and indignation mixed with admiration at the challenge required a conscious control of body expression and speech. A blending of philosophical, theoretical and ethical assumptions seems to have informed my response, as I reflexively thought to remain open, value the person and work with the process in order to turn this into a learning experience. The creativity in this was in the act of regulating my instinctively defensive response and realigning it with an enabling, developmental intent, without being certain where the process would lead. The need for deeper reflection and re-action had to be put on hold, in order to render myself available at that moment in time to focus on group learning.

I was trying to turn the 'crisis' we were experiencing into potential for 'transformative action'.

'Stop, take stock, think again'

The final line of the poem summarises our position. We had *stopped*; *we took stock* and offered choice in relation to continuing with the programme. We explored this at some length and everyone opted to stay, a self-determining action. In line with Fay's (1987) theory of education, we then reconsidered and redefined the purpose of the programme and identified the enabling and inhibiting factors. We redrafted the ground rules and evaluated the day. Although extremely painful, as a group we felt we had made significant progress. Angela said:

> I liked being able to speak about those issues in a very constructive manner without getting aggressive or angry. I also liked having had the opportunity to be quite open and honest about not only that but other things too and just having the time to take stock really.

To achieve emotional closure, we each identified how we were feeling. Angela reported 'I feel relieved and I feel empowered'. What arose as a potential barrier to group survival in terms of high challenge and opposing perspectives became a catalyst for new insights and subsequent growth for us all, through learning about self, power relations and social behaviours. Attention to the process and working collaboratively through person-centred and honest engagement enabled the transition, whilst for me (Liz), deep introspective critical reflection afterwards challenged my own 'false consciousness' (Fay, 1987) and proffered much personal (and painful) learning around my subconscious use of power and control.

However, in thinking reflexively with the above story, I could hear the need for 'prizing' within the group (Rogers, 1983). By constantly challenging practice and being exposed to others' and self-scrutiny, there was real danger of internalising feelings of inadequacy. We needed to *think again* about the approach taken, to look for and highlight the inherent good in our practice, in order to generate further growth and development.

Making use of care stories

Valuing nursing expertise

In response to this, the following month the CNS agreed to recount a clinical situation in which they had made a difference to patient care. After each narration, we engaged in critical dialogue to explicate embedded and embodied professional craft knowledge (Titchen, 2000).

The attributes of nursing expertise (RCN, 2003) provided an extremely useful tool in helping the CNS understanding of their clinical practice expertise. There are elements of Fay's 'education' theory here, in that I was helping the CNS investigate their own practice and through an appreciative response to their story telling provide a nurturing climate in which they began to understand and value their expertise.

We also challenged each other as to what the added value of CNS might be, since many generalist nurses have expertise. This really made us *think again* in order to better understand and reappreciate the role, and to render visible the small things that make a huge difference to patients. Care stories as inquiry became a significant feature during the past 6 months of the programme, with an increasing willingness to question our own practice and in so doing release tacit knowledge embedded in our experience and bodies. The taped stories as well as the critical dialogue were transcribed verbatim and narrative analysis subsequently undertaken. Key phrases identified in individual stories were grouped to form sub-themes from which overarching themes were agreed (Figure 11.3).

Evaluating the impact of the programme

Towards the end of the 2 years, we spent time reviewing the data and engaging in reflective dialogue to evaluate the overall impact of the programme. The group story previously outlined illustrates *how we sought to maximise our role potential.* This next section considers *the impact of the programme* which relates to three main areas:

1. Findings from care narratives: how CNS engage in clinical practice;
2. PD initiatives;
3. Increased personal and professional effectiveness (human flourishing).

Findings from care narratives

How CNS engage in clinical practice

Hannah's care story

I met John and Elsie at the beginning of the year when John was diagnosed with lung cancer and brain secondaries. I had built up a good relationship with them over the last few months. But when I went into the ward last week, I sensed a lot of tension between the staff and Elsie. The staff were avoiding her as she was constantly complaining about things not done. I sat down to speak with her and

---

was sure enough that she had a list of complaints, but I felt that wasn't really what she was angry about. I said to her, I sense there is a lot of anger about John's care but I'm wondering if there is something more? It was just the catalyst, the floodgates opened and she said 'you're going to get it all now ... I'm sorry it's you but you are going to get it all' and she just launched into ... Yes she was focusing on his pain control and his care whatever, but the whole thing was really about that she felt that people didn't see him as a person, that he had lost his individuality. She said 'they just see him as a thing in this bed, but he's my soul mate' ... then it came round, they had lost all they'd hoped for – the future. Everything had gone out of the window, she had been struggling to look after him at home and she could no longer do it, she lost all of that, so we must have spent about an hour and a half where she just talked through all of that, we acknowledged the losses, I listened, and just showed her I understood and cared. Afterwards, I went back to the staff, and we did a reflection on it all, and how she was feeling ... And it really helped, the relationship between the staff and Elsie changed totally, the tension went and they were able to relate again. We were eventually able to put a package in and John got home.

The above vignette and Susan's narrative on her poem at the commencement of the chapter are but mini-illustrations of the type of care story heard from the CNS, all of them evident examples of nursing expertise. After each story, we engaged in critical dialogue to explore in depth how the CNS engaged in such practice. In listening to each other's narratives of care, we began to appreciate that using self therapeutically is core to our practice. On the other hand, it is also clear that this is not restricted to CNS. The difference emerging from our data is illustrated under the 'role-specific elements' in the connecting part of the diagram (Figure 11.3). By being positioned outside of the ward setting, we are able to *bring to the situation a fresh or wider perspective*. We *know the system* and how to navigate it. We see the gaps and act to *bridge those gaps*, *linking* and connecting elements up. We constantly act as a go-between and find that we need to be prepared to do whatever is required for the person's well-being. This often necessitates us *challenging others*, which can be *personally challenging*. We frequently struggle to overcome barriers *and troubleshoot* to resolve issues.

Unpacked in this way, each activity can look quite trivial, but when taken as a whole, it makes a significant statement not only about our contribution but also about barriers and weaknesses in the health care context. Finding ways to overcome these and practising in this way necessitates us having personal resilience and a stereoscopic perspective, which culminates in our *attending to the whole situation*.

Initially, we thought care stories were hardly worth recounting, viewing them simply as the normal things we do in everyday practice. But after listening to each other, and engaging in critical dialogue, we began to gain a new perspective on things and a fresh appreciation of the value of our work and contribution to care. The systematic way we did this (taping the dialogue and theming the transcriptions) has also enabled new practice knowledge and understanding to emerge and a language to make our contribution clear. We have revealed the hidden,

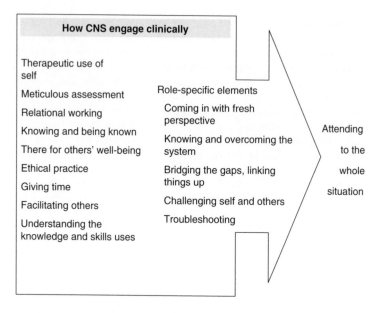

Figure 11.3 Themes from the care stories.

taken-for-granted aspects of our work that make a significant contribution to patient care, and to the governance agenda. The care stories clearly identify our effectiveness in minimising and reducing complaints and demonstrate that through holistic, personal, interpersonal and system-related interventions, we play a key role in reducing risk and contributing to improvements in the standard of care and quality of service. This was subsequently fed back to the advisory group.

PD initiatives

A second outcome of the programme is evidenced through the implementation of our work-based objectives, listed in Table 11.2. These deliberate attempts to fulfil the various domains of the CNS role were informed by the shared vision we developed for the role, activity analysis, individual role clarification exercises and the advisory group feedback.

Personal growth and increased professional effectiveness (human flourishing)

Reflecting on the outcomes of this programme from a critical creativity perspective, I can see that this section may be linked with the notion of 'human flourishing'. However, as the concept of 'human flourishing' is not yet delineated in PD literature, it is taken here to simply mean personal growth and development which results in increased personal and professional effectiveness. In a creative evaluation at the end of the programme, the majority of participants chose roses or leaves to symbolise the 'blossoming' and 'flourishing' that they believed had occurred. Even though individuals emphasised different things, there was an overarching

Table 11.2   PD outcomes

Participant	Developments in practice outcomes	Referenced to CNS role components
Individual participants	• Enabling patient expression through the medium of poetry	Clinical leadership
	• Use of patient poetry to develop a more person-centred ethos at the multidisciplinary team meeting	Leadership
	• Contribution to patient pathway mapping	Education/learning leadership and education
	• Use of structured reflection with ward staff	
	• Development of protocols for reviewing patients at a nurse-led clinic for use by others	
	• Facilitating a clinical leader to improve communication among the multiprofessional team using a PD approach	Leadership
Small group of participants	• Production of a resource pack for staff	Education/learning
	• Taking a lead in patient pathway mapping	Leadership
	• Audit of patient waiting times	Leadership
	• Mapping availability of patient information	Leadership
	• Development of a research proposal into carer and user experience of the service in negotiation with a charitable organisation	Research
Larger group of participants	• Facilitating learning in various wards throughout the Trust in relation to particular clinical issues. Rather than stand and 'teach', the CNS applied PD learning gained on the programme to work with staff's values and beliefs, in order to enable new insights	Education/learning

sense that each person had gained something from the experience, and an acknowledgement that the thorns (painful times), whilst unpleasant, were as necessary for growth as the easy enjoyable times. Indeed, pain and personal angst are potential manifestations of perspective transformations (Mezirow, 1981) and have been reported in other PD work (e.g. Binnie & Titchen, 1999; McCormack & Wright, 2000).

Key to our growth and development is the learning that occurred. We learnt by engaging in group work and by listening to each other, learning how to engage in new processes and to work creatively. We learnt new skills such as facilitation, questioning, listening and reflecting, and being systematic when seeking to develop practice. We have learnt to think differently and have developed a language to describe what we do.

We have also gained new knowledge and understanding about workplace culture, how we are embedded in it, contribute to it and are influenced by it. We see a huge difference between the nourishing culture within the group, compared with the culture of criticism and power struggles 'out there' in the workplace.

But one of the significant outcomes of the programme is increased self-awareness, and new insights about self in relation to others. For example, Angela reported, 'I have become more aware of who I am and what I am.' Ruth said that her achievement was 'becoming more open to myself and about myself and aware of my effect on other people'. Colette reported being 'more consciously aware of myself and what I'm doing ... and more aware of my behaviours". This increased self-awareness in turn gave rise to increased self-confidence. Again Colette stated, 'I have observed other people coming out of themselves and developing and becoming more confident.'

What is the relevance of all of this to practice? First of all, the fact that nurses are constantly establishing and working in relationship with patients and carers (as well as members of the health care team) shows the importance of knowing self before seeking to know others. They must be aware of their own values and prejudices so that these do not interfere with their caring practice. Given that 'therapeutic use of self' is core to how we practice, it is reasonable to assume that increased knowledge of self can only enhance the therapeutic relationship and provide a basis for positive relationships within the health care team. Furthermore, the new skills gained in terms of listening, facilitative questioning, and providing support and challenge are directly applicable to clinical practice, not only whilst engaging with patients or carers, but equally so with members of the health care team.

There is also evidence that the programme has impacted on how we operationalise our role, albeit through small role changes. For Bernie, the change was in 'starting to say no ... recognising that not all things are as important'. Colette was more aware of 'how aspects of my role have changed' and of being 'much more consciously aware of what I am doing in it'.

Whilst Angela observed the real achievement realised through the programme was 'the opportunity to really explore the components [*of the role*] and look at what the vision is, and ... enable us to approach it in a way that we might try to spread ourselves throughout those components a bit more evenly. We have done that.'

In summary, our collective evaluation can be summarised as 'human flourishing', manifest through:

- increased personal insight and growth;
- increased self-confidence (which includes the ability to challenge);
- increased cultural awareness;
- ability to interact better with others;

- an increased ability to reflect and to question our practice;
- increased ability to think laterally;
- enhanced focus;
- greater appreciation and understanding of our own skill, knowledge and expertise;
- more effective role functioning.

Conclusion

This chapter has outlined the journey undertaken by participants and facilitator during a 2-year PD programme. The explicit intent of the programme was to enable CNS to develop their practice through maximising their role, part of which was enabling them to recognise, value and articulate their nursing expertise. In looking back, we can see that the programme provided a space amidst the busyness of practice to stop, to look critically at self in practice and at the practice culture, to listen to and learn from each other, and through person-centred engagement, to re-energise, grow and develop. As facilitator, I too developed during the course of the programme, gaining experiential knowledge through facilitation practice and critically reflecting on it. Then as the knowledge became increasingly embodied in who I am as a person and facilitator, my professional artistry was refined. Critical creativity as a new paradigmatic framework for PD has helped me to make sense of the experience.

Critical creativity is a world view in which critical consciousness (cognition) and creative imagination and expression engage in a synergistic dance. It is clear to me now that the programme described fits within the critical creativity paradigm. The praxis spiral is the central spiral of the critical creativity framework (Titchen & McCormack, 2007). It represents the journey towards human flourishing as both the means and the end of the PD work, brought about by processes of blending, reflecting, connecting, practising, learning, re-energising and becoming. Praxis is thoughtful intentional doing, with moral intent. The explicit intent of the programme was to enable the CNS to fulfil their role potential and we engaged in processes of reflexive action to identify and overcome barriers to their achieving this potential. My role in the endeavour was to facilitate understanding and learning from the process. In developing as a facilitator, professional artistry was demonstrated through the blending of knowledge, personal qualities and creative imagination in order to engage in ways appropriate to the moment. Professional artistry is the dynamic energy in an ongoing spiral of blending, reflecting, learning and practising (Titchen & McCormack, 2007). Part of the blending, in this case, incorporated Fay's critical theories, as we drew upon them to help inform and transform our practice. As a facilitator, I was also blending these theories with others as shown in Figure 11.2.

Critical creativity is not merely a method of using creative arts or tools, it is an approach to PD that builds on the assumptions of emancipatory PD but adds its own nuances. The concept of human flourishing is a central focus of critical creativity and is viewed not only as the ultimate purpose of PD but also as the way of bringing it about. In other words, it is claimed that by paying attention to and creating the conditions (culture) within the workplace in which people can flourish and grow, the achievement of more effective person-centred health care will be enabled.

The last word of the chapter goes to Angela, who in summing up our collective programme evaluation selected a rose as a symbol and said, 'Listening this morning it's evident people have blossomed in their role. I've been one of the big cynics, but I do feel that there has been some growth and blossoming.'

Acknowledgement

I wish to acknowledge the programme participants Bridie Conway, Anne Finn, Fiona Madden, Susan Piggott, Ann Robinson, Lesley Rutherford and Edna Wilson for their wholehearted engagement and contribution to the programme, and in particular to the unique contribution of our esteemed colleague and friend, the late Pauline O'Connor. I would also like to acknowledge Susan Piggott and Lesley Rutherford for agreeing to the use of their poetry in this chapter. Acknowledgement and thanks are also due to Professor Brendan McCormack and Professor Angie Titchen for their invaluable, critically creative challenge and support (Brendan's during the programme and Angie's in writing this chapter).

References

Belenky, M., Clinchy, B., Goldberger, N. & Tarule, J. (1986) *Women's Ways of Knowing*. Basic Books, New York.

Benson, J.F. (2001) *Working More Creatively with Groups*. Routledge, London.

Binnie, A. & Titchen, A. (1999) *Freedom to Practise: The Development of Patient-Centred Nursing*. Butterworth-Heinemann, Oxford.

Fay, B. (1987) *Critical Social Science*. Polity, Oxford.

Froggatt, K. & Hoult, L. (2002) Developing palliative care practice in nursing and residential care homes: the role of the clinical nurse specialists. *Journal of Clinical Nursing* **11**(6), 802–808.

Garbett, R. & McCormack, B. (2002) The qualities and skills of practice developers. *Nursing Standard* **16**(50), 33–36.

Gibson, F. & Bamford, O. (2001) Focus group interviews to examine the role and development of the clinical nurse specialists. *Journal of Nursing Management* **9**(6), 331–342.

Hardy, S., Garbett, T., Titchen, A. & Manley, K. (2002) Exploring nursing expertise: nurses talk nursing. *Nursing Inquiry* **9**, 196–202.

Henderson, L (2004) *Critical Application of Johari Window in the Development of Clinical Nurse Specialist Practice Using Existentialist Narrative Inquiry*. Unpublished MSc Thesis, University of Ulster.

Heron, J. (2002) *The Complete Facilitator's Handbook*, 3rd edn. Kogan Page, London.

Johns, C (1992) Ownership and the harmonious team: barriers to developing the therapeutic nursing team in primary nursing. *Journal of Clinical Nursing* **1**, 89–94.

Johns, C. (1995) Framing learning through reflection within Carper's fundamental ways of knowing in nursing. *Journal of Advanced Nursing* **22**, 226–234.

Luft, J. (1970) *Group Processes: An Introduction to Group Dynamics*, 2nd edn. Mayfield Publishing Company, CA.

Manley K., Hardy, S., Titchen, A., Garbett, R. & McCormack, B. (2005) *Changing Patients' Worlds through Nursing Practice Expertise*. A research report. Royal College of Nursing, London.

Manley, K. & McCormack, B. (2003) PD: purpose, methodology, facilitation and evaluation. *Nursing in Critical Care* **8**(1), 22–29.

Mezirow, J. (1981) A critical theory of adult learning and education. *Adult Education* **32**(1), 3–24.

McCormack, B. (2004) Person-centredness in gerontological nursing: an overview of the literature. *International Journal of Older People Nursing*, in association with the *Journal of Clinical Nursing* **13**(Suppl. 1), 31–38.

McCormack, B. & Henderson, L. (2007) Critical reflection and clinical supervision. In: *Clinical Supervision in Practice* (ed. V. Bishop). Palgrave, Basingstoke.

McCormack, B. & Titchen, A. (2001) Patient-centred practice: an emerging focus for nursing expertise. In: *Practice Knowledge and Expertise in the Health Professions* (eds J. Higgs & A. Titchen). Butterworth-Heinemann, Oxford.

McCormack, B. & Titchen, A. (2006) Critical creativity: melding, exploding, blending. *Educational Action Research* **14**(2), 239–266.

McCormack, B. & Wright, J. (2000) Achieving dignified care for older people through PD. *Nursing Times Research* **4**, 340–352.

Rogers, C. (1983) *Freedom to Learn for the 80's*. Merrill, Ohio.

Royal College of Nursing (RCN) (2003) *Expertise in Practice Project: Final report*. RCN, London.

Titchen, A. (2000) *Professional Craft Knowledge in Patient-Centred Nursing and the Facilitation of Its Development*. D.Phil., Linacre College, University of Oxford. Ashdale Press, Tackley, Oxfordshire.

Titchen, A. (2003) Critical companionship: part 1. *Nursing Standard* **18**(9), 33–40.

Titchen, A. & Higgs, J. (2001) Towards professional artistry and creativity in practice. In: *Professional Practice in Health, Education and the Creative Arts* (eds J. Higgs & A. Titchen), pp. 273–290. Blackwell, Oxford.

Titchen, A. & McCormack, B. (2007) A methodological walk in the forest: critical creativity and human flourishing. In: *PD in Nursing: International Perspectives* (eds K. Manley, B. McCormack & V. Wilson), Blackwell, Oxford.

Skilbeck, J. & Seymour, J. (2002) Meeting complex needs: an analysis of Macmillan nurses work with patients. *International Journal of Palliative Nursing* **8**(12), 574–582.

Section Three

Methods and Resources for Revealing Practice Expertise

12. Developing Expertise through Nurturing Professional Artistry in the Workplace

Angie Titchen

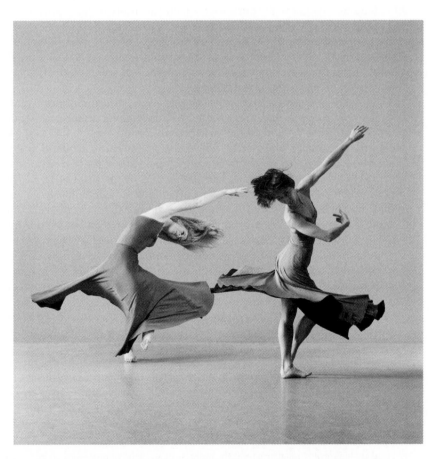

Figure 12.1   Professional artistry symbolised as dance. Photo © Lois Greenfield 1985 (Lar Lubovitch Dance Company).

Introduction

This book is a celebration and articulation of nursing expertise. It brings to life, through accounts from the Expertise in Practice Project (EPP) (Manley *et al.*, 2005) and beyond, how this articulation can be enabled by critical companionship (Titchen, 2004). Critical companions 'walk' alongside nurses with expertise to help them on reflexive, learning journeys towards investigating their own expertise and professional artistry. This book is evidence that the facilitation processes, strategies and professional artistry of critical companionship are effective in helping nurses to become practitioner researchers able to engage in the analytical and critical thinking necessary for research. Doing practitioner inquiry, as the nurses' chapters show, results in further development of expertise, possibly due to their enhanced capacity to analyse and critique their own and others' practices (e.g. see Chapter 4). The portfolios of evidence presented to the critical review panel in the EPP demonstrated how the nurses were using a variety of conceptual frameworks (e.g. Benner, 1984; Manley & McCormack, 1997; Titchen, 2001a) to unravel, unpick and put back together again their own and others' experiences of their expertise. Chapters by the critical companions reveal that they engaged in a parallel process by using the critical companionship conceptual framework (Titchen, 2001b) to investigate their facilitation practices.

These were new processes for the majority of nurses and critical companions, so it is not surprising that they seemed to miss talking about and naming their professional artistry. Professional artistry, we claim in this book, is the essence, hallmark or pinnacle of expertise whether it is clinical or facilitation expertise[1]. However, I am not surprised that it wasn't talked about for two reasons. The first is that when I ask professionals and researchers at the peak of their practice to describe their professional artistry, they often look at me blankly. Even visual and performing artists sometimes do. So people are not used to talking about it. The second reason is that, apart from my own work above and that with Joy Higgs (Titchen & Higgs, 2001), virtually nothing had been written about it in the nursing literature at the time of the EPP. Building on more recent empirical and scholarly research (McCormack & Titchen, 2006; Titchen *et al.*, 2007) and my review of nursing literature of the dimensions of professional artistry, this chapter is the first attempt to deepen an explication of professional artistry.

Professional artistry is difficult to describe because it is embedded and embodied in our practices, but when we see and experience it, we know it. Even nurses with expertise need space and help to reveal and articulate their expertise and its essence, as this book has shown. If professional artistry is so deeply hidden, even to those who have expertise, how much more difficult it is for those of us who are trying to develop it. Given that professional artistry appears to cross clinical and professional fields of practice (see Manley *et al.*, 2005; Titchen *et al.*, 2007),

---

[1] It is likely that professional artistry is the pinnacle of any kind of professional practice, for example practice development (McCormack & Titchen, 2006), education, research (Titchen *et al.* 2007), leadership and management.

this chapter attempts to look at what is necessary to nurture and develop, in the workplace, the professional artistry of any field of practice.

Before we can nurture and develop professional artistry in ourselves and others, we have to know what it is, so the chapter begins with an account of professional artistry emerging from the literature reviewed in Chapter 3. There, professional artistry was defined as the hallmark of expertise and involving processes of blending and interplay. Here I expand on these processes to show the synthesis, balancing and synchronising of diverse but interconnected dimensions, symbolised as dance (see Figure 12.1). These dimensions are qualities, practice or praxis skills, intelligences, different knowledges, ways of knowing, creative imagination, multiple discourses or 'languages', artistic and cognitive critique and therapeutic use of self. Bit of a mouthful, but professional artistry is essentially the processes that put all these dimensions together to create the 'dance' of fluent and seamless practice. As a patient once said to me when describing a nurse with expertise, 'That nurse moves on wheels.' Such practice has an elegant simplicity that seems easy to the onlooker, but is enormously complex and skilled.

Fluency comes from praxis enabled by professional artistry. Praxis is mindful, intentional action, with the moral intent of human flourishing for the givers and beneficiaries of, in our case, nursing care or facilitation of learning and inquiry. Previously, praxis has been presented as a spiral to suggest evolving and continuing growth towards human flourishing (see McCormack & Titchen, 2006; Titchen *et al.*, 2007). I continue that idea here, with the spiral symbolising the reflexive journey undertaken by individuals, teams, workplaces and organisations as they develop professional artistry and/or the conditions for it.

However, merely articulating and understanding the nature of praxis enabled by professional artistry is not enough. To enable expertise to grow and flourish, we need to create the right conditions in our workplaces and organisations. This means developing cultures, systems, strategies for work-based learning (WBL) and facilitation skills to nurture them. This chapter, therefore, draws on two recent concept analyses (Manley *et al.*, in press; unpublished) to set out what is necessary for organisations, workplaces, leadership, management, education and practitioners to do.

Professional artistry dimensions

The dimensions of professional artistry are set out in Figure 12.2 in the black praxis spiral[2]. The spiral image and the white arrows show that the relationships between the dimensions are not linear or sequential. As in jazz improvisation (Schon, 1983), professional artistry emerges through a 'conversation' or as a 'dance' with all these dimensions of self. The processes of this dance, attunement, interplay,

---

[2] The parallel grey praxis spiral represents the elements necessary for nurturing professional artistry in the workplace, which are considered later in the chapter.

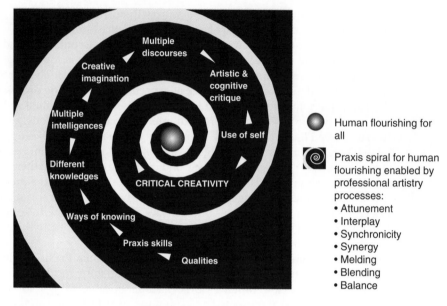

Figure 12.2 Facilitation of professional artistry.

synthesis, melding, blending, synchronicity and balance, are shown beside the spiral and in Figure 12.3. Each 'dance' is unique, depending on the context, situation, people involved, problem, and issue to be worked with, and yet, these processes can be discerned in each 'dance'. This section is my elaboration of Titchen *et al.*'s (2007) earlier description of professional artistry and is relevant to expertise in clinical practice, facilitation and practitioner research, although most of the examples and text refer to the nurse with expertise. In descriptions of the dimensions, I sometimes refer to inquiry. This term refers to learning as inquiry, as promoted in WBL (Manley *et al.*, in press), and practitioner research. Support for the dimensions of professional artistry from the nursing research and educational literature, where available, were given in Chapter 3. As pointed out there, there is only little support yet for the dynamic relationships between the dimensions, probably due to the fact that contemporary nurse researchers tend to focus on the components of expertise, rather than looking at it as a whole. This is an area ripe for research.

Artistic qualities

Spiralling out of, and into, human flourishing are the artistic qualities of the nurse with expertise as a practitioner, inquirer or facilitator. Such qualities encourage nurses with expertise to step into the reflexive, meaning making, living spaces of the praxis spiral. Examples of qualities that are central to praxis that is both critical and creative include a *disposition to what is good* and *audacity*. Boldness and sticking power are required to transgress boundaries and go the extra mile towards human flourishing, for example Manley *et al.*'s (2005) attribute of creative and challenging

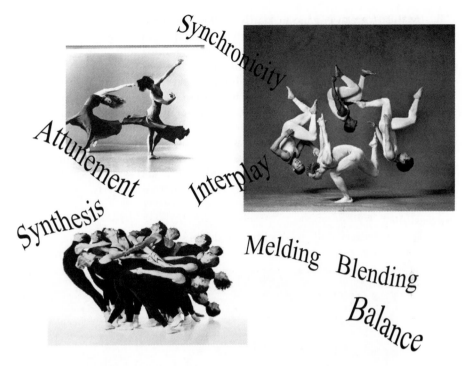

Figure 12.3 Processes of professional artistry. Photos © Lois Greenfield 1985, 1993, 1995.

behaviour. Making the new for a particular and creative intervention with a patient or within a nursing inquiry requires *discernment*; for example, it means sifting and sorting through old traditions or alternative interventions and judging what should be kept for melding or blending, and what should be set aside. Discernment also leads to insight. *Critical and creative appreciation* enables the practitioner or inquirer to evaluate the resulting meld or blend through qualities of *connoisseurship* and *discrimination*. For example, Liz Henderson (in Chapter 11) shows these qualities in action when she says:

> The attributes of nursing expertise . . . provided an extremely useful tool in helping the CNS' understanding of their clinical practice expertise. There are elements of Fay's 'education' theory here, in that I was helping the CNS investigate their own practice and through an appreciative response to their story telling provide a nurturing climate in which they began to understand and value their expertise.
>
> *Henderson, Chapter 11*

Such qualities may also enable the use of Benner's (1984) qualitative graded distinctions. Another quality is a *commitment* to understand deeply, the philosophical, theoretical or methodological traditions, conventions, rules and dominant practices that nurses with expertise have found they need to transcend.

By this, I mean engage in Hardy *et al.'s* (2006) maverick practices for the best interests of their patients, as shown by Margaret Conlon in Chapter 6.

Practice and inquiry concerned with human flourishing attract nurses with expertise who are *hopeful, compassionate* and *ethical*. They are people who display not only *sensibility*, artistic sensibility, but also sensibility in terms of *deep feeling*. *Passion* enables nurses with expertise to work in ways that enable human flourishing for all (e.g. especially for those who are disempowered and unheard). They display *humility*; a genuine respect for what others have to say, express or do and try not to get in others' way, rather accompanying them on a journey towards healing or effective working together. Passion and humility whirl these nurses towards critical, creative edges, which requires *playfulness* and *suppleness of mind*. *Creativity* emerges through rational, intuitive and imaginative interplay.

Praxis skills

The key praxis skills for melding and blending the dimensions of professional artistry are, as symbolised in Figure 12.4, the capacities to interplay, unravel,

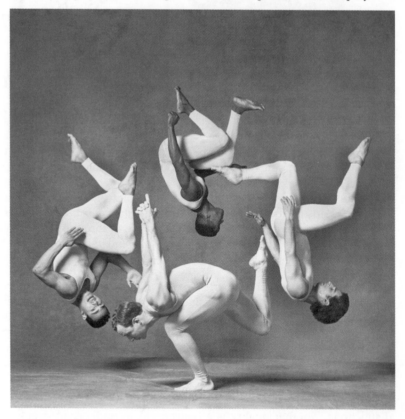

Figure 12.4 Interplay and balance. Photo © Lois Greenfield 1993 (Chris Harrison, Andrew Pacho, Flipper Hope, Harrison Beal/ANTIGRAVITY).

reveal, interweave, imagine, symbolise, harmonise and balance. These skills enable nurses with expertise to disclose what has been observed, perceived and done and to imagine and achieve personalised, unique outcomes for their patients, colleagues, co-learners and inquiries. They intertwine the four ways of knowing, that is, pre-cognitive (embodied, intuitive), cognitive, metacognitive and reflexive, as these ways influence and challenge each other during peak performance and integration, as in this example from Maeve McGinley's chapter:

> Using Johns's (1998) model of structured reflection on an incident within one of the sessions in the 360° feedback, enabled me to begin to understand what made my clinical practice 'expert' compared to other practitioners. It raised my consciousness of the knowledge which Titchen (2000) argues is largely tacit and embedded in practice and of my pre-cognitive way of knowing. I became aware of the types of knowledge (propositional, personal and professional craft knowledge) that I used and how I blended them in practice in an almost seamless way and even how I created new knowledge. I became very aware of my use of the three knowledge domains of person-centred care that Titchen (2000) described in the skilled companionship conceptual framework. I was able to evaluate the strengths and balance of each of my knowledge domains, when working with my patients. I could also see where my colleagues' skilled companionship domains required strengthening, for example, where they were not enabling a patient to share in decision-making about care, and how I could raise their consciousness, that whilst saying they engage in person-centred care, their actual care did not match what they said they did.
>
> *McGinley, Chapter 4*

Different ways of knowing

Pre-cognitive knowing is ineffable knowing without mental representation. Practitioners with expertise know about particular situations pre-cognitively, through the senses, that is, through perceptual awareness (intuition, aesthetics and the embodied knowing), emotions and spiritual awareness. Moreover, this knowing may be embedded in their practice and in their qualities, such as the compassionate making of a patient's bed in a caring way that is relaxing and healing for the patient. Some researchers, such as Benner (1984), see this knowing as unarticulated, but shared, meanings within situational and relational background practices. Such knowing can sometimes be observed, for instance, in looks, facial expressions and body comportment and in meanings shared between people. Pre-cognitive knowing can also be seen in the way people may tell a story that follows on from tacit, shared meanings.

Cognitive knowing means seeking to bring our embodied, pre-cognitive, 'heart' knowledge to thought and to words, to know for one-self, and to communicate with others. Cognitive knowing is the owned and conscious journey into knowing or meaning making that effective health care epitomises. Cognitive knowing occurs, for example, when nurses with expertise name their practices and professional artistry, when they 'map out' what they know and what they want to know in order to frame their development or inquiry direction and questions, when they craft their care interventions, evaluations and inquiry strategies, when they analyse the evidence emerging from their assessments, interpret their findings, and shape them into emergent interventions. The combination of cognitive and pre-cognitive knowing is evident when a nurse with expertise seeks to articulate pre-cognitive knowing when engaging in a self-inquiry to enable others to access and understand the meaning of a particular situation or episode of care.

Metacognitive knowing refers to practitioners with expertise being aware of their cognitive processes and exerting control over these processes; it includes the cognitive skills that are necessary for the management of knowledge and other cognitive skills (Biggs, 1988). 'High quality human performance inevitably requires metacognitive as well as cognitive components. To perform well, one needs to be aware not only of the knowledge and algorithms required for the task, but of one's own motives and resources, the contextual constraints, and to plan strategically on that knowledge' (Biggs, 1986, p. 143). In choosing and using a particular care intervention, for instance, the nurse with expertise makes conscious choices about many aspects of the patient and situation that are likely to best fit the goals of care. The nurse enacts these choices knowingly at cognitive, metacognitive and reflexive levels and thus makes considered decisions that are monitored, as well as the outcome of these decisions and the actions in relation to them:

> For me, assessing a new patient is an infinitely variable interpersonal process; not a predetermined procedure. The process is adapted according to the patient's condition and how he responds to me, and according to other demands within the ward. But in some way or other, I spend time being with the patient and, at some stage, his family too. I listen to his story, as he presents it, encouraging or empathising in whatever way seems helpful at the time. I try to discover 'where he is at' and what his perceptions and concerns are. As I listen, my nursing observational skills are at work, partly at a rational, partly intuitive level. I pick up cues that my professional knowledge enables me to recognise as significant and worthy of further exploration. As the conversation proceeds, or maybe at a later stage, I ask questions that arise from the patient's story or from what I have observed or sensed. In this way, I begin to get to know the patient and his family and build a relationship with them.
>
> *Titchen, 2000, pp. 80–81*

Reflexive knowing is self-knowledge and self-awareness as a person and as a professional in interaction with others (as the above example also shows). Angela Brown, an EPP critical companion, reveals her reflexive knowing:

> My revelation now is that whilst listening and questioning are powerful strategies to make what was hidden revealed, I missed the opportunity to deepen my questioning through observing [Gill] at work. I realise now that observing in a

hospice was an issue for me and that by not reflecting upon my statement that observation could detract from the work done so far, I let myself off the hook. I remember feeling relieved that I did not have to observe in a palliative care setting.

Brown and Harrison, Chapter 5

Reflexive knowing includes awareness of the impact of that interaction on self and others, as Alison Greggans, another EPP critical companion, shows:

Challenge came in a variety of ways and any potential anxiety managed by our shared respect and prior knowledge of each other's ways of working. As an outsider, I had permission to ask almost daft questions which for Margaret was challenging in that she had to clearly explain the layers of practice – some of which were obvious – others were not so. Moreover, my constant inquiry pro- moted her to consider how these layers of practice integrated into a composite whole which could be accessed and understood by a potential novice. My ap- preciation of her expertise was helped by my own personal memories of nursing within adult intensive care units. Although a very different professional world of nursing in terms of clinical context, the espoused values and approaches she demonstrated chimed loud and clear with my own. This resonance of values and beliefs came about because we occupied familiar ground. This helped me to rapidly grasp the significance of the work and the risks Margaret took on be- half of her clients which in turn accentuated the clarity of the picture of her own expertise. How her espoused beliefs and values were translated in her practice provided opportunities for us to seek out the unique nature of this expertise and what the consequence of this expertise was on those she comes into contact with – parents, children and colleagues alike.

Greggans and Conlon, Chapter 6

Different types of knowledge

Different types of knowledge, as entwining entities (interconnected and in- terdependent propositional, professional craft[3], participant, local, political and "othered"[4] knowledge), are merged, woven together and balanced (see Higgs & Titchen, 1995; Titchen, 2001a; Rycroft-Malone *et al.*, 2004). For example, propo- sitional knowledge informing nursing care, such as philosophical, theoretical or research knowledge is individualised for the particular health care context, per- son(s) and situations. This particularisation requires attunement, as symbolised in Figure 12.5, and is a form of alchemy brought about by the nurse with exper- tise drawing on the other types of knowledge, professional judgement artistry

---

[3] For an articulation of professional craft knowledge which includes experiential, aesthetic, intu- itive and embodied knowledge, for example, and its development, see Titchen and Ersser (2001).
[4] "Othered" knowledge includes, for example, the different kind of knowing of people with a dementia or with a learning disability.

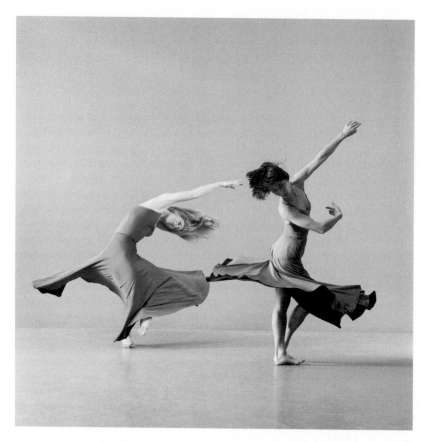

Figure 12.5 Attunement. Photo © Lois Greenfield 1985 (Lar Lubovitch Dance Company).

(Paterson *et al.*, 2006) and her or his qualities. It is shown in the following example of a skilled companion helping a staff nurse to interplay research knowledge with professional craft knowledge:

> *AB*: 'You've probably heard of Dave Thompson's work... When he measured anxiety levels in patients after coronaries, the spouse has a significantly higher anxiety than the patient themselves which is always worth bearing in mind... I often think it's worth offering the spouse some time on their own because they may be worried about things that they don't want to say in front of their husband because they think they may worry him more. But you've got to do that in such a way that you've got permission from the patient. What's quite a good idea is to ask him, "How's your wife coping?", "Does she seem anxious about all this?" and then, if he says, "She does seem a bit worried or whatever", then try to get round to saying, "Would it be helpful if I had some time with her by herself, so she can ask me questions on her own?", so that you've got the patient's permission.'

Barbara: 'Mmh. And they know that you're not going behind their backs.'
AB: 'And they know you're doing it to help the wife, rather than to go behind his back and tell him things he's not allowed to know'
(Titchen, 2000, pp. 139–140).

Professional artistry mediates different types of knowledge, ways of knowing and intelligences into the complexity and messiness of doing critical creative, human flourishing care. Propositional knowledge of research (philosophical, theoretical and methodological knowledge) is transformed, by the professional artistry of the nurse with expertise through experience and over time, to become professional craft knowledge or practical knowledge of caring for patients. As in the example above, this practical knowledge, along with other non-propositional forms of knowledge (personal, local and political knowledge), enables de-contextualised or abstract propositional knowledge to be used to guide patient care or facilitation practice in specific contexts as shown by Maeve McGinley:

> My reflective piece of evidence had provided an action plan, which I hoped to use to help work colleagues develop their expertise. Compiling the portfolio made me conscious of the new knowledge, skills and tools I was now using to examine my practice expertise and that of other practitioners. I realised that the language of expertise and the conceptual frameworks [multiple discourses – see below] that I once found impossible to understand had become embedded in my knowledge and practice such that they were now a vital and integral part of my professional craft knowledge. My understanding of the attributes of expertise had developed so much that I no longer thought of them as separate entities to the conceptual model of skilled companionship. Rather, when I thought of *knowing the patient* and *moral agency* I linked them to Titchen's (2000) relationship domain, because I understood that to really know the patient I had to realise the concept processes within that domain. I was already beginning to evaluate my own and others' practice, using tools such as the attributes and then linking them to the conceptual framework. In doing so, I was identifying how I could develop and improve practice and, at the same time, showing an aspect of professional artistry, that is, being aware that I was blending different types of knowledge in practice [metacognition].
>
> *McGinley, Chapter 4*

Using different types of knowledge is also shown by Liz Henderson:

> [In relation to painful growth for learners and herself as facilitator] On this occasion I was again drawing on many knowledge sources. Knowledge of the co learners and reading what was going on identified that there was a problem. Practice development knowledge, facilitation theory, group theory and previous experience helped me to handle it, personal knowledge gave me the confidence to so act, whilst professional artistry helped mediate the theory into action and prompted the timing ... In terms of personal knowledge I was very self aware in the midst of the situation. By remaining calm, composed and present

[embodied and emotional intelligence – see below], and by interpreting what was happening I was aiming to give the group confidence that the process was being attended to. This is another example of praxis enabled by professional artistry within a critical creativity worldview, but this time in the midst of a painful situation, yet one that resulted in growth for us all.

Henderson, Chapter 11

Multiple intelligences

As symbolised in Figures 12.4 and 12.5, different types of knowledge and ways of knowing work together or synchronise in a choreographed dance of theory into action and meaning making through the interplay, seemingly, of *four intelligences* (embodied, artistic, emotional and spiritual). Professional artistry also involves the blending and interplay of a variety of intelligences and the use of self as person, practitioner and inquirer. Intelligence is taken to mean a capacity for, and quickness of, understanding or sagacity (*Concise Oxford Dictionary*, 1982) or as the organisation of the mind (Gardner, 1993). Complementary to Gardner's theory of multiple human intelligences, four intelligences appear relevant to nursing expertise; these are embodied, emotional, artistic and spiritual intelligences (Titchen & Higgs, 2001). These intelligences provide the capacity and background wisdom that facilitate different ways of knowing. Higgs and Titchen (2007) 'hypothesise that these intelligences contribute to the rapid blending of the different types of knowledge discussed above and the ability to switch quickly and effortlessly from one level of knowing to another as appropriate to the context and situation' (p. 18).

Embodied intelligence is the wisdom of the body that enables nurses with expertise to engage in body-situated, reflexive analysis of their practice. The body holds hidden knowing or insight that is usually overshadowed by our cognitive knowing. This hidden knowing can be accessed and expressed through embodied intelligence, that is, our capacity and quickness to gain understanding of pre-cognitive knowledge of ourselves and others. Drawing on ideas from creative arts therapies, nurses with expertise may develop their embodied intelligence through enactment (role-playing), engaging the body through gesture and physical expression as critical reflection (Coats, 2001), dynamic gesture or image theatre (Boal, 1982), and authentic movement (Pallaro, 1999). It seems that embodied intelligence is developed through embodied learning and through paying attention to the body.

Although *artistic intelligence* (Cowan, 2002) in nursing practice is central to the aesthetically satisfying care and multidisciplinary working, I argue that it is also central to the process of artistic critique in critical and creative practice and its development. Building on Gardner's work (1993), it is proposed that artistic intelligence is the capacity to create, to perform and to appreciate artistic expression. Working synergistically with embodied intelligence, artistic intelligence facilitates the sensing of the unconscious and brings it to consciousness through artistic expression. The use of creative arts media is helpful, not only in helping us to do this, but also in enabling others to surface and then critique their knowledge and wisdom artistically, cognitively and metacognitively. Many others use Art (with a capital A) to access ontological knowing or experiencing (e.g. Silva *et al.*, 1995; Stephens *et al.*, 2004). Artistic intelligence also helps us, often in an instant, to judge whether some new thing is expressed in exactly the right way. It shows us whether the expression is enough, satisfying, fulfilling, whether there is balance, beauty, synchronicity, interplay and form. The synergy of embodied and artistic intelligences can be seen in this following example from my research:

> By not rushing Pam and by being graceful in her movements, Alison [nurse with expertise] appeared to create a therapeutic, healing environment around Pam. The pace and mood were set by her relaxed posture, fluent, unhurried movements and a patient, warm, but energetic tone of voice. She tried to create as little noise as possible as she lifted furniture or equipment and seemed aware when she banged equipment inadvertently.
>
> *Fieldnote*: Alison helped Pam, who was agitated and disoriented, onto the commode and told her that she was going to make the bed. She gave Pam a lot of time to take it all in and kept reassuring her that she was still there and that she was not going to leave her for now. Alison kept returning to the front of the commode to give Pam eye contact and to hold both her arms. She explained that Pam was getting better and kept reminding her to try to use the commode. This re-iterative, flowing pattern of movement, almost poetic in nature, epitomised for me the gracefulness of Alison's movements that relaxes her patients. I am constantly struck by the graceful way in which she makes a bed, smoothes a patient's pillow or strokes a patient's cheek [aesthetic knowing].
>
> *Titchen, 2000, p. 90*

Emotional intelligence gives nurses with expertise awareness of, or attunement to, their own and others' feelings, facilitating social adeptness, empathy, compassion, motivation, caring and appropriate responses to pain or pleasure. Gardner (1993) refers to this as intra- and interpersonal intelligence. This intelligence enables practitioners to use their professional craft knowledge, as shown above in the skilled companionship example, or in relation to knowing the patient or colleague as a person and knowing ourselves in relationship with them (personal knowledge), for instance. A capacity and quickness in picking up cues, in ourselves and others, is central to practice with a concern for human flourishing and transformation. For example, Liz Henderson, in her Chapter 11 account of helping clinical nurse specialists to develop their expertise, demonstrates her capacity to respond quickly to cues from her nursing colleagues and by immediately engaging emotionally and genuinely with them as people, with the whole of herself as a person, the group crisis is resolved and learned from. Emotional intelligence serves us well as we engage with our other intelligences, which are likely to challenge and take us out of our comfort zones. It is also central to critical thinking (metacognition) as feelings and emotions are inherent in critical thinking (e.g. Kuiper & Pesut, 2004), and if negative emotions arising from critical reflection are handled intelligently, then critical thinking will be promoted.

Spiritual intelligence (Zohar & Marshall, 2000) enables us to address and solve problems of meaning and value and place our actions, lives and pathways in wider, richer meaning-giving contexts. It gives us our moral sense and allows us to discriminate, to aspire, to dream and to uplift ourselves. Whereas embodied and emotional intelligences allow us to work *within* the boundaries of our situation and context and be guided by the same, artistic and spiritual intelligences, let us work *with* the boundaries and shape and transform the situation. However, embodied intelligence may lead to the awakening of spiritual intelligence. We also invoke spiritual intelligence when we are creative, using our deep, intuitive sense of meaning and value to guide us when we are at the boundary of order and chaos, that is, at the very edge of our comfort zone. Thus, artistic intelligence and spiritual intelligence are very closely linked.

If nursing, facilitation and inquiry expertise are like dancing a choreographed piece, but with the freedom to let go, improvise and be creative, then it is the four intelligences that give us the capacity to dance. The intelligences work in harmony, responding to each other, facilitating synthesis and interplay of all aspects of self (our being, knowing, doing and becoming), and creativity emerges (see Figure 12.6). Capacity and quickness develop through reflexive, creative journeying and through critical and creative conversations with others on the way. These intelligences have the potential to enable speedy, effective responses to care, inquiry and learning situations and open the way for meaning making.

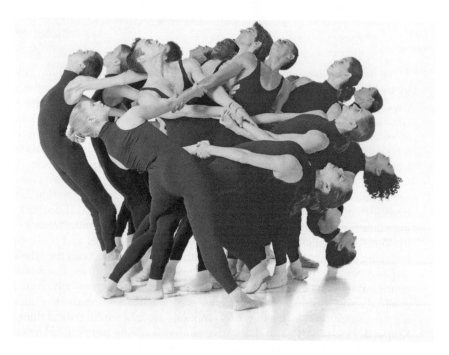

Figure 12.6 Synthesis and blending. Photo © Lois Greenfield 1995 (Ballet Tech).

Creative imagination

Creative imagination, so it is reported, was considered by Albert Einstein to be more important than knowledge. Overall, it seems to be metacognitive skills that action imagination with ways of knowing, knowledge and intelligences in the uniqueness of relationships and in all aspects of practice. Metacognition in this capacity is shown in Liz Henderson's (Chapter 11) account of using postcards to help a group of clinical nurse specialists to symbolise their thoughts about where they were at as a group:

> This is an example of being critically creative. The postcard images were the tool used. But as facilitator I was consciously drawing on and blending knowledge sources, whilst using my creative imagination, and engaging in creative expression with the intent of intensifying the conditions for human growth and flourishing (i.e., I was engaging in professional artistry).
>
> *Henderson, Chapter 11*

Metacognition also manages the fine interplay between intuition, meditation, contemplation, practical reasoning and rational reasoning. It also works with the pre-cognitive, creative imagination and artistic expression and reflexivity to enable artistic and cognitive critique. Moreover, creative leaps and moments of inspiration are often a result of metacognition doing its work. Imaginative and creative approaches inform and are informed by rational understandings and meaning making.

Professional artistry provides the synergy and power to blend. It allows nurses with expertise to dance between imagination, conventions, 'truths' and the local situation. It means seeing the macro- and micro-pictures at the same time or being able to see the whole and the parts of some aspect of practice or experience. The trick is to move between them and get the balance and form right. Thinking creatively, imaginatively and diversely allows multiple choices, explanations and solutions to emerge.

Multiple discourses

As well as all the above capacities and flexibility to interplay, juxtapose and mediate, the practitioner with expertise is also able to dance between the different discourses used at different interfaces in the workplace and organisation. So the nurse is able to speak the language of diverse colleagues in the multiprofesssional team, the patient and their families, senior managers and policy makers, for example. This capacity and skill enables the nurse to mediate and influence and make things happen for the benefit of the patient.

Artistic and cognitive critique

The synergy between artistic and cognitive critique occurs through a re-iterative, reciprocal dialogue between words and art forms. A few nurses with expertise in the EPP engaged in such critique and were able to turn their emerging understanding of their own expertise into informed, transformed and transforming

233

action with moral intent human flourishing for themselves and those they worked with and cared for as shown in Chapter 5 and in the EPP report:

> During one of those defining moments with my critical companion, we recognised something in my daughter's old home-made painting pinned over my desk. It was an abstract wheel that threw out paint streaks as the paper had revolved around a turntable. It epitomised the nature of the nurse-patient expert interaction. Without movement there would still be a painting but only random dots and splashes although the very same actions had taken place. Movement had created cohesion, patterning and beauty.... The difference [between expertise and non-expertise] is in the heart of the action, the underpinning movement itself and at the moment of its creation (portfolio evidence).
>
> *Manley et al., 2005, p. 27*

This kind of critique enables the continual reconstruction of theory in and on practice. This is an area in need of research to test and elaborate.

Transformative, creative use of self

Being personal is fundamental to work that is concerned ultimately with human flourishing. Being critical and creative is personally transforming, creative, person centred, relationship based; bringing who I am – mind, body, imagination, spirit, into my practice and practice relationships. Being person centred and heart based in relationships means dancing with our multiple selves to transform individuals, teams, organisations, communities, cultures and practices. Knowing one's self (reflexive knowing) is paramount to intentional use of self in person-centred care, inquiry and facilitation. 'Dancing' with others means engaging the whole of ourselves with patients, families, colleagues as individual people. This 'dance' requires creative approaches to ensure that genuine person-centred relationships can be formed. These are relationships in which those with whom the professional works feel comfortable, safe, valued and known as an individual and person. In addition, they feel cared for and about and really met by the professional on their terms. In each intervention, by getting to know others as people, the professional with expertise is able to design a unique approach by melding and blending.

Creating the conditions

You may be thinking that this professional artistry is a tall order! And so it is, as expertise is not easily developed. Facilitation of its development using the processes and strategies of critical companionship and any other holistic facilitation approach is likely to work, as this book shows, but it is not the only thing. Without the conditions for human flourishing and professional artistry in place (i.e. a supportive culture and systems), the use of facilitation processes and strategies will simply not be enough. As Patricia Benner (1984) recognised all those years ago, there is a need for creating and sustaining the conditions for expertise development in your team, workplace, organisation or community. Since then, new understandings about how to create and sustain these conditions have been developed through collaborative research in the new field of practice development. Now, I draw on two pieces of this work to suggest how the conditions for professional artistry development can be provided through creating cultures, systems, strategies and learning opportunities at work that promote human flourishing (see Figure 12.2).

Creating cultures and systems for human flourishing

Much has been written in the practice development literature about creating transformational cultures of effectiveness (e.g. Manley, 2004; Dewing & Titchen, 2007). Until recently, human flourishing has not been openly espoused as one of the outcomes of such a culture, but now it has in two concept analyses, one of workplace culture which is examined here and the other of WBL which guides our thinking in the next section.

Based on an extensive literature review, Manley *et al.* (unpublished) differentiated the enabling factors, attributes and outcomes of an effective workplace culture. Five key attributes were identified (see Box 1.4). The first is that specific values are promoted in the workplace and that these values are person-centredness, lifelong learning, support and challenge, leadership development, involvement and participation by stakeholders, evidence use and development, positive attitude to change, open communication, and teamwork. The living of these values is partially explicated in the above description of professional artistry, particularly in relation to being a person-centred nurse, inquirer or facilitator, and to using evidence (different types of knowledge) and developing it (through blending, synthesis, interplay and balance, and the use of different ways of knowing). The second attribute is that these values are really lived and that there is a shared vision and mission in the workplace and individual and collective responsibility. Thus, to nurture professional artistry, there would need to be a common vision and mission about the development of expertise in the workplace and its development would be the responsibility of individual practitioners, managers and leaders. There would be a collective responsibility within the governance of the organisation.

The third attribute is that adaptability, innovation and creativity maintain workplace effectiveness. It could be argued that if practitioners, leaders, managers and facilitators intentionally develop and refine their own professional artistry, especially their ways of knowing, intelligences, creative imagination and transformative, creative use of self, then this attribute would be seen in their workplace. The fourth attribute is that appropriate change is driven by the needs of patients, users and communities. Nurses with expertise, as shown in this book, are skilled at getting to *know the patient* (professional craft knowledge) and thus what their needs are (the patients' personal knowledge). Such nurses also possess local knowledge about the context and community and propositional knowledge about how to involve stakeholders' participation in decision-making. The interaction of these knowledges occurs through professional artistry and this blended knowledge use enables stakeholders, which include patients and clients, to feel genuinely involved, listened to and valued and so, possibly, to flourish. The final and fifth attribute is that formal systems exist to foster and evaluate learning, performance and shared governance. In a workplace that intentionally promotes the development of expertise of its staff, diverse WBL opportunities are going to be in place, such as clinical supervision support, action learning, active learning and reflexive learning strategies, in addition to opportunities for critical review, career progression, recognition and/or accreditation.

Building on this concept analysis, the enabling factors for nurturing professional artistry are likely to be transformational leadership, skilled facilitation, role clarification, flattened and transparent management, organisational readiness, and human resource management support. Drawing next on the concept analysis of WBL, organisational readiness is further explored before articulating the attributes of an effective facilitator of active learning within a WBL context. But first, a contemporary understanding of WBL is offered.

Developing professional artistry through WBL

Arising from a recent concept analysis of WBL (Manley *et al.*, in press), again from an extensive literature review, WBL is defined as:

> Everyday work of healthcare is the basis for learning, development, inquiry and transformation in the workplace. WBL requires skilled facilitators who are able to integrate multiple organisational agendas and draw on a wide range of appropriate skills and resources for simultaneous learning, development, inquiry and transformation. WBL is also recognised by active learners who learn with, and from, each other in a variety of formal and informal learning situations and approaches. Systems are in place in the workplace for providing assessment, feedback and support and for enabling learners to investigate, evaluate and transform their practice and work environment. WBL is enabled by organisation-wide learning philosophy and a supportive infrastructure. The consequences of WBL include individual/personal, interdisciplinary/team and organisational effectiveness. WBL aspires to enable all those involved in WBL, and those benefiting from it, to flourish and grow.
>
> *Manley et al., in press*

According to this review, the WBL literature demonstrates that in the past, the contextual focus of learning and work has tended to be on *using the work context for learning*. Thus, learning has occurred at a distance from the work context, for example, problem-based learning or distance learning. Alternatively, learning is seen as an integration of practice experiences with the broader goals of an undergraduate curriculum. More recently, and the EPP is an example, there has been a shift to a contextual focus of *learning at/in work* where practitioners, in partnership with practice development consultants/internal or external facilitators/colleagues, undertake WBL to improve patient care, create cultures of effectiveness, meet government targets, and contribute to their organisation's innovation, service improvement, and implementation and evaluation of clinical, shared and research governance agendas.

In this book, our vision of developing expertise through nurturing professional artistry is located in the *learning at/in work* focus and is concerned with the creation of an active learning culture and developing systems and partnerships that support active learning in the workplace. Active learning revolves around reflection, dialogue with self and others and engaging in learning activities in the workplace that make use of the senses, multiple intelligences and doing things (i.e., workplace learning activities) together with colleagues and others (Dewing, 2008). Thus, active learning engages learner and facilitator in all the dimensions of professional artistry set out above. For this vision to live, organisational readiness is paramount. It is likely that this readiness is displayed when there exists an organisation-wide learning philosophy, as described by Manley *et al.* (in press). This philosophy would include a learner-centred approach, education outcome directly related to the needs of the organisation as well as the needs of learners, a workplace active learning culture in place, nurturing creativity and reflexivity to develop professional artistry, and collaborative learning towards shared goals. Organisation readiness is also demonstrated by a supportive organisation-wide infrastructure that might include partnership working between practitioners, academic and health care organisations and communities, professional and academic accreditation, locally delivered programmes tailored to the workplace, preparation of supportive facilitator roles, strategic direction for learning, and time and financial resources.

Active learners have motivation and potential for learning and development. They are willing and prepared to *learn at/in work* as adult, lifelong learners. They are likely to have different potential for learning and development. This potential may vary on a spiralling continuum in relation to their starting points and their movements along the continuum (see Box 12.1).

Whilst most of the literature refers to individual learners, there is sufficient evidence, as implied above, that learning does not just happen on an individual basis, but can also be achieved through group or team-based processes.

Learning from and with others. Health care work involves interaction with others. These interactions can be used as a basis for learning and development involving others, specifically:

- Learning *from* others who have health care expertise, experiences of care, workplace culture and communities of practice. This may occur informally and formally.
- Learning *with* others in small groups such as action learning or clinical supervision.
- Learning *with* a facilitator in a one-to-one relationship such as mentorship, supervision, critical companionship, sponsorship and coaching.

The facilitation processes of active learning are presented in Box 12.2.

Box 12.1   Characteristics of active learners

At one end of the spiralling continuum, active learners have potential for the following characteristics:
- listen and learn from others;
- take the initiative in identifying self-deficits;
- set their own learning objectives and goals;
- learn from their own work experience.

Along the continuum, active learners have potential to:
- appreciate the integral and reciprocal roles of learning and inquiry;
- investigate and advance their own work skills and practices;
- develop their reflexivity;
- identify contradictions and opportunities for innovation and transformation;
- develop different ways of thinking, that is, pre-cognitive, cognitive, metacognitive and reflexive;
- become mindful doers who are competent and confident;
- work with complexity;
- recognise, expose, critically review and evaluate the different types of knowledge underpinning work (practice epistemology) and purposefully integrate them;
- collaboratively test current knowledge and co-construct new knowledge through learning and inquiry;
- undertake practitioner research to develop new understandings and to transform work practices simultaneously.

At the end of the continuum, active learners have the potential to develop professional artistry which, as the pinnacle of professional practice, encompasses all the above.

The development of professional artistry is a spiralling continuum and it is not only for people like the nurses with expertise in the EPP. This development can become a way of life in the workplace with practitioners moving along different parts of the continuum. Not all will, or will want to, reach the pinnacle of professional artistry, but understanding its nature, and that developing it is a journey, will enable leaders, managers, facilitators and practitioners to work together to create the conditions for human flourishing and thus for professional artistry.

Concluding remarks

This chapter has re-emphasised the importance of skilled facilitation of active learning in the development of practice expertise. It has built on the assumption that professional artistry, often hidden and embedded in practice, is the essence, pinnacle and hallmark of expertise, whatever a person's field of clinical, inquiry or facilitation practice. As a resource for practitioners, inquirers and facilitators, the dimensions and processes of professional artistry have, therefore, been set out, building on empirical and scholarly research. The necessary conditions (culture,

Box 12.2   Active learning facilitation processes

At one end, active learners have potential for the following characteristics:
- Adopts an internal or external role.
- Prepares and develops the learning and inquiry/practitioner research culture and learners for adult learning and WBL.
- Negotiates learning contracts and actions to be taken to achieve goals.
- Optimises the use of appropriate resources.
- Helps people to learn opportunistically in the midst of everyday work and in one-to-one and group learning situations.
- Helps learners to achieve the attributes of active learner as appropriate to the person, group and context (see above attributes of active learner).
- Role-models and articulates own professional craft knowledge about the professional artistry of being an active learner, facilitating active learning, and being a person-centred, effective health care worker.
- Enables the development of all the dimensions of professional artistry and their integration within praxis through using approaches that are cognitive and creative.
- Uses a wide range of styles, processes and skills that match where learners are at and the contexts in which they are working.
- Enables a working relationship/partnership built on mutual trust and high challenge and high support through paying attention to the whole person, processes as well as outcomes.
- Facilitates rigorous organisational, cultural and practice change at individual, team, organisational and community levels through practice development or practitioner research.
- Project administration/management.

systems, structures and facilitation) to promote the growth of expertise and professional artistry in the workplace have been discussed. It has been proposed that WBL and skilled facilitation are central to promoting active learning as an inquiry process along a continuum of expertise development towards professional artistry. The attributes of active learning and its facilitation have been set out and it has been suggested that learning and inquiry can be integrated and enabled simultaneously.

Within the context of increasing demand for finite health care resources and a greater emphasis being placed on value for money, learning approaches such as WBL that can meet the integrated learning needs of the individual, the health care team and the organisation should be considered. It is also concluded that the development of expertise through WBL is an organisation-wide responsibility. Whilst the key research upon which this book is based (i.e. Manley *et al.*, 2005) has shown convincingly that active learning and expertise development can be facilitated through action learning, practitioner research and critical companionship in the workplace, these learning approaches are insufficient in themselves. Implications in relation to the enabling factors and attributes of WBL and an effective workplace culture need to be considered, recognised and acted upon by the organisation, workplace, team and individual. This may mean that organisational, practice and professional development needs to take place.

The implications for organisations are as follows:

- Expertise development can meet the needs of individuals as well as teams and the organisation and should be built into the strategic direction of the organisation.
- Organisation-wide cultures of effectiveness, learning and inquiry can be created through systematic practice development approaches.
- Organisation-wide systems, learning support structures and skilled facilitation development need to be in place.
- Leaders and managers are supported in taking WBL forward across all levels of the organisation.
- Higher education providers can be commissioned to support WBL programmes that promote simultaneous learning and inquiry for expertise development in the workplace itself.
- Time for WBL learning and inquiry must be provided for staff if they are to become more efficient and effective.
- Expertise development can be recognised, valued and rewarded by the organisation through career development opportunities and accreditation.
- Academic and/or professional accreditation can be offered.

These implications for the organisation impact on the workplace:

- Workplace cultures of effectiveness, learning and inquiry can be created by those who work in the workplace using systematic practice development approaches.
- Leaders and managers in the workplace:
  - overtly value expertise development;
  - are genuinely transformational in the way they work with staff (this may require some fundamental changes in leadership and management styles and ways of working) (see Dewing, 2008);
  - ensure that they and others in the workplace develop the skill sets for effective facilitation of WBL and expertise development;
  - re-frame the common perception and assumption that there is no time for learning in and from work by learning how to facilitate others and their own learning during the work itself and to role-model it;
  - demonstrate, through their actions, that inquiry into practice is a professional responsibility and that time must be made available for evaluating performance and impact on patients/clients and for providing evidence of expertise.

The implications for educators are as follows:

- There is a move away from historical models of learning and development provision towards a contemporary conceptualisation of WBL.

- A focus on developing skilled facilitators in the workplace to support expertise development and professional artistry.

Implications for individual practitioners are that they:

- commit to active learning as inquiry along a continuum;
- gather evidence from their practice and analyse it in relation to conceptual frameworks of expertise and professional artistry to identify their gaps and document their journeys towards expertise.

References

Benner, P. (1984) *From Novice to Expert: Excellence and Power in Clinical Nursing Practice.* Addison-Wesley, London.

Biggs, J. (1988) The role of metacognition in enhancing learning. *Australian Journal of Education.* **32**, 127–138.

Biggs, J.B. (1986) Enhancing learning skills: the role of metacognition. In: *Student Learning: Research into Practice – The Marysville Symposium* (eds J.A. Bowden), pp. 131–48. Centre for the Study of Higher Education, The University of Melbourne.

Boal, A. (1982). *The Theatre of the Oppressed.* Routledge, London.

Coats, E. (2001) Weaving the body, the creative unconscious, imagination and the arts into practice development. In: *Professional Practice in Health, Education and the Creative Arts* (eds J. Higgs & A. Titchen), pp. 251–263. Blackwell, Oxford.

Concise Oxford Dictionary (1982) (eds A.L. Hayward & J.J. Sparkes). Omega Books, London.

Cowan, D. (2002) *Artistic intelligence and leadership framing: Employing the wisdom of envisioning, improvisation, introspection and inclusion.* Presented at The Art of Management and Organization Conference, King's College, London.

Dewing, J. (2008) Implications for nursing managers from a systematic review of practice development. *Journal of Nursing Management* **16**, 134–140.

Dewing, J. & Titchen, A. (2007) *Workplace Resources for Practice Development.* Royal College of Nursing, London.

Gardner, H. (1993) *Multiple Intelligences: The Theory in Practice.* Basic Books, New York.

Hardy, S., Titchen, A., Manley, K. & McCormack, B. (2006) Re-defining nursing expertise in the United Kingdom. *Nursing Science Quarterly* **19**(3), 260–264.

Higgs, J. & Titchen, A. (1995) The nature, generation and verification of knowledge. *Physiotherapy* **81**(9), 521–530.

Higgs, J. & Titchen, A. (2007) Qualitative research: journeys of meaning-making through transformation, illumination, shared action and liberation. In: *Being Critical and Creative in Qualitative Research* (eds J. Higgs, A. Titchen, D. Horsfall & H.B. Armstrong), pp. 11–21. Hampden Press, Sydney.

Johns, C. (1998) Opening the doors of perception. In: *Transforming Nurses through Reflective Practice* (eds C. Jones & D. Freshwater), pp. 1–20. Blackwell, Oxford.

Kuiper, R.A. & Pesut, D.J. (2004) Promoting cognitive and metacognitive reflective reasoning skills in nursing practice: self-regulated learning theory. *Journal of Advanced Nursing* **45**(4), 381–391.

Manley, K. (2004) A transformational culture: a culture of effectiveness. In: *Practice Development in Nursing* (eds B. McCormack, K. Manley & R. Garbett), pp. 51–82. Blackwell, Oxford.

Manley, K. & McCormack, B. (1997) *Exploring Expert Practice* (NUM65U). Royal College of Nursing, London.

Manley, K., Titchen, A. & Hardy, S. (in press) Work based learning in the context of contemporary healthcare education and practice: a concept analysis. *Practice Development in Health Care.*

Manley, K., Sanders, K., Cardiff, S., Garbarino, L. & Davren, M. (unpublished) Workplace culture of effectiveness: a concept analysis. *International Practice Development Collaborative.*

Manley, K., Hardy, S., Titchen, A., Garbett, R. & McCormack, B. (2005) *Changing Patients' Worlds through Nursing Practice Expertise: A Research Report.* Royal College of Nursing, London.

McCormack, B. & Titchen, A. (2006) Critical creativity: melding, exploding, blending. *Educational Action Research: an International Journal* **14**(2), 239–266.

Pallaro, P. (1999). *Authentic Movement: Essays by Mary Starks Whitehouse, Janet Adler and Joan Chodorow.* Jessica Kingsley, London.

Paterson, M., Wilcox, S. & Higgs, J. (2006) Exploring dimensions of artistry in reflective practice. *Reflective Practice* **7**(4), 455–468.

Rycroft-Malone, J., Harvey, G., Seers, K., Kitson, A., McCormack, B. & Titchen, A. (2004) An exploration of the factors that influence the implementation of evidence into practice. *Journal of Clinical Nursing* **13**, 913–924.

Schon, D.A. (1983) *The Reflective Practitioner: How Professionals Think in Action.* Temple Smith, London.

Silva, M.C., Sorrell, J.M. & Sorrell, C.D. (1995) From Carper's patterns of knowing to ways of being: an ontological philosophical shift in nursing. *Advances in Nursing Science* **18**(1), 1–13.

Stephens, G., Titchen, A., McCormack, B. *et al.* (2004) *Creative Arts and Humanities in Healthcare: Swallows to Other Continents.* The Nuffield Trust, London.

Titchen, A. (2000) *Professional Craft Knowledge in Patient-Centred Nursing and the Facilitation of Its Development.* University of Oxford DPhil Thesis. Ashdale, Oxford.

Titchen, A. (2001a) Skilled companionship in professional practice. In: *Practice Knowledge and Expertise in the Health Professions* (eds J. Higgs & A. Titchen), pp. 69–79. Butterworth Heinemann, Oxford.

Titchen, A. (2001b) Critical companionship: a conceptual framework for developing expertise. In: *Practice Knowledge and Expertise in the Health Professions* (eds J. Higgs & A. Titchen), pp. 80–90. Butterworth Heinemann, Oxford.

Titchen, A. (2004) Helping relationships for practice development: critical companionship. In: *Practice Development in Nursing* (eds B. McCormack, K. Manley & R. Garbett), pp. 148–174. Blackwell, Oxford.

Titchen, A. & Ersser, S. (2001) The nature of professional craft knowledge. In: *Practice Knowledge and Expertise in the Health Professions* (eds J. Higgs & A. Titchen), pp. 35–41. Butterworth Heinemann, Oxford.

Titchen, A. & Higgs, J. (2001) Towards professional artistry and creativity in practice. In *Professional Practice in Health, Education and the Creative Arts* (eds J. Higgs & A. Titchen), pp. 273–290. Blackwell, Oxford.

Titchen, A., Higgs, J. & Horsfall, D. (2007) Research artistry: dancing the praxis spiral in critical-creative qualitative research. In: *Being Critical and Creative in Qualitative Research* (eds J. Higgs, A. Titchen, D. Horsfall & H.B. Armstrong), pp. 282–297. Hampden, Sydney.

Zohar, D. & Marshall, I. (2000) *SQ: Spiritual Intelligence the Ultimate Intelligence.* Bloomsbury, London.

13. Revealing the Hidden Treasures of Practice Expertise

Sally Hardy

Principal methods for transformation

Within this chapter, several principal methods for promoting, capturing and enabling practice transformation are presented. It is my intention to explore and explain the theoretical background alongside practical ways of adapting and utilising methods to ensure participants, in the inquiry process, are learning, developing and flourishing, whether that be in a personal way (e.g. in terms of increased or improved self-confidence), or in a professional sense (e.g. further understanding and articulating their expertise). I have titled this chapter, revealing the hidden treasures of practice expertise, as it is often difficult for expert practitioners to readily articulate their practice wisdom and professional artistry. However, the following choice of methods have all been tried, tested and written about in the literature to reveal that they can provide a structured process for helping practitioners gain insight and understanding of tacit knowledge and habitualised daily expert practices. I have concentrated on the experiences gained through the Expertise in Practice Project (EPP) (Manley *et al.*, 2005). Using direct practice observation, developmental feedback and critical reflexivity to further understand and articulate practice expertise will together form a foundation from which to reveal nursing's hidden treasures.

Additional resources

At the end of this chapter is a list of additional resources. The more complete the resource, the more useful it will be to more people. However, using educational programs (e.g. workbooks) and resources (e.g. videos, fact sheets and interactive CD's) do not adequately prepare people to utilise the methods, it is through facilitative support and adapting to the specific contexts (as identified by Jill Down's account of an emancipatory action research project at Addenbrooke's Foundation

Trust (Cambridge, UK) outlined in the narratives section in this chapter) that most lasting effect is achieved.

One resource that provides a versatile collection is from the Royal College of Nursing's *Workplace Resources for Practice Development* (Dewing & Titchen, 2007). This pack provides an excellent resource for any practice developer bringing together templates, workshop outlines and other activities, for example, undertaking a values clarification exercise through to protocols for obtaining staff and patient feedback.

Qualitative 360° feedback

Alimo-Metcalffe (1996) suggests that

> The process [of 360 degree feedback] is about getting people who work together to share their perceptions of each other, citing specific evidence and examples of what appears to them as effective behaviour or perhaps a problem.
>
> *Alimo-Metcalffe, 1996, p. 15*

Feedback tools in the literature tend to address aspects of leadership and/or managerial behaviour. Models of 360° feedback appear to have been developed in organisations where workers can anticipate contact with a large number of co-workers. An example of this more traditional form of 360° feedback remains in use by the UK's RCN's Clinical Leadership project (Cunningham & Kitson, 2000).

Drawing on the clinical leadership experience, 360° feedback was used in the EPP, as part of a repertoire of approaches used by practitioners to collect a varied portfolio of evidence. The rationale for using a 360° approach within the EPP was to gather corroborative evidence, looking to understand and articulate individual practitioner's practice expertise.

Garbett *et al.* (2006) explore the literature and influences that informed the process for using qualitative 360° feedback as part of the EPP (Manley *et al.*, 2005). Redwood *et al.* (2007) used a process of 360° feedback as part of an evaluation of the consultant nurse role. Other authors give various and technical accounts of the utility of 360° feedback with a variety of groups such as managers (Dalton, 2005), health care administrators (Garman *et al.*, 2004), an entire local health department (Swain *et al.*, 2004), and as a process for assessing medical competency (Rodgers & Manifold, 2002).

What are the ethical implications of working with 360° feedback?
One of the ethical considerations for using 360° feedback is whether anonymisation is necessary to improve the validity of 'authentic' feedback (Lepsinger & Lucia, 1997; Tornow & London, 1997; Ward, 1997). Anonymous feedback is based on an assumption that people will only offer honest feedback if they believe the

person in receipt of that feedback will not know who the feedback is coming from. The EPP project team wanted to contest the notion that anonymity was a necessary precondition to obtaining feedback, in order to consider the wider value of feedback as a process for improved organisational communication and teamwork (Tornow & London, 1997).

In health care, however, feedback is often experienced in a very negative way, and received only when something is perceived to be going wrong, rather than seen as an expectation of balanced and ongoing developmental opportunity.

A second major aspect of ethical consideration is the process of inclusion, particularly for people with direct experience of health care (i.e. service users) as significant role set members. Hardy *et al.* (2007) describe the issues involved in gathering feedback from service users, as people with experience of health care, and the impact that had on the EPP nurse participants. The need for multicentre ethical approval for this aspect of the EPP proved a convoluted process which impacted on allowing adequate time within the project time frame to meaningfully complete the process.

What are the challenges associated with 360° feedback?
Another challenge of engaging in 360° feedback was participants' ability to identify a role set (that represented the range of stakeholders with experience of different aspects of practice). The role set was considered to potentially comprise of representation from:

- *Peers*: Work colleagues of similar grade/level.
- *Junior colleagues*: Other nurses who the participant leads, supervises or otherwise models good practice to.
- *Senior colleagues*: Managers or professional leaders who have an influence on the participant's clinical practice.
- *Colleagues from other disciplines*: Including, for example, members of the various allied health professionals and medical staff.
- *Service users*: The complex and sensitive nature of the process of collecting feedback from service users was deemed to be an activity in its own right. Nonetheless, it is acknowledged that a true '360° view' should incorporate the view of the service user.

An example matrix, used to facilitate the choice of role set members, based on their knowledge of the person seeking feedback and their own capacity to provide feedback as used in the EPP, is outlined below (Box 13.1). Within the EPP, role sets ranged in size from three people to a maximum of ten. From the information gathered in participants' portfolios of evidence, role set members consisted of 6 service users, 27 'senior colleagues', 25 'junior', and 44 'peers'. The remaining five role set members either were unidentified or did not fit within the identified in the matrix (i.e. union representative).

Box 13.1 A matrix for ensuring coverage of the scope of practice and different types of feedback

Role set		Understanding of specialist issues	Interpersonal skills	Clinical knowledge	Able to provide challenging feedback	Willing to provide supportive feedback
Peer	Clinical nurse specialist A	✓		✓	✓	
Senior colleague	Manager E				✓	
Senior colleague	Doctor B		✓			✓
Peer	Occupational therapist C		✓			
Junior colleague	Nursing auxiliary D	✓				✓
Service user	Client/patient/user	✓	✓		✓	✓

Three methods were used in the EPP for gathering feedback from role set members:

(a) *Feedback gathered in interviews by the critical companions.* Interviews provide rich data but are time consuming to organise and produce large quantities of data that need to be processed and analysed. Producing and distributing a questionnaire may be more manageable and less threatening but the detail of feedback may be less.

(b) *Both critical companion and expert participant involved in gathering data.* This approach appeared to be a highly successful strategy, in that a larger role set was engaged, due to two people gathering the feedback. The critical companion was most often used in this approach when the participant was concerned about obtaining biased feedback (e.g. with patients and junior colleagues).

(c) *Data gathered using an anonymised questionnaire.* This approach was able to reach a large number of potential role set respondents but yielded only minimal response rates (33%). Four participants designed their own questionnaires. Two participants used the same instrument that was designed initially by another participant in their action learning set. In three cases, there was an overt attempt to anonymise the feedback. The attributes and enabling factors of expertise (Manley & McCormack, 1997) were used to shape the questions posed. This was particularly true of the questionnaire, used in the EPP (see Box 13.2).

A critical companion to one participant described the difficulties experienced using the questionnaire. Initially, she described considerable resistance to providing feedback (even though it was anonymous). Her initial response was to 'badger people' but realised that trying to understand why they were not responding would be more fruitful.

A variety of approaches were used to help make sense of the feedback. These can be summarised as follows:

- The critical companion analysed the feedback and then presented a summarised thematic form to the expert participant for further discussion. However, this reduced the potential for feedback to be detailed and specific.
- The critical companion and expert participant jointly analysed the data. This process provided the greatest learning opportunities for both parties involved.

What are the benefits for engaging in 360° feedback?
A number of participants reported feeling affirmed by the nature of the feedback they received. For some, this was tempered by a degree of disappointment that the feedback was not challenging enough. They were also left with doubts as to the completeness or authenticity of the feedback received. This was especially true for those who did not receive feedback from every role set member approached. Nonetheless, even where the degree of challenge was apparently low, it still provided a stimulus for self-critique and reflection.

Box 13.2   Example of 360° questionnaire: using attributes and enabling factors of practice expertise (Manley & McCormack, 1997)

---

1. Holistic practice knowledge
   How far do you think my practice involves:
   - looking at all aspects of patient need?
   - appreciating the range of influences in each person's life that need to be taken into account?
   - looking at things from the patient's perspective?
   - utilising and integrating different forms of knowledge and applying them appropriately to individuals and circumstances?
2. Saliency
   What feedback would you offer on my ability to:
   - prioritise?
   - manage conflict effectively?
   - getting to the heart of the matter quickly?
3. Knowing the patient
   To what extent do you think I demonstrate:
   - empathy;
   - accessibility;
   - individualised care;
   - rapport building;
   - negotiation skills within the therapeutic relationship?
4. Moral agency
   How far do you think my relationship with the client respects their personhood, dignity, values and beliefs, and safety, and is based upon openness, being genuine and non-judgemental?
5. Skilled know-how
   How well do you think I demonstrate both interpersonal as well as technical skill, intuitive decision-making and the use of evidence and reflection to influence my practice?
6. Reflective ability
   Do I demonstrate how I systematically learn from my practice and apply that learning to new situations?
7. Organisation of practice
   How far do you think that the way in which delivery of care is organised helps or hinders my ability to demonstrate expertise in my practice?
8. Interpersonal relationships
   What feedback would you offer on my ability to develop relationships with others in the work setting?
9. Authority and autonomy
   To what extent do you think I demonstrate autonomy in my practice?

Those participants on the EPP that did manage to obtain service user feedback found the process very challenging, but most rewarding. Detail of this is offered in the discussion to follow, looking at including narratives as a tool for transformation.

What are the facilitation issues around working with 360° feedback?
It was a combination of the critical companion and expert participant working together that provided the best opportunity for in-depth discussion of feedback data. As outlined in the previous chapter (Chapter 11) on facilitating expertise, it remains imperative that all transformational activity is skilfully facilitated, otherwise the purpose and intention, let alone the approach and outcomes, will mean that increased insight into an individual's role may not articulate itself into a change in practice.

Recommendations

From the experience gained from working with a qualitative approach to 360° feedback, the following three aspects are essential elements to using and working with this tool:

1. *The purpose of the exercise*. To ensure that the aspects of practice feedback required are clarified. This can be achieved with the practitioner, team or stakeholders
2. *Role set selection*. To clarify the rationale for selecting role set members. For example personal qualities, values and beliefs; knowledge base; and experience of working with the recipient of the feedback
3. *Approaches*. Making judgements about the approaches used, based on contextual decisions about colleagues' availability and willingness to participate. Negotiating the means of collecting data may be of value. If the process is not progressing well, approach participants to identify what concerns they have to help find strategies to address any of their issues as early into the feedback process as possibl.

Observations of practice

The elusive nature of knowledge used by practitioners in their practice expertise has been the source of considerable creative concern for researchers. In her research into professional craft knowledge, Titchen (2000) developed the strategy of 'observing, listening and questioning', initially, as a data collection method, and subsequently, as a component of the critical companionship model (Titchen, 2001). Titchen describes how the strategy was used to help her colleague Alison Binnie (whose practice was the focus of the research) 'to surface unreflective knowing in a cognitive form' (p. 119).

Benner *et al.* (1999) used a protocol of questions and probes (e.g. *what are you noticing in this situation?*, p. 559) directly following periods of observation. Titchen

(2000) similarly ensured observation was followed as closely as possible by an opportunity to ask questions about what had been seen, both during the observation itself and later in a reflective interview/conversation. She relates how 'observation gave us a shared experience and a set of specific nursing events to discuss'.

Titchen (2001) details the various exploratory strategies in her work on critical companionship through, for example, asking detailed questions about the rationale for actions, intuitions, choices, options, decision, and so on. It was this form of direct questioning that Alison Binnie found productive (if challenging):

> The questions I've had difficulty answering – that have taken me further – is usually just, 'Why did you do that?' I mean, that's all. There are several times on the tape where there has been a long silence when I've been trying to think and it's been when answering the question 'Why'?
>
> *Titchen, 2000, p. 119*

Titchen's (2000) work provided a background structure for participant observation as an appropriate method for the EPP participant to:

(a) provide a naturalistic communicative context, where common human (nursing) practices could be observed and questioned;
(b) access constructions of nursing practice situations through consideration of observed nursing activity;
(c) gain a shared experience (with the nurse under observation) for understanding the rationale for nursing actions;
(d) provide recorded evidence of interactions and activities for retrospective detailed analysis with the observed nurse.

There are many publications relating to the use of observation to further understand and articulate nursing practice. Benner (1984) and Benner *et al.* (1996) write about their theory of nursing expertise, from observations of nursing practice. Allen (2001) used a sociological approach to understanding the *Changing shape of nursing practice* through the use of observations. Strange (1996) used an ethnographic approach to observe and study nursing's use of rituals. Additionally, interrogatory frameworks such as that outlined in Benner *et al.* (1999) could also be used or adopted to help guide discussion about practice (refer to Box 13.3 below). McCormack *et al.* (2006) have devised a cultural assessment tool utilising observation as the main process for informing practice change for entire teams.

What are the ethical implications for observing practice?
When using observation of team activities, obtaining ethical approval for observing practice can prove difficult, particularly if an individual on the unit does not wish to take part in the activity. Being well informed and ensuring participants that the observations are on specific issues (i.e. to improve workplace practices and culture) can help to allay fear and anxiety associated with perceptions of surveillance.

Box 13.3 Questions and probes for clinical observations from Benner *et al.* (1999, p. 559)

What are your concerns about this patient?
What are you noticing in this situation?
What is going on at this point?
What hunches do you have about this patient?
What do you anticipate with this patient?
What are your priorities at this time?
What did you learn from the shift report that helped care for the patient?
I noticed that you did _____. Tell me about this.
How is this situation similar to other situations you have experienced?
How is it different?
Is this situation familiar to you? In what ways?
What are you thinking about in this situation?
What are you watching out for in this situation?
What are you feeling about this situation?
Is the situation going as you expected?
What are the typical interventions for situations like this?
What interventions do you anticipate needing for this patient?
In this situation, what do you expect this intervention to do for this patient?
Have your priorities changed during this situation? How?
What was your primary source of learning about interventions like this?
Were there things you learned from books/lectures that guided you with this problem?
What guidelines would you give other nurses for managing this situation?
If you had to do it all over again, would you do anything differently?

It would seem that observation of practice requires similar levels of planning and critical debate that other activities practitioners engaged with for the EPP undertook (e.g. 360° feedback and narrative). Identifying aspects of practice that could be observed, when they occur, whether there are ethical frameworks, and, crucially, identifying time and strategies for discussing the observed practice, in depth, soon after the observation has taken place, are all important aspects to clarify with practitioners in order to obtain informed consent to participate.

What are the challenges associated with observation of practice?
For the EPP critical companions, observing their colleagues in practice presented a range of hurdles. Whilst some could legally attend ward-based activities because of their existing relationship with the practitioner (e.g. as manager, colleague or educator) and legitimately spend time with them in practice settings, others could not. For these critical companions, arranging to attend and observe the nurse in practice settings raised considerable ethical and legal questions.

The observation itself (i.e. where it took place) was not necessarily the greatest challenge but more about the practical difficulties of arranging observations around competing work priorities. Even when an observation session had been agreed and organised, last minute issues meant that, on occasion, being observed was deemed to be inappropriate (e.g. concerns around ward/patient safety). From the experiences of the EPP, it was easier to find and plan for observational opportunities when the participant and their critical companion worked in the same organisation. This was easier still if there was an existing working relationship. Where this was not the case, logistical problems became an issue, for example the ethical issue of permission to enter into clinical areas and indemnity insurance cover for non-health authority staff.

There was not evidence enough to suggest, from all the accounts of observation undertaken as part of the EPP, that full advantage was taken of the opportunity to delve into practitioners' use of different forms of knowledge as they negotiate their way through complex practice issues. The key issue is to use a rich source of material and to employ a range of questions and techniques to search for the strategies and forms of knowledge being used. However, without in-depth critique, no amount of material will render useful insights.

Organising the process of observing practice plus the need for a follow-up period for debriefing and feedback, both posed considerable logistical difficulties for participants. The delay caused by waiting for ethical clearance cannot be discounted as another hindrance to enabling the nurse participants to experience an 'outsider' observing their daily practice.

What are the benefits for undertaking observation of practice?

Evidence from the EPP portfolios alludes to both the initial discomfort of the experience and the ultimate usefulness of receiving meaningful feedback from the observations. One nurse participant welcomed the opportunity of being directly observed in practice. Previous experience, due to her senior position, meant that obtaining feedback on her performance was difficult, as colleagues were reluctant to provide any critique. Therefore, having a critical companion observe, provide feedback on and ask questions about practice was described as 'something of a luxury' and recognised as extremely useful for professional and personal development. This level of critique could not have been achieved in any other form, as feedback was specific and directly related to what had occurred during the observation, rather than on 'second hand' or 'here say' based evidence. However, for some, this direct approach made the evidence feel 'raw', or 'too close to the bone', as the process of being observed occurred in real time, under real circumstances. Those EPP nurses, who did take part, relished the chance of getting a different perspective on their daily practice from someone they trusted and respected.

Engaging in a process of critical dialogue about what was observed will promote high levels of challenge as well as new insight into practice behaviour, values, and beliefs, which in turn increase practitioner's ability to be reflexive. Observation requires the practitioner undertaking the observation to be aware of their own expectations, whilst also remaining open and responsive to new experiences, as they come into mind and into view. The observer identifies questions in relation to what they observe to take back to the individual as part of the debriefing. The purpose is to check out what is being seen or observed and how that relates to the person being observed, what they were thinking or intending through their actions. This process aims to help the practitioner surface their tacit knowledge that emerges from habitualised, almost subconscious, levels of practice.

What are the facilitation issues around observation of practice?
The facilitation process of observations of practice, in the EPP, was provided through the critical companion role. The EPP practitioners were aiming to use the evidence and reflections for assembling a portfolio of evidence to demonstrate expertise. The facilitation of the process of observing practice will need to take into consideration how to prepare the entire clinical environment for the observers' presence and purpose. Identifying the aspects of practice that are being observed and preparing for how the observations are to be meaningfully feedback to the practitioner being observed can all fall to the facilitator. As outlined clearly in the WCCAT tool (McCormack *et al.*, 2006), it is important for the facilitator not to be seen as 'sitting in judgement' of what they have observed, and it is far more important to be working with the participants, utilising graceful care in a collaborative process of giving and receiving feedback through high support, balanced with high challenge.

Recommendations

Future projects (or research) that aim to incorporate observation for the identification of new insights into nursing practice expertise need to consider sufficient time be included in the project design to incorporate the following practical, ethical and conceptual barriers to achieving observation of practice:

- Obtaining prompt ethical clearance;
- Discussing practical implications for clinical areas (e.g. indemnity, confidentiality, etc.);
- Providing practical and experiential opportunities for 'trying out' the process;
- Outlining and supporting the observer's role.

Compared to other suggested approaches to evidence collection, observation of practice was used relatively little by participants[1]. It is difficult to ascertain how far the exercise was used as an opportunity to explore the observed practice in depth as a means to uncovering hidden knowledge. The feedback from critical companions tended to reflect back what they had seen, using either the attributes and enabling factors of expertise (Manley & McCormack, 1997), or the domains and strategies of skilled companionship (Titchen, 2000).

However, there does not seem to have been critical discussion of these observations. For example, in the portfolio of one nurse participant with regard to the

---

[1] However, comparing the response rate expected from survey design (33%), the take-up of both observation (45%) and user narratives (40%) is comparable, if not significantly higher.

demonstration of saliency in her morning's care of two patients that she had not previously cared for, the critical companion writes:

> Through your assessment from a variety of sources, you were able to identify the pertinent issues for each of the patients and were able to consider the priorities for each.

The last paragraph from one of the EPP nurse participants not only hints at the value of the observation exercise, but perhaps also implicitly suggests that deeper exploration may have proved more useful still:

> From the feedback I received from the observation it would appear that attributes of expertise could be identified. Some of these I was more conscious of than others but they seemed to show I function at different levels and use a range of skills, some acquired through conscious study, some perhaps more innate. I am now more aware of the need to examine these and subject them to challenge in order to refine them further.

Using narratives (patient and staff stories)

According to Harden (2000), one of the most significant developments in nursing has been a growing recognition of the wide utility of narratives in health care. She argues that for researchers, understanding more about language use offers a process through which nurses, in particular, can further understand and capture a person's subjectivity, which, in turn, can inform health care practice. Harden (2000) goes on to describe how the life story of an individual, as a patient, represents him or her to the nurse and is in turn responded to through the care that individual subsequently receives.

As a research tool, narrative methodology has been employed extensively to explore the stories of those suffering from a variety of illnesses although these narratives have tended to describe the experience of a specific disease or the journey travelled from sickness to health. Leight (2002) states that approaching people as narrators and their stories as text allows for a rich source of material that can enhance almost any form of practice inquiry. Overcash (2004) argues that narrative-based research can be integrated into clinical nursing practice as nurses are often uniquely situated as story gatherers for the health care team. By listening carefully to a patient's individual story, nurses can identify themes and issues which affect that patient's life experiences and thereby develop appropriate clinical and therapeutic interventions as a result.

Cunningham and Kitson (2000) used patient stories as part of the clinical leadership program. The process of narrative research is varied and influenced by many theoretical stances that can be found in the literature and textbooks (see Section *Additional resources for developing practice expertise* at the end of this chapter). Hardy *et al.* (2007) outline the issues of using patient-based stories as part of the EPP, whilst another paper by Hardy *et al.* (2009) explores more of the theoretical components of narrative-based inquiry. Some examples of collaborations through the use of narratives can be found on the Internet, where research participants take control of the data collection, presentation and content (cf. mental health blogs).

What are the ethical implications of using narratives?
Mishler (1986a) warns how analysing narratives are open to personal interpretation, which in turn are effected by the very process of gathering the narrative. Mishler suggests a process of co-construction when undertaking research interviews, which occurs in the gathering of narratives; as the speaker and listener engage in the process of talking (whether that be in an unstructured or structured interview format), they jointly create a reality that is agreed and constructed between them. His main area of concern is how the researcher then uses these gathered narratives.

> Interpretations will differ depending on how we {the researcher} view the separate episodes (of the story).
>
> *Mishler, 1986b, p. 73*

According to Connelly and Clandinin (1990), when analysing narratives, the researcher works to actively find the voice of the participant in a particular time, place or setting. Mishler identifies concern about traditional roles for interviewers and interviewees, where power relationships often exist, with the researcher placed in a position of authority, which is again often found in health care settings. He proposes a more collaborative relationship between the information gatherer and the informant, where the informant is engaged in all stages of the research process where possible. However, for most research, the aims and approaches, lines of analysis and interpretation, and final report writing are all under the control of the researcher.

Whatever the chosen approach to analysing narratives (e.g. coding, categories, themes and taxonomy), it remains necessary to maintain the feedback loop (through, e.g., the 360° system), as can be seen from an example given here from the work at Addenbrooke's NHS Foundation Trust in Cambridge.

The experience of developing a patient stories protocol at Addenbrooke's NHS Foundation Trust

Jill Down was the lead practice development nurse at Addenbrooke's during a 3-year action research-based practice development project (2003–2006).

Jill writes, 'The importance of putting patients at the centre of our work is an admirable aspiration that most health care professionals would aspire to, supported by policy directives (Department of Health, 2000, 2001, 2004; Lygon & Hittinger, 2003).' However, the challenge faced in everyday practice by many practitioners is working with the tension that arises between:

- meeting short-term goals and national (externally set) targets;
- using outcome indicators to demonstrate a patient-centred approach;

and

- identifying changes needed in practice from the patients' actual experience;
- focusing on changing the culture of clinical areas to enable sustainable change.

As the practice development project was a Trust wide initiative, an important evaluation question guiding the project was: What is the culture as experienced by the patient? Central to this evaluation objective was the need to develop staff skills, systems and processes (experienced through the protocol development) to help staff understand the patient's experience and then to use the information gathered to inform and make changes in practice, plus to share good practices throughout the Trust.

Material presented is based on one complete action cycle of gathering and analysing patient stories from across the Trust and supplemented with evidence from a second action cycle.

Developing a protocol (first cycle)

As many staff as possible were involved in the developmental phase of the protocol. As the project began, there were no available protocols (in the public domain) that would enable a robust, standardised method of undertaking patient stories across a Trust, so this became the starting point for 'the PD group'. First, the project group identified key stages of the process:

- Preparation of self;
- Preparation of ward staff;
- Selection and preparation of patients.

Following this, the group performed a 'facilitated dramatisation' of the process to further develop a protocol that could be used readily across the Trust. The facilitated dramatisation literally meant several people acting out the process of gathering the patient stories from start to finish, observed by others. Each participant, whether actor or observer, was able to stop the enactment whenever any issues arose that would help to discuss and clarify the emergent process. Issues highlighted during this developmental process were concerned with very practical matters (how to introduce oneself to the patient), ethical matters (how and when to obtain consent, when is the best time of day to approach people) and process matters (what to do if or when...). Eventually, the process was re-enacted from start to finish with all those involved clear as to the steps to be incorporated into a first draft protocol. The patient stories protocol was then tested in the ward areas and some minor revisions made at the end of the first phase of the action research cycle.

This preparatory work had the effect of actively involving staff and using an approach that was inductive and practical whilst highlighting the ethical and moral issues that might be encountered in clinical areas when taking stories. In addition, skills in active listening were developed in staff undertaking the stories together with skills in thematic analysis of the interviews once the stories had been collected, which all worked towards ensuring a robust validation process for the protocol.

During the second cycle, there were several additional changes, largely due to personnel changes, who had not been initially involved in the preliminary phase of the protocol development.

As a result, all ward areas have undergone patient stories, with a second phase being considered. Our work has invested in the training and development of processes using a systematic and robust approach within an action research framework. The work identified has produced a protocol for use by practitioners in practice refined and developed in an ongoing manner.

What are the facilitation issues associated with using narratives?
The need to give and receive effective feedback was highlighted as crucial to the work and that was an area that required additional development. Guidelines were developed, again using an inductive approach, which would support practitioners to be more effective in providing feedback to one another and to other departments involved in the care of patients (e.g. catering, pharmacy, estates).

Skilled facilitation appears to be a crucial element to the successful implementation of these transformational processes. Time taken to navigate the narrative protocol through the governance and ethical procedures and then for nurse participants to assimilate their ideas and put into practice the processes outlined, all added to nurse participants' anxiety and concerns. Yet, it also helped to focus attention to the core elements of the activity. However, as seen from the final portfolios of evidence and captured in the patient feedback, what can be gained from the commitment is greater clarity and insight into the 'swampy lowlands' of clinical practice (Schön, 1983) so that future practitioner researchers might continue to challenge their personal assumptions. Additionally, work was undertaken to facilitate action plans with ward teams setting objectives that were specific, measurable, achievable, realistic and time scaled in direct response to the issues raised by the patient stories.

Evaluation has taken place at each stage of the process and the learning has been fed back to inform the next stage, resulting in refinements to protocols, development of facilitation skills, development of achievable objectives and widening participation of clinical teams. Most importantly, the initiative generated and uses evidence from patients and integrates it within everyday practice and provides a practical tool for evaluation of practice. (For a copy of the Addenbrooke's protocol refer to Section *Additional resources for developing practice expertise*; RCN Workplace Resources.)

What are the benefits of using narratives?
Utilising narratives in exploring the process and outcomes of practice expertise, from the EPP, revealed how, for individual practitioners, using narrative enabled them to work from a heightened level of awareness, around their communication with patients, listening, not working from assumptions, ethical principles of obtaining a sensitive process for obtaining informed consent. Using an inductive approach, practitioners were able to become engaged with and to think in action. They experienced a process that enabled them to engage in a process of collaboration, a 'doing with rather than doing on patients' (EPP nurse participants' portfolio of evidence).

258

What are the challenges to using narratives?

For the EPP, a common decision by the nurse participants was to use their critical companion as interviewer in the gathering of the narrative. This arrangement aimed to provide an element of impartiality to the feedback and to decrease any risk of patients feeling that they could not criticise someone actively involved in their treatment or care. Within the narrative protocol, the interviewer was encouraged to consider the narrative as an opportunity for the person to talk about their experiences of the particular nurse participant's care. Therefore, the interviewer was encouraged to offer minimal prompts and to actively listen. Questioning was open and responsive to the conversation, rather than following any pre-constructed format to enable negotiation and a mutual sharing of ideas. In addition, the interviewer was encouraged to check that they had understood the person's feedback, thereby ensuring that meaning was agreed. Following the initial narrative, further opportunities were offered, and additional meetings arranged to clarify the issues emerging from the narrative that would then be feedback directly to the nurse in question by either the critical companion, or if desired, by the patient themselves.

All interviews were audio taped and a copy given to the patient participant to keep. Mostly, the critical companions, who generally feedback salient issues to the nurse participant, then transcribed the tapes. In one case, feedback was given directly by the patient participant to the nurse for consideration in uncovering and exploring their personal practice expertise from the patient's perspective.

How the nurse participants' presented these narratives in their final portfolios of evidence varied greatly:

- Three nurse participants included a full transcript of their narratives as part of their portfolio of evidence.
- Two others presented an overview of what occurred, summarising the process in their own words.
- One nurse presented an inductive thematic analysis.
- Two completed a deductive thematic analysis and presented direct quotations under the headings of 'attributes of expertise' derived from the Manley and McCormack (1997) framework.
- Three nurse participants included a reflective piece written in response to the experience.

In particular, the EPP nurse participants identified and expressed initial concern and discussed an 'overwhelming sense of vulnerability' when first considering engaging people receiving care directly from them. One nurse participant further defined this sense of vulnerability as 'fear', associated with not knowing how to deal with what she described as *raw patient data*.

Having had the experience of involving people receiving services, the nurse participants' initial reservations were transformed, particularly during the final critical review process of the portfolios and in debates within action learning sets. The nurse participants largely agreed that it was this element of the project that had been the most valuable. For example, one nurse wrote:

A tense time being scrutinised by a patient. I felt vulnerable and quite uneasy at the prospect, as this patient is known for having a frank approach. But an enlightening experience, to be valued by those people who in my eyes really matter. I was uncomfortable with the prospect of involving patients in this study but it has been invaluable to view me as others do. I express my gratitude for their keenness to be involved.

Fear, vulnerability and uncertainty at being challenged about one's working practice are considered by most people as only natural. Yet, overcoming that fear can be achieved through supportive and facilitative relationships in a workplace that offers space to consider and reframe potential barriers (Manley, 2004; Manley *et al.*, 2004).

The collaborative development of the EPP narrative protocol enabled nurse practitioners to consider the implications of approaching their patients for direct feedback on the care experience. The patient participants were able to engage in voicing their opinions and offered sophisticated levels of feedback that left an impact on the nurse participants. One patient identified the specifics of their recognised expert nurse as follows:

I knew by the looks and tut-tutting when I came to clinic that I began to dread attending and I think that has also made me terrified of problems arising. I think this is why I didn't go to the clinic or phone very often. You were less judgmental than anyone else. It was really only you I could show my monitoring diary too.

You have suffered these things with me. If your name ever comes up, people just go, say no more!

Many nurse participants concluded in their final portfolios that 'patients were able to remain impartial in their feedback', and were also able to identify and offer comparative examples of care given by others, which the nurse participants found extremely useful. Those nurse participants who engaged with their patients as co-participants provided the opportunity for the 'singing up' of the patient voice in illuminating and evaluating practice expertise. Engaging people receiving services as research participants in the process of evaluating the health care, they experience offers an opportunity for nurse participants to uncover and develop their practice. The process of inquiry also provides an authentic space for people receiving services to voice their opinions and offer their own expertise on what is effective, person-centred health care practice.

Reflexivity (reflection into critically appraised action)

According to Hardy and Blomfield (2000), reflective practice has been explored at length in nursing literature and draws largely from the work of Schön's (1983) text, *The Reflective practitioner*. Schön (1983) identified the importance of 'tacit' knowledge that is gathered through a person's work experience but is difficult to articulate and explain to others. From work of authors such as Boyd and Fales (1983), Kolb (1984), Boud *et al.* (1985), for example, reflective practice has been further defined as a process that professionals use to explore their experiences in order to bring about changes in their understanding. Benner (1984) wrote that a value of reflective practice is its natural phenomenological focus and that through a collaborative research approach with practitioners', through an exploration of their practice, that new insights can be derived from nursing knowledge that lies embedded in everyday practitioner's working lives.

A criticism of reflection is that it only takes place after the event, with limited impact on how a practitioner then acts, thinks or responds to a situation in the future. However, it has been widely applied to nursing practice, through group reflection (cf. Getliffe, 1996), critical incident techniques (cf. Minghella & Benson, 1995), or using writing and art (cf. Holly, 1989; Cruickshank, 1996) as a starting point for professional development. It has been argued that the considerable effort expended in promoting and facilitating reflection has not had a demonstrable effect on patient care (cf. Newell, 1994). Such a critique does not entirely negate reflection as contributing to the development of praxis, nor on the ability for practitioners to learn from experience.

Maeve (1994) argues that there is a difference between the ways in which improvements can be made at both macro- and micro-levels. She associates reflection with micro-level improvements, as she considers reflection a shared activity between practitioners working together, and therefore sharing the impact that has on patient care. She asserts:

> [T]he immediate consequence of this sharing may foster the physical or psychological well being of a particular patient. However, in the longer view, each improvement or improved understanding has a positive effect on the practice of nursing by individuals and on nursing collectively.
>
> *Maeve, 1994, p. 14*

Reflection in action involves questioning assumptions about practice and results in on-the-spot evaluation and experimentation in response to new information. In expert practitioners, such reflection may be subtle and may occur without the practitioner being able to articulate the knowledge that underpins their action, as in the practitioners, knowing in action is embedded in a socially constructed context, in which their practice takes place. This is where observation of practice can help practitioners identify their practice expertise and ability to utilise their multiple knowledge, as they demonstrate their expertise and professional artistry.

It is this reflection in action that Rolfe (1997) identifies as the basis for arguing for a stage of expert practice performance he terms reflexive practice. He draws a distinction between the intuitive aspects of expert practice as described by Benner (1984) and prefers a more deliberate form of theorising on and from practice, based on Schön's work. Rolfe argues that the significance of reflexion is that it solves problems in practice through the construction of informal theories which are constantly being tested, modified and retested in a process of on-the-spot experimentation. As distinct from the reflective practitioner, who works in an unconscious way, the reflexive practitioner is someone able to work as almost the antithesis to Benner's description of expert. The reflexive practitioner is described as working with intense concentration, thinking about their actions, and relating their knowledge to the particular instance at hand. This way of working, according to Rolfe, synthesises personal academic and scientific knowledge into a unique formal theory that can be tested and modified.

> Theory and practice are one and the reflexive practitioner is both researcher and theory builder.

Rolfe, 1997, p. 97

Manley and McCormack (1997) describe the evolution of models for reflection. Drawing particularly from the work of Johns (1996) and Johns and Freshwater (1998), they suggest a model (shown in Box 13.4 below) that builds on assumptions concerning the philosophical roots of nursing as a caring activity, the importance of reflexivity and the centrality of the relationship between nurse and patient.

An example taken from an expert nurse participant in action learning helps to explain the process of reflexivity (alongside that of working in a critical companionship relationship) and how that process had clarified and crystallised her notions of expertise through an improved ability to reflect in and on her actions.

Box 13.4   A model for structured reflection

Asthetics	Ethics
What was I trying to achieve?	How did my actions match my beliefs?
Why did I respond as did?	What factors made me act in incongruent ways?
What were the consequences of that for the patient, others and myself?	Empirics
How was this person (people) feeling?	What knowledge did or should have informed me?
Personal	**Reflexivity**
How did I feel in this situation?	How does this connect with previous experiences?
What internal factors were influencing me?	Could I handle this better in similar situation?
	What would be the consequences of alternative actions for the patient, others and myself?
	How do I now feel about this experience?
	Can I support myself and others better as a consequence?
	Has this changes my way of knowing?

Source: From Johns and Freshwater (1998).

Lots of people work at the level I do, as effectively as I am, but not many are consciously considering it at the same level. The project has made me bring it [expertise in practice] up even further. Sometimes that has been uncomfortable. It's because it involved talking about the self, that makes people feel uncomfortable and produces anxiety.

Reflexivity is the process of using reflection in an active state, for example, within a practice context. Koch and Harrington (1998) discuss reflexivity in terms of hermeneutics, associating reflexivity with critical discussion and debate, opening up the possibilities. They also suggest feminist theory has influenced reflexivity in terms of positioning, of the politics of location, and attempting to remain open to these constraints on perspective and understanding. For Webb (1996), reflexivity requires that practitioner researchers write about the process of carrying out the project from their points of view as a means of exploring and identifying tacit understanding. Working from this level of honesty, about how and why choices are made and resulting actions, enables others to benefit from the process as much as from the findings, as the interpretation of issues is clearly expressed and laid bare.

Burman (2006) writes of how engaging with reflexivity inevitably returns to consideration of self, but this runs the risk of hearing only about the researcher, taking focus and attention away from participants' views of their self(s). She proposes a reminder to practitioners that reflexivity is not an indulgent selfish act, nor reductive, but should be seen as a part of the process or actions of a project. She quotes Parker's (2005) proposal for 'radical research' where reflexivity is 'undertaken alongside and in collaboration with co-researchers (and they then have some reflexive work to do with you as well)' (Parker, 2005, p. 35).

For expertise, reflexivity is not only all of these things, identifying self and locating self to others in any activity, but also taking into consideration the wider context of actions and behaviours, and the impact of those actions on others we work alongside. Koch and Harrington (1998) describe this as signposting, so that others will 'be able to travel easily through the worlds of the participants' (Koch and Harrington, 1998, p. 887).

What are the challenges associated with reflexivity?
A central theme when looking at the challenges of engaging in reflexivity is the temptation and sometimes eloquent retreat people make towards 'naval gazing'. This process becomes counter to the intention behind reflexivity, which is focused on considered action. In a recent qualitative research text (Higgs *et al.* 2007), there are many examples of the challenges of working with reflexivity (cf. Chapter 2, p. 16; Chapter 8, p. 79; Chapter 14, p. 158). As previously stated, one's ability to be reflexive is often linked to the critical companionship relationship available, or the facilitation of the reflexive process.

What are the benefits of reflexivity?
Increased reflexive ability was from the nurse participants' evaluative feedback, recognised as a positive experience and identified as part of the process of being

engaged in the EPP. Both the nurse participants and their critical companions expressed how their reflexive skills had been greatly advanced through being part of the project. It is concluded therefore that working with action learning and a critical companionship framework in a practice research programme can offer positive benefits for research participants, through advanced skills of reflection in and on their action. Remaining reflexive requires a broad understanding of different theoretical stances, a meta-theorising ability that is immediately doubled when working with a critical companion, or quadrupled when drawing from different stakeholders understandings.

What are the ethical implications?
Familiar experiences may produce an unexpected result that it may not be possible to resolve using familiar strategies. Even if the problem has been resolved, there may be something different about the results. Consequently, practitioners can either choose to dismiss the incident as a novel experience, or they can reflect and learn from the specifics. It could be argued therefore that not engaging in reflexive practice is indeed unethical, as a practitioner who does not think in action could be a liability in terms of choosing to ignore, or not being consciously aware of the implications of their actions.

What are the facilitation issues?
Working with a critical companion, supervisor or mentor can aid the process of moving from reflection into reflexivity. Diaries are useful tools for capturing reflections of daily experiences. The daily discipline of a diary can help reveal patterns of thinking, behaviour, responses and activities that might otherwise go unseen, or unnoticed. Patterns may reveal concerns or issues that recur over time. Like diaries, journals are extremely common reflection tools. Unlike keeping a diary, which requires a daily routine and generally captures 'what happened,' journaling is a much more free-form tool and has taken on a new interest through the home computer. Journals offer the time and space for capturing observations, feelings and emotions, quotes, stories and drawings, as well as dated experiences. However, taking these reflections further into reflexivity requires engaging in a critical dialogue with another person about those reflections.

Harvesting learning and recording it in a learning log requires the writer to ask probing questions in addition to 'what happened?' Those questions might include, 'What did I expect in this situation?', 'What surprised me about this situation or event?', 'What do I see or know now that I didn't see or know before?', or 'What would I say to someone who asked what I learned in this situation?' Once again, a practice portfolio and learning log cannot on their own move a practitioner into reflexive practice. This needs to be facilitated through taking the evidence of the practice portfolio onto a deeper level of learning, mapping and reflexivity. As described above, working with a critical companion can aid that process considerably.

Within the EPP, participants were invited to develop a portfolio of evidence that identified multiple sources of evidence about their practice. It was most meaningful to participants when these entries had been deconstructed and reconstructed following a period of reflexivity and then synthesised into their daily practice and professional craft knowledge. It was not however the production of the portfolio that had meaningful impact on the practitioners themselves, it was the process of engaging with others during the EPP that enlightened and transformed their thinking, being and understanding of their practice expertise.

Recommendations

At the outset, the EPP aimed to provide a research approach that enabled transformation for nurse participants and their critical companions. To conclude this chapter on tools for transformation, I will present some of the claims and issues that arose in the EPP project.

1. *The nurse participant and transformation.* The EPP provided an opportunity for practitioners to engage in facilitative and developmental relationships in the workplace (e.g. through critical companionship and obtaining feedback from people receiving services). Arising from the nurse participants and critical companions' experiences, key processes necessary for transforming practice were identified as:
   (a) the maintenance of effectiveness and continuing competency through professional supervision and
   (b) providing opportunities for nurse participants to be reflexive and consider how to overcome barriers associated with challenging and changing their practices.

Through a process of high challenge and high support, nurse practitioners became more explicit about the different knowledge that underpinned their practice. They gained confidence, were able to articulate their practice expertise to others, and, as a result, achieved increased recognition for the value and significant contribution they provide to health care. For example, two participants were able to renegotiate their role and clinical grade as a result of the substantial evidence provided in their project portfolios.

Conclusion

There is a risk then, when considering processes for transformation, in wanting to explore, deconstruct and re-synthesise practice behaviours, as the practitioner will potentially be offering a challenge to conventional ways of seeing, doing and thinking about health care practice. Yet, the potential to 'change people's lives', whether that be colleagues, patients or indeed an entire organisation, is achievable (Manley *et al.*, 2005) with strategic thinking, and rigorous systematic processes of inquiry and critical support.

Working with processes for transformation requires a practitioner be mindful of the purpose, intention and potential outcomes of any investigation. By that,

I mean entering into the research or inquiry process with an explicit intention to engage self and others in a process of reflexive action (a deconstruction and reconstruction of practice situations), exploring not only the obvious, but also taking into consideration the unexplored, so that the future can be responded to in ways previously unimagined.

Any practitioner undertaking transformation needs high levels of reflexive abilities, engagement in all forms of intelligence, to be a transformational leader and engage in collaborative practices. Most importantly, the objective of any transformation is not to set out to achieve set targets or goals, but instead to concentrate on the process of building the capacity, energy, excitement and commitment to move towards bold visions for the future (cf. van Wyk, 2003). Yet, that visioning and the courage to move into new waters, leaving behind the comfort and security of the familiar shores, need extensive planning, infrastructures of support, principles of collaboration and inclusion, all mixed together with rigorous and systematic, transparent processes. I wish you all the best, and to hear more about your explorations into the sea of possibilities that is transformation.

References

Allen, D. (2001) *The Changing Shape of Nursing Practice. The Role of Nurses in the Hospital Division of Labour*. Routledge, London.

Alimo-Metcalffe, B. (1996) 360 degree feedback and leadership development. *International Journal of Selection and Assessment* **6**(1), 35–44.

Benner, P. (1984) *From Novice to Expert: Excellence and Power in Clinical Nursing Practice*. Addison Wesley, Menlo Park, CA.

Benner, P., Hooper-Kyriakidis, P.L. & Stannard, D. (1999) *Clinical Wisdom and Interventions in Critical Care. A Thinking in Action Approach*. Springer, New York.

Benner, P., Tanner, C.A. & Chesla, C.A. (1996) *Expertise in Nursing Practice Caring: Clinical Judgement and Ethics*. Springer, New York.

Boud, D., Keogh, R. & Walker, D. (1985) *Reflection: Turning Experience into Learning*. Kogan Page, London.

Boyd, E.M. & Fales, A.W. (1983) Reflective learning: key to learning from experience. *Journal of Humanistic Psychology* **23**, 99–117.

Boykin, A. & Schoenhofer, S.O. (1993) *Nursing as Caring. A Model for Transforming Practice*. National League for Nursing, New York; Jones & Bartlett (Re-release), Boston.

Burman, E. (2006) Emotions and reflexivity in feminized education action research. *Educational Action Research* **14**(3), 311–314.

Connelly, F.M. & Clandinin, D.J. (1990) Stories of experience and narrative inquiry. *Educational Researcher* **19**(5), 2–14.

Cruickshank, D. (1996) The 'art' of reflection: using drawing to uncover knowledge development in student nurses. *Nurse Education Today* **16**(2), 127–130.

Cunningham, G. & Kitson, A. (2000) An evaluation of the RCN Clinical Leadership Development Programme: Part 1. *Nursing Standard* **15**(12), 34–37.

Dalton, F. (2005) Using 360 degree feedback mechanism. You can harness their power and utility by following these seven best practices. *Occupational Health & Safety* **74**(7), 28, 30.

Department of Health (2000) *The NHS Plan: A Plan for Investment, A Plan for Reform.* DH, London.

Department of Health (2001) *Essence of Care: Patient Focused Benchmarking for Healthcare Professionals.* The Stationary Office, London.

Department of Health (2004) *Standards for Better Health: Healthcare Standards for Services under the NHS.* DH, London.

Garbett, R., Hardy, S., Manley, K., Titchen, A. & McCormack, B. (2006) Developing a qualitative approach to 360 degree feedback to aid understanding and development of clinical expertise. *Journal of Nursing Management* **15**, 342–347.

Garman, A.N., Tyler, J.L. & Darnall, J.S. (2004) Development & validation of a 360 degree feedback instrument for health care administrators. *Journal of Healthcare Management* **49**(5), 307–322.

Getliffe, K.A. (1996) An examination of the use of reflection in the assessment of practice for undergraduate nursing students. *International Journal of Nursing Studies* **33**(4), 361–374.

Harden, J. (2000) Language, discourse and the chronotype: applying literary theory to the narratives in health care. *Journal of Advanced Nursing* **31**(3), 506–512.

Hardy, S.E. & Blomfield, R. (2000) Evidence based nursing. In: *Evidence Based Practice. A Critical Guide* (eds S. Pearce & L. Trinder).Blackwell, Oxford.

Hardy, S., Garbett, R., Titchen, A. & Manley, K. (2002) Exploring nursing expertise: nurses talk nursing. *Nursing Inquiry* **9**(3), 196–202.

Hardy, S., Gregory, S. & Ramjeet, R. (2009) An exploration of intent for narrative methods of inquiry in health care research. Accepted for April 2009 publication in *Nurse Researcher* (N10).

Hardy, S., Titchen, A. & Manley, K. (2007) Patient narratives in the evaluation of practice expertise. *Nursing Inquiry* **14**(1), 80–88.

Higgs, J., Titchen, A., Horsfall, D. & Armstrong, H. (2007) *Being Critical and Creative in Qualitative Research.* Hampden, Sydney.

Holly, M.L. (1989). *Reflective Practice in Nursing: The Growth of the Professional Practitioner.* Blackwell Scientific, London.

Johns, C. (1996) Visualising & realizing caring in practice through guided reflection. *Journal of Advanced Nursing* **24**(6), 1135–1143.

Johns, C. & Freshwater, D. (1998) *Transforming Nursing through Reflective Practice*, 2nd edn. Blackwell, Oxford.

Koch, T. & Harrington, A. (1998) Reconceptualising rigour: the case for reflexivity. *Journal of Advancced Nursing* **28**(4), 882–890.

Kolb, D.A. (1984) *Experiential Learning: Experience as the Source of Learning and Development.* Prentice Hall, Englewood Cliffs, NJ.

Leight, S.B. (2002) Starry night: using story to inform aesthetic knowing in women's health nursing. *Journal of Advanced Nursing* **37**(1), 108–114.

Lepsinger, R. & Lucia, A.D. (1997) *The Art and Science of 360 Degree Feedback.* Jossey-Bass/Pfeieffer, San Francisco.

Lygon, M. & Hittinger, R. (2003) Editorial: patient and public involvement. *Clinical Governance Bulletin* **4**(4), 1.

Maeve, M.K. (1994) The carrier bag theory of nursing practice. *Advances in Nursing Science* **4**(9), 9–22.

Manley, K. (2004) Workplace culture: is your workplace effective? How would you know? *Nursing in Critical Care* **9**, 1–3.

Manley, K. & McCormack, B. (1997) *Exploring Expert Practice* (NUM65U). Royal College of Nursing, London.

Manley, K., Hardy, S.E., Garbett, R., Titchen, A. & McCormack, B. (2004) *Changing Patients' Worlds through Nursing Practice Expertise. A Research Report.* Royal College of Nursing, London.

Manley, K., Hardy, S., Titchen, A., Garbett, R. & McCormack, B. (2005) *Changing Patients' Worlds through Nursing Practice Expertise. Exploring Nursing Practice Expertise through Emancipatory Action Research and Fourth Generation Evaluation.* A Royal College of Nursing Research Report 1998–2004. RCN, London.

McCormack, B., Henderson, E., Wright, J. & Wilson, V. (2006) Workplace Culture Critical Analysis Tool (WCCAT). Contact the authors for access and use of this tool.

Minghella, E. & Benson, A. (1995) Developing reflective practice in mental health nursing through critical incident analysis. *Journal of Advanced Nursing* **21**(2), 205–213.

Mishler, E. (1986a) The analysis of interview-narratives. In: *Narrative Psychology: The Storied Nature of Human Conduct* (ed. T. Sarbin), pp. 233–255. Praeger, New York.

Mishler, E.G. (1986b) *Research Interviewing. Context and Narrative.* Harvard University Press, New York.

Newell, R. (1994) Reflection: art, science or pseudo-science. *Nurse Education Today* **14**(2), 79–81.

Overcash, J.A. (2004) Using narrative research to understand the quality of life of older women with breast cancer. *Oncology Nursing Forum* **31**(6), 1153–1159.

Parker, I. (2005) *Qualitative Psychology: Introducing a Radical Research Approach.* Open University Press, Buckingham.

Redwood, S., Lloyd, H., Carr, E., Hancock, H., McSherry, R., Campbell, S. & Graham, L. (2007) Evaluating nurse consultants work through key informant perceptions. *Nursing Standard* **21**(17), 35–40.

Rodgers, K.G. & Manifold, C. (2002) 360-degree feedback: possibilities for assessment of the ACGME core competencies for emergency medicine residents. *Academic Emergency Medicine* **9**(11), 1300–1304.

Rolfe, G. (1997) Beyond expertise: theory, practice and the reflexive practitioner. *Journal of Clinical Nursing* **6**(2), 93–97.

Schön, D. (1983) *The Reflective Practitioner. How Professionals Think in Action.* Basic books, Harper Collins, New York.

Sparkes, A.C. (2005) Narrative analysis. In: *Qualitative Research in Healthcare* (ed. I. Holloway). Open University Press, Maidenhead.

Strange, F. (1996) Handover: an ethnographic study of rituals in nursing practice. *Intensive and Critical Care Nursing* **12**, 106–112.

Swain, G.R., Shubot, D.B., Thomas, V., Baker, B.K., Foldy, S.L., Greaves, W.W. & Monteagudo, M. (2004) 360 degree feedback: program implementation in a local health department. *Journal of Public Health Management & Practice* **10**(3), 266–271.

Titchen, A. (2000) *Professional Craft Knowledge in Patient Centred Nursing and the Facilitation of Its Development.* D.Phil. Thesis, University of Oxford. Ashdale Press, Kidlington, Oxfordshire.

Titchen, A. (2001) Critical companionship: a conceptual framework for developing expertise. In: *Practice Knowledge and Expertise in the Health Professions* (eds A. Higgs & A. Titchen). Butterworth Heinemann, Oxford.

Tornow, W.W. & London, M. (1997) *Maximising the Value of 360 Degree Feedback.* Institute of Personnel and Development, London.

Ward, P. (1997) *360 Degree Feedback*. Institute of Personnel and Development, London.

Webb, C. (1996) Caring, curing, coping: towards an integrated model. *Journal of Advanced Nursing* **23**(5), 960–968.

van Wyk, B. (2003) Exploring the notion of educational transformation: in search of constitutive meaning. *International Journal of Special Education* **18**(2), 1–17.

Additional resources for developing practice expertise

Belenky, M.F., Clinchy, B., Goldberger, N. & Tarule, J. (1986) *Women's Ways of Knowing: The Development of Self, Voice, and Mind*. Basic Books, New York.

Binnie, A. & Titchen, A. (1999) *Freedom to Practice: The Development of Patient Centred Nursing*. Butterworth Heinemann, Oxford.

Bogdan, R.C. & Biklen, S.K. (1982) *Qualitative Research for Education: An Introduction to Theory and Methods*. Allyn Bacon, Inc., Toronto, ON.

Bruner, J. (1987) Life as narrative. *Social Research* **54**(1), 11–32.

Bruner, J. (1990) *Acts of meaning*. Harvard University Press, Cambridge, MA.

Bruner, J. (1994) From communicating to talking. In: *Language Literacy and Learning in Educational Practice* (eds B. Stierer & J. Maybin), pp. 59–73. Multilingual Matters Ltd, Bristol, PA.

Campbell, S.M., Roland, M.O. & Buetwo, S.A. (2000) Defining quality of care. *Social Science and Medicine* **51**(11), 1611–1625.

Coates, E., Dewing, J. & Titchen, A. (2006) *Opening Doors on Creativity: Resources to Awaken Creative Working. A Learning Resource*. Royal College of Nursing, London. Available from http://www.rcn.org.uk.

Coher, J. (1999) Exploring the meaning of dissatisfaction with health care: the importance of personal identity threat. *Sociology of Health and Illness* **21**(1), 95–124.

Dewing, J. & Titchen, A. (2007) *Workplace Resources for Practice Development*. Royal College of Nursing, London.

Egan, G. (1977) *You and Me: The Skills of Communing and Relating to Others*. Wadsworth, Belmont, CA.

Eisner, E.W. (1988) Aesthetic modes of knowing. In: *Learning and Teaching and the Ways of Knowing* (ed. E.W. Eisner), pp. 23–36. 84th Yearbook of the National Society for the Study of Education. University of Chicago Press, Chicago.

Ferdman, B.M. (1990) Literacy and cultural identity. *Harvard Educational Review* **60**(2), 181–204.

Fox, C. & Feasey, S. (2001) *RCN Research into Child Health Group. Evidence Based Care Benchmark*. Royal College of Nursing, London.

Garaway, G. (1996) The case-study model: an organizational strategy for cross-cultural evaluation. *Evaluation* **2**(2), 201–211.

Guideline Evaluation: Appraisal of Guidelines for Research Evaluation (AGREE) tool Agree Collaboration (2001).

Guba, E. & Lincoln, Y. (1989) *Fourth Generation Evaluation*. Sage, Newbury Park, CA.

Hardy, S., Garbett, R., Titchen, A. & Manley, K. (2002) Exploring nursing expertise: nurses talk nursing. *Nursing Inquiry* **9**(3), 196–202.

Hardy, S., Titchen, A., Manley, K. & McCormack, B. (2006) The attributes and enabling factors of practice expertise. *Nursing Science Quarterly* **19**(3), 260–264.

Hathaway, P. (1998) *Giving and Receiving Feedback: Building Constructive Communication.* Crisp Publications, Menlo Park, CA.

Higgs, J. & Titchen, A. (2001a) *Practice Knowledge and Expertise in the Health Professions.* Butterworth Heinemann, Oxford.

Higgs, J. & Titchen, A. (2001b) *Professional Practice in Health, Education and the Creative Arts.* Blackwell, Oxford.

Hopkins, R.L. (1994) *Narrative Schooling: Experiential Learning and the Transformation of American Education.* Teachers College, New York.

Jude-York, D. & Wise, S. (1997) *Multipoint Feedback: A 360 Degrees Catalyst for Change.* Crisp Publications, Menlo Park, CA.

Lauritzen, C. & Jaegar, M. (1997) *Integrating Learning through Story: The Narrative Curriculum.* Delmar, Albany, NY.

Long, V. (1996) *Communication Skills in Helping Relationships: A Framework for Facilitating Personal Growth.* Brooks/Cole, Pacific Grove, CA.

Marshall, C. & Rossman, G.B. (1995) *Designing Qualitative Research,* 2nd edn. Sage, Thousand Oaks, CA.

Maurer, R. (1994) *Feedback Toolkit: 16 Tools for Better Communication in the Workplace.* Productivity Press, Portland, OR.

McGill, I. & Beatty, L. (2001) *Action Learning: A Guide for Professional, Management & Educational Development.* Kogan Page, London.

Dr Mark L. Merickel of Oregon State University offers a very useful "sequence for self-reflection," at http://oregonstate.edu/instruction/ed555/zone1/mezirow.htm, which is based on Jack Mezirow's work in transformational learning theory and practice.

Merriam, S.B. (1988) *Case Study Research in Education: A Qualitative Approach.* Jossey-Bass, San Francisco.

Mishler, E. (1986) The analysis of interview-narratives. In: *Narrative Psychology: The Storied Nature of Human Conduct* (ed. T. Sarbin), pp. 233–255. Praeger, New York.

Mishler, E. (1999) *Storylines: Craftartists' Narratives of Identity.* Harvard University Press, Cambridge, MA.

Murray, K. (1986) Literary pathfinding: the work of popular life constructors. In: *Narrative Psychology: The Storied Nature of Human Conduct* (ed. T. Sarbin), pp. 276–292. Praeger, New York.

Pawson, R. & Tilley, N. (1997) *Realistic Evaluation.* Sage, London.

Polkinghorne, D. (1988) *Narrative Knowing and the Human Sciences.* State University of New York Press, Albany, NY.

Rich, P. & Copans, S.A. (1998) *The Healing Journey for Couples: Your Journal of Mutual Discovery.* John Wiley & Sons, Inc., New York.

Ricoeur, P. (1988) *Time and Narrative, Vol 3.* University of Chicago Press, Chicago.

Rubin, I.M. & Campbell, T.J. (1997) *The ABCs of Effective Feedback.* Jossey-Bass, San Francisco.

Rumelhart, D.W. (1980) Schemata: the building blocks of cognition. In: *Theoretical Issues in Reading Comprehension* (eds R.J. Spiro, B.C. Bruce & W.F. Brewer), pp. 33–58. Erlbaum, Hillsdale, NJ.

Stake, R.E. (1988) Case study methods in educational research: making sweet water. In: *Complementary Methods for Research in Education* (ed. R.M. Jaegar), pp. 253–265. American Educational Research Association, Washington, DC.

Stephens, G., Titchen, A., McCormack, B., Odell-Miller, H., Sarginson, A., Hoffman, C., Francis, S., Petrone, M.A., Philipp, R., Naidoo, M. & McLoughlin C. (2004) *Creative Arts and Humanities in Healthcare: Swallows to Other Continents.* The Nuffield Trust, London.

Sutton-Smith, B. (1971) Piaget on play: a critique. In: *Child's Play* (eds R.E. Herron & B. Sutton-Smith), pp. 326–336, 340–345. John Wiley & Sons, Inc., New York.

Titchen, A. (2001) Critical companionship: a conceptual framework for developing expertise. In: *Practice Knowledge and Expertise in the Health Professions* (eds A. Higgs & A. Titchen), Butterworth Heinemann, Oxford.

Titchen, A., Dewing, J., McCormack, B. & Manley, K. (1999) *Realising Clinical Effectiveness and Clinical Governance through Clinical Supervision.* Royal College of Nursing Open Learning Pack, Radcliffe Medical Press, Abingdon.

Upsher, R.E.G., VanDenKerhof, E.G. & Goel, G. (2001) Meaning and measurement: an inclusive model of evidence. *Journal of Evaluation in Clinical Practice* 7(2), 91–96.

Warfield & Manley, K. (1990) Nursing development unit: developing a new philosophy in the NDU. *Nursing Standard* 4(41), 27–30.

Wolcott, H.F. (1990) On seeking and rejecting validity in qualitative research. In: *Qualitative Inquiry in Education: The Continuing Debate* (eds E.W. Eisner & A. Peskin), pp. 121–152. Teachers College, New York.

Concluding Remarks

14. A Final Turn of the Kaleidoscope

Sally Hardy, Angie Titchen, Kim Manley and Brendan McCormack

Interrelated journeys

This book has brought together the work of many practitioners over many years, in a complicated interplay towards improved understanding and articulation of the challenging beauty that is the professional artistry of nursing practice expertise. There are different examples presented that aim to reveal, reflect, refract and refine nursing practice expertise. What is common to all of these practitioners is their heartfelt desire to enable others, whilst at the same time refining and honing their own professional artistry.

Professional artistry and practice expertise

We have seen commonalities emerging from both the literature and contributors' chapters that support the notion of professional artistry as lying at the heart of expertise.

Professional artistry shares some characteristics with nursing artistry, particularly in terms of practice skills imbued with aesthetic knowledge and the use of self within therapeutic relationships. However, we propose that professional artistry goes further not only epistemologically, in detailing pre-cognitive, cognitive, metacognitive and reflexive ways of knowing, but also ontologically, in setting out multiple intelligences and use of creative imagination and expression – again witnessed and evidenced in each chapter of this book. Professional artistry does not separate being artistic with being scientific. A nurse with expertise, we propose, needs to be both, blending, melding and 'dancing' simultaneously between the two.

Professional artistry appears to be generic to a wide range of nursing specialities and, we believe, health care professions, except perhaps for domain specific knowledge where the clinician needs to apply propositional, personal and professional knowledge in a particular context. This proposition, however, needs to be further tested.

A systematic approach to practitioner research can further demonstrate the potential for transformation in collaborative, participatory and inclusive ways that will continue to contribute to theory development – theory about nursing practice expertise and its effectiveness. Developing critically creative methodologies that integrate established philosophical, theoretical and methodological perspectives is crucial to the engagement of practitioners in research. This is essential within a health care arena that is increasingly pressurised, economically driven and professionally challenging, which tends to further remove, even dehumanise, the human element of nursing practice within the context of health care delivery. As chapters in this book illustrate, drawing on practitioner research methodologies enables 'critical spaces' to be created within which windows of opportunity can be opened for the growth of human potential. In Chapter 12, we focused on work-based learning as a form of inquiry or practitioner research and as a means for nurturing professional artistry in the workplace.

Critical creativity is an approach to practice development (PD) that builds on the philosophical, theoretical and methodological assumptions of emancipatory PD (see Chapters 1, 2 and 11) but adds its own nuances. The concept of human flourishing is a central focus of critical creativity and is viewed not only as the ultimate purpose of transformational PD, but also as the way of bringing it about. In other words, it is claimed that by paying attention to, and creating, the conditions (culture) within the workplace in which people can flourish and grow, the achievement of more effective person-centred health care will be enabled.

Given the hidden nature of professional artistry, it is imperative that nurses are able to articulate their expertise, to broaden a current health care discourse that, as previously stated, values a quantitative, technical reliance on clinical guidelines and protocols for patient care. We are concerned that this discourse downplays other types of knowledge and ignores the importance of the complex processes of professional artistry. We propose, therefore, that it is important that nurses (and other health care professionals) are guided and supported to become aware of and articulate attributes of their expertise and professional artistry. This will enable practitioners to not only further develop their own expertise and professional artistry, but also help to enable others to develop theirs and further enlarge contemporary health care discourse.

Oscar Wilde suggests that the acceptance of a prevailing moral discourse is itself 'immoral' and, in the context of this book, we believe that the acceptance of a dominant scientific discourse is in itself 'disabling' of the kaleidoscope that is the professional artistry of nursing expertise. We hope this book has gone some way towards challenging that discourse and providing methodologies and methods for expertise in all its many forms to flourish.

Index

279